COMMUNITY AND PUBLIC HEALTH NURSING

COMMUNITY AND PUBLIC HEALTH NURSING

An Active Learning Approach

Cindy Farris and Denise McEnroe-Petitte

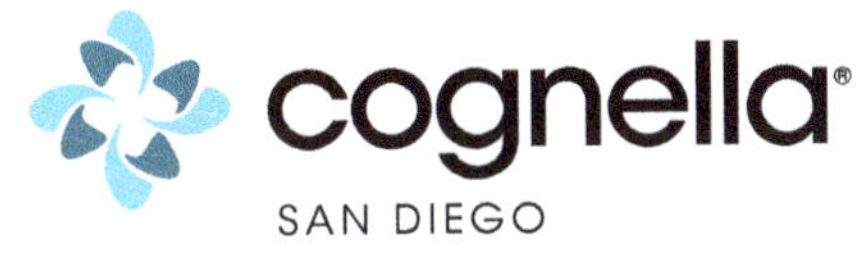

Bassim Hamadeh, CEO and Publisher
Amanda Martin, Executive Publisher
Zoe Flores, Project Editor
Jeanine Rees, Production Editor
Jess Estrella, Senior Graphic Designer
JoHannah McDonald, Licensing Coordinator
Natalie Piccotti, Director of Marketing
Kassie Graves, Senior Vice President, Editorial
Alia Bales, Director, Project Editorial and Production

Printed in the United States of America.

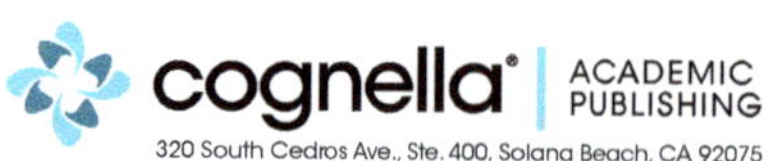

This book is dedicated is to my parents, William and Therese McEnroe. They have always encouraged me to strive in my education and excel in my life. Although I have the loving memory of my father, he would have been proud of me for this accomplishment, and my mother has wholeheartedly supported me from the beginning to the completion of this book. In addition, I want to thank my husband, Kevin, for realizing that this accomplishment was important for me. He has always pushed me to reach for the stars.

I would like to include my children, Cory, Danielle, and Zachary, and grandchildren Daniel, Avery, Jackson, Whitley, and Jameson, as they have given me joy and happiness.

For the readers of this book, consider the importance of the profession of nursing and the numerous ways that nursing can be utilized. Community and Public Health nursing roles are just some examples, and they need to be seen as specializations that impact the community and the world. With the presentation of this book, nursing can be enhanced through further inclusion in nursing curriculums and future practice.

—Denise McEnroe-Petitte

Brief Contents

Detailed Contents

Preface

Many changes are occurring in global healthcare, especially in the nursing field. Adequate preparation for nursing students on community, public health, and population-based concepts is essential. With expertise in undergraduate academic teaching of community and public health, the authors stress that clients transitioning from acute to outpatient/community care has become common practice. Today's nursing students require more education and exposure to succeed. Clients and families who need additional support and resources must continue to have their needs addressed. Nurses can reach many populations concerning their specific needs by involving community members. Those working in community and public health must be fully aware and educated on how to meet the needs of these diverse individuals through multidisciplinary interactions with other professionals. Much support is needed regarding care and developing policies and procedures, guidelines, management, health equity, education, addressing the social determinants of health (SDOH), and financial, local, state, national, and international collaboration to enhance many areas and provide proper health promotion and disease prevention.

Community and Public Health Nursing: An Active Learning Approach provides significant information on various topics, such as levels of prevention, the SDOH, healthcare delivery, epidemiological principles, communicable diseases, emergency preparedness, community nursing roles, evidence-based practices, critical thinking, practical application, and clinical judgment skills. These topics can be used at all levels of nursing education as nurses have become more active in the community and public health settings; hence, they have a greater need to focus on all types of nursing education fields.

This book uses active learning reflection activities, intervention wheel activities, and case studies linked to the American Association of Colleges of Nursing *Essentials* (2021).[1] An instructor's manual with suggested answers to the active learning activities, intervention wheel activities, and case studies is present for each chapter. Additional active learning exercises for each chapter and potential answers accompany this book.

1. American Association of Colleges of Nursing. (2021). *The essentials: Core competencies for professional nursing education*. https://www.aacnnursing.org/Portals/0/PDFs/Publications/Essentials-2021.pdf

CHAPTER 1

Community, Public Health, and Population-Based Nursing

"Every nurse is an angel with a key for a healthy community! All in caring for patients—it's part of a nursing soul."

—Aleksandra Radenovic

Learning Outcomes

After reading this chapter, students should be able to:

1. Understand the concepts of community health, public health, and population-based nursing
2. Compare and contrast community health, public health, and population-based nursing
3. Compare and contrast acute care nursing with community health, public health, and population-based nursing
4. Understand the history of community health, public health, and population-based nursing
5. Apply the intervention wheel at systems-focused, community-focused, and individual-focused levels
6. Understand the history of community/public health (Nightingale and Wald)
7. Understand the functions/purpose of the Council of Public Health Nursing Organizations (CPHNO)
8. Apply objectives from Healthy People (HP) 2030
9. Apply community health, public health, and population-based nursing using active learning exercises
10. Use case studies to enhance learning related to community health, public health, and population-based nursing
11. Understand the concept of a community health needs assessment (CHNA)
12. Apply the characteristics of a windshield survey

Keywords and Concepts

Acute care nursing, community health needs assessment (CHNA); community health nursing; Healthy People 2030; intervention wheel; population-based nursing; public health nursing; Quad Council; windshield survey

Definitions of the Keywords

Acute care nursing: Primary responsibility is to deliver the necessary care that clients require increasing the likelihood of positive outcomes from medical treatment in an acute care setting (Indeed, 2022)

CHNA: State, tribal, local, or territorial health assessment identifying health needs/issues through data collection and analysis (Centers for Disease Control and Prevention [CDC], 2022)

Community health nursing: Works to promote health and prevent disease in groups and families to improve health in a certain geographical area (Public Health Nursing, n.d.)

Council of Public Health Nursing Organizations (CPHNO): Formally known as the *Quad Council* (QC); made up of seven nursing organizations (CPHNO, 2023)

HP 2030: Data-driven national objectives to improve health and well-being over a designated decade (Office of Disease Prevention and Health Promotion [ODPHP], n.d.a.)

Intervention wheel: A framework to plan and evaluate practice, responding to issues such as emergency preparedness; control measures for emerging contagious disease outbreaks; and promoting population-based lifestyle changes/health improvement related to population health improvement (Minnesota Department of Health, 2019)

Population-based nursing: Works to advance the health outcomes of a group of individuals, including distribution to the group (Ariosto et al., 2018)

Public health nursing: Practice of promoting and protecting the health of populations using knowledge from public health, social sciences, and nursing with application to where they work, play, live, and learn (American Nursing Association [ANA], n.d.; Association of Public Health Nursing [APHN], 2022)

Windshield survey: Observational tool used in community needs assessment (Guin, 2020)

Introduction

Nursing practice continues to evolve as the world's health needs change. Various global issues have evolved since the times of Florence Nightingale and Lillian Wald. The education of today's nursing students will need to be expanded as social issues now affect the health outcomes of individuals, families, communities, and populations (Valentine-Maher et al., 2021). Understanding the world of community, public, and especially population-based health must be a priority for future nurses.

The chapters in this book will allow for many opportunities to enhance the understanding of community and public health nursing concepts. Changes in the nursing curriculum will need to be directed toward preparing future nursing students with more insight and knowledge of various practice settings. Nursing programs must produce nursing students who provide care addressing determinants of health for individuals and populations (Valentine-Maher et al., 2021). As effective health practices become more complex, the nursing curriculum will need enhanced instruction and teaching about caring for these populations. Nursing students need to become strong leaders who advocate for what affects the community and public health by better understanding the population's demographics, environment, relationships, and critical issues (Kent, 2018).

Background of the Concepts

Nursing remains the most trusted profession (Walker, 2024). With trust comes the understanding that the nurse will be prepared for all levels of care, including in all settings. Knowing about the client's, family's, and population's physical, emotional, mental, and social needs is crucial to effective patient-centered care.

Providing a continuum and effective transition with respect is critical for the client and family. Safe primary care is needed to provide continuity between acute and community care (World Health Organization [WHO], 2016). Change in care from acute to community continues to expand. Seeing the client in the community, especially at home, allows the nurse to build trust (Conway et al., 2022). The client and family feel more comfortable in the home environment, allowing for assessment of the environment and social determinants of health (Conway et al., 2022; Box 1.1).

Nursing education must change to encompass societal changes. *The Future of Nursing 2020–2030: Charting a Path to Health Equity* promotes health for all, no matter the setting (National Academy of Medicine [NAM], 2021). Nurses live and work at the intersection of health, education, and community (NAM, 2021). The achievement of health equity in the United States is built on nursing capacity and expertise (NAM, 2021).

BOX 1.1 ACTIVE LEARNING REFLECTION ACTIVITY

Video on Understanding and Application of Community and Public Health Nursing

Watch the following video to understand community and public health nursing: https://www.youtube.com/watch?v=X2uolyrA8vc.

1. What are two things you learned from the video that you did not know about community and public health nursing before watching it?
2. What are two ways you could implement what you learned from the video in your future nursing practice?

American Association for Colleges of Nursing (AACN) *Essentials* (2021): Domains: #1; #3; #7; #10

- Competencies: 1.1; 1.3; 3.1; 7.1; 10.2
- Subcompetencies: 1.1a; 1.1b; 1.3a; 1.3c; 3.1a; 3.1e; 7.1c; 10.2a; 10.2d

Spheres of Care: Wellness/Disease prevention

Concepts: Clinical judgment; Evidence-based practice; Compassionate care

Source: CPHNO, 2020.

In 2021, the AACN updated professional competencies. The new addition of *The Essentials: Core Competencies for Professional Nursing Education* combined with professional nurse education at all levels (AACN, 2021). The change is based on the need for more competency-based education principles to bridge the gap between education and practice (AACN, 2021).

Previously, the focus was on clinical education in acute care, but the new essentials focus on the future of healthcare delivery. The changes will occur within four spheres of care: 1) disease prevention/promotion of health and well-being (promotion of physical and mental health in all clients and management of minor acute and intermittent care needs in generally healthy clients); 2) chronic disease care (management of chronic diseases and prevention of adverse outcomes); 3) regenerative or restorative care (critical/trauma care, complex acute care, acute exacerbations of chronic conditions, and physiological treatment); and 4) hospice/palliative/supportive care (end-of-life care as well as palliative and supportive care for individuals requiring extended care (AACN, 2021; Figure 1.1).

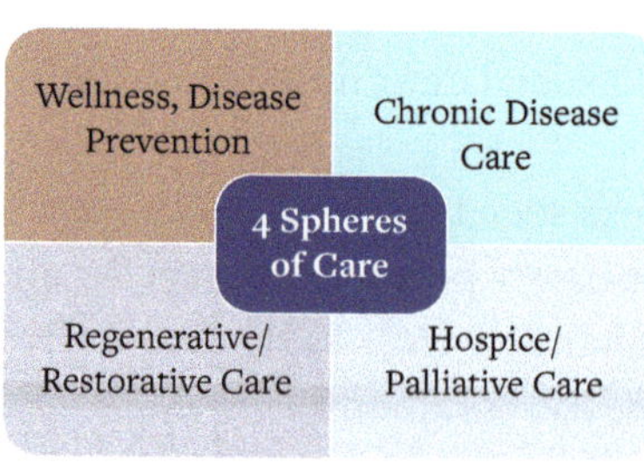

FIGURE 1.1 The Essential Four Spheres of Care

Further changes include domains and integrated concepts. There are a total of 10 domains noted in the new essentials (AACN, 2021). These domains are critical for effective nursing practice. Each domain has designated competencies and subcompetencies at the entry and advanced levels. Eight concepts are interwoven and threaded throughout the 10 domains (AACN, 2021; Table 1.1).

The inclusion of a new focused domain—population-based—is at the center of community and public health nursing. Population-based nursing entails all local, regional, national, and global care in many settings (public health, acute care, ambulatory care, and long-term care). Population-based nursing involves stakeholders, collaborative activities, and strategies (AACN, 2021; Table 1.2).

TABLE 1.1 Essentials: Ten Domains and Eight Concepts

Domains	Concepts
• Knowledge for nursing practice • Person-centered care • Population health • Scholarship for nursing practice • Quality and safety • Interprofessional partnerships • System-based scholarship • Information and healthcare technologies • Professionalism • Personal, professional, and leadership development	• Clinical judgment • Communication • Compassionate care • Diversity, equity, and inclusion (DEI) • Ethics • Evidence-based practice • Health policy • Social determinants of health (SDOH)

Source: AACN, 2021.

TABLE 1.2 Elements of the Essentials: Population Domain #3

Descriptor: "Population health spans the healthcare delivery continuum from public health prevention to disease management of populations and describes collaborative activities with both traditional and non-traditional partnerships from affected communities, public health, industry, academia, health care, local government entities, and others for the improvement of equitable population health outcomes" (AACN, 2021, p. 10).
Competencies: 3.1 Manage population health 3.2 Engage in effective partnerships 3.3 Consider the socioeconomic impact of the delivery of healthcare 3.4 Advance equitable population health policy 3.5 Demonstrate advocacy strategies 3.6 Advance preparedness to protect population health during disasters and public health emergencies

Source: AACN, 2021.

History of Community and Public Health Nursing

Many individuals have been instrumental in the history of community and public health nursing. Florence Nightingale and Lillian Wald were two of the most influential community and public health nursing figures. Both women were pioneers in establishing the importance of community and public health nursing care.

Florence Nightingale

Nightingale's legacy regarding home care is noted in the concept of district nursing (Bates & Memel, 2021). She worked alongside William Rathbone to establish a model of community care. As a member of the wealthier class, her beginnings with this type of work were in upper-class charitable home visiting (Bates & Memel, 2021). Nightingale's ideal home vision of care was the element of attachment to a local community subscribing to the self-help model, in which responsibility lay on poor householders to improve their environment through appropriate and effective guidance. In creating district nursing systems, she implicitly assigned much more commitment to the broader community to provide (or at least fund) home-based care and sanitary advice, both locally and nationally (Bates & Memel, 2021).

Nightingale was often known for her persistence in outcomes that transformed nursing education and practice. She influenced care worldwide with many public health ideals that remain relevant today. She noted the importance of health promotion, public health sanitation, proper nutrition, and infection control (Matthews et al., 2020). Similar to language consistent with the SDOH, she considered the importance of housing, social support, access to healthcare, employment, and education crucial and interrelated to a person's health and well-being (Matthews et al., 2020; McDonald, 2020). Nightingale also noted the importance of tracking progress, mimicking today's meaning of *surveillance* (McDonald, 2020).

Lillian Wald

Wald's exposure to the poor Upper West Side immigrant population in New York City was the catapult to her public health service (Nursing-Theory.org, 2023). She proposed immersion into the community to serve the population's needs better. She developed Henry Street Settlement, where the origin of district nursing began in the United States (Nursing-Theory.org, 2023; Box 1.2).

Advocacy for all, especially immigrants, was critical to Wald's agenda. She focused on education, access to care for all, school boards, children's rights, and fair work through unions (AAHN, 2018). She was also the founder and first president of the National Organization for Public Health Nursing (AAHN, 2018).

BOX 1.2 ACTIVE LEARNING REFLECTION ACTIVITY

Henry Street Settlement; Lilian Wald

Watch the following video on Lillian Wald and the history of the Henry Street Settlement: https://www.henrystreet.org/. Scroll down to the video on the house on Henry Street/baptism by fire.

Reflect on the importance of Lillian Wald and her conception of the Henry Street Settlement. Answer the following questions:

1. How has the overall concept of Henry Street Settlement changed over the years? Name at least three ways.
2. What aspects of how Wald viewed district nursing are still the same today? How are they different? Name at least two for each aspect.

AACN *Essentials* (2021): Domains: #1; #2; #3; #6

- Competencies: 1.1; 1.3; 2.3; 3.1; 6.4
- Subcompetencies: 1.1a; 1.1b; 1.1c; 1.3a; 1.3b; 1.3c; 2.3f; 3.1c; 3.1e; 6.4d

Spheres of Care: Wellness/Disease prevention

Concepts: Clinical judgment; Compassionate care; Evidence-based practice

Source: Henry Street Settlement, 2023.

Council of Public Health Nursing Organizations

Initially formed in 1991 as the Quad Council of Public Health Nursing Organizations (QC), the organization focuses on unifying public health nurses (PHNs). In 2020, the name became the Council of Public Health Nursing Organization (CPHNO, 2023). Today, there are seven members of the CPHNO (CPHNO, 2023; Table 1.3).

A focus of the CPHNCO is to advocate locally, regionally, and globally for equitable health policies. The organization's mission is to bring all areas of community and PHNs together to influence and affect the population's health (CPHNCO, 2023). Having a collective voice concerning public health nursing and its role is vital for the future of this type of nursing.

TABLE 1.3 Members of the CPHNO

• Association of Community Health Nurse Educators • Alliance of Nurses for Healthy Environments • American Nursing Association (ANA) • American Public Health Association (APHA) Public Health Nursing Section • American Public Health Nursing (APHN) • National Association of School Nurses • Rural Nurse Organization

Source: CPHNO, 2023.

Types of Nursing

Nursing comes in many different forms and styles. Most clients feel more comfortable in their homes and can form more trusting bonds with nurses (Conway et al., 2022). More care has been delivered safely at home in the past two decades. More providers are being held accountable for high-quality care and lower costs, which is conducive to settings outside of the hospital (Conway et al., 2022; Box 1.3).

BOX 1.3 ACTIVE LEARNING REFLECTION ACTIVITY

Introduction to Types of Nursing Care Settings

Watch the following video about community and public health nursing: https://www.youtube.com/watch?v=pdTvSHAcQ1s. Reflect on the video by answering the following questions:

1. What two principles of community and public health nursing will you apply?
2. What do you see as the differences between community and public health? Name at least two.
3. How is community health different from acute care settings? Name at least two ways.
4. How will you apply what you learned for this reflection in your future nursing practice? Discuss at least two.

AACN *Essentials* (2021): Domains: #1; #3; #4; #10

- Competencies: 1.1; 1.3; 3.1; 4.2; 10.2
- Subcompetencies: 1.1b; 1.1d; 1.3a; 1.3b; 1.3c; 3.1a; 3.1c; 3.1h; 4.2a; 4.2c; 10.2a; 10.2d

Spheres of Care: Wellness/Disease prevention; Chronic disease management

Concepts: Evidence-based practice; Clinical judgment

Source: Karen Teeley, 2016.

Acute Care Nursing

In acute care nursing, the focus is on treatment rather than prevention. *Acute care* is a level of healthcare in which a patient is treated for a brief but severe episode of illness, for conditions resulting from disease or trauma and during recovery from surgery. Acute care is generally provided in a hospital by various clinical personnel using technical equipment, pharmaceuticals, and medical supplies (CT.gov, 1999; Hirshon et al., 2013).

Acute care is time sensitive. Usually, there is a critical need for individual-focused immediate care (Hirshon et al., 2013). The term *acute care* encompasses a range of clinical healthcare functions (Figure 1.2).

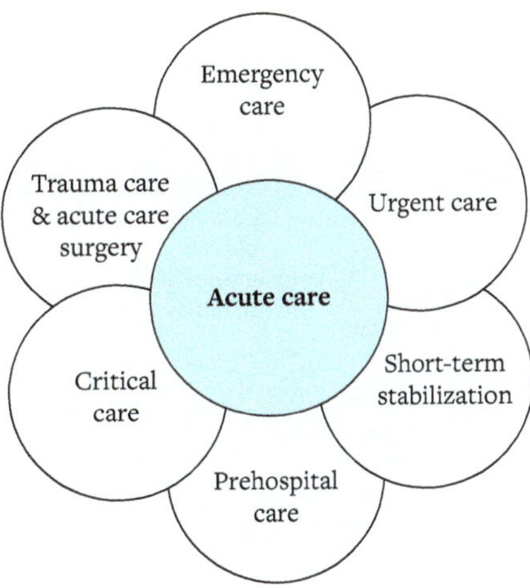

FIGURE 1.2 Domains of Acute Care

As healthcare continues to change, providers must address the complexity of care. More value-based care is needed to avoid the treatment of a client when it arises. Providers must address the overall risks, trajectory of needs, and social challenges that lead to acute care (Hirshon et al., 2013). The key is to think more about prevention long before the issue arises. Understanding the differences between public health, community health, and population-based health is critical.

Public Health

Public health promotes the health of people and communities where they live, work, and play (APHA, 2021b). The goal is to advance health and wellness by encouraging healthy behaviors. Public health is about advocacy, education, surveillance, health policy, and improving quality of life (APHA, 2021b).

Public health's foundation is built on the three core functions of assessment, policy development, and assurance. These core functions are essential for assessing health conditions and potential threats to communities, developing policies to protect the health of individuals and communities, and ensuring the health and safety of individuals and communities (CDC, 2023; Goodwin.edu, 2022). Further, specific core services provide more precise public health activities (CDC, 2023).

The 10 essential public health core services describe the public health activities communities should use (CDC, 2023). The framework originated in 1994 and was updated in 2020 to align with changes in the public health arena (CDC, 2023). The differences are noted in protecting and promoting health for all communities (Figure 1.3).

Public health nursing is defined as promoting and protecting populations' health using knowledge from nursing, social, and public health sciences (APHA, 2021b). Public health nursing practice focuses on population health, promoting health, and preventing disease and disability. PHNs provide healthcare to people and communities who cannot seek assistance (APHA, 2021b; Box 1.4).

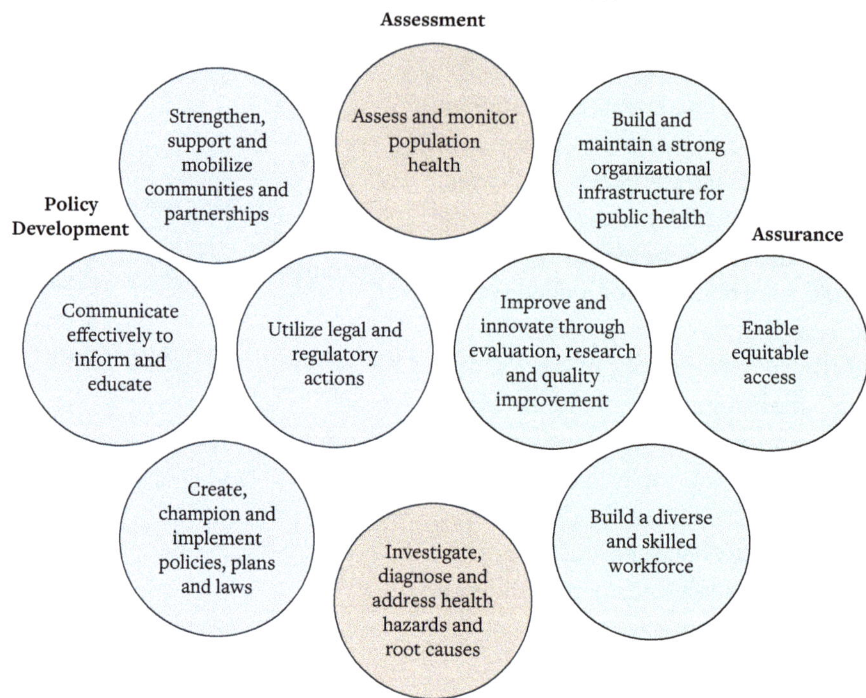

FIGURE 1.3 Ten Essential Public Health Core Services (2020 Version)

BOX 1.4 ACTIVE LEARNING REFLECTION ACTIVITY

What Is Public Health?

Watch the following video from the APHA and reflect on the following questions: https://www.youtube.com/watch?v=ig2cnOLFBR4.

1. Name three aspects of the video demonstrating public health's role in today's world.
2. Apply the three core functions of public health to items noted in the video.
3. Reflect on three ways to implement the role in your future nursing practice.

AACN *Essentials* (2021): Domains: #1; #3; #4; #5; #7; #10

- Competencies: 1.1; 1.3; 3.1; 3.4; 4.2; 5.1; 7.2; 10.2
- Subcompetencies: 1.1b; 1.3a; 1.3b; 1.3c; 3.1a; 3.1c; 3.1e: 3.4b; 3.4c; 4.2c; 4.2d; 5.1a; 7.2b; 10.2a; 10.2d

Spheres of Care: Wellness/Disease prevention

Concepts: Evidence-based practice; Clinical judgment; SDOH

Source: APHA, 2021c.

Public health nursing is the largest segment of the professional public health workforce. PHNs collaborate with the individuals and families who compose the communities and systems that affect them. They work in various settings, such as health departments, schools, homes, community health centers, clinics, correctional facilities, and worksites (APHN, 2022).

The knowledge and skills of PHNs enable them to make significant contributions to public health. PHNs use their clinical expertise and unique relationships with those whom they serve to assist in designing and implementing programs and policies to meet the needs of vulnerable populations. Combining a clinical nursing background with public health and social sciences knowledge provides a sound basis for public health leadership positions (APHN, 2022).

Community Health

Community health efforts promote health within a geographically or culturally defined group (Maraccini et al., 2017). These initiatives use evidence-based strategies to engage and collaborate with communities, providing culturally appropriate interventions (Maraccini et al., 2017). The progress and success of these initiatives originate from the community members who are collectively empowered to address self-identified vulnerabilities (e.g., education, employment, public safety, and environmental issues; Table 1.4).

TABLE 1.4 Comparison of Acute Care and Hospital Nursing Versus Community Health, Public Health, and Population-Based Nursing

Acute Care and Hospital Nursing	Community Health, Public Health, and Population-Based Nursing
Single focus on the individual/unit hospitalized clients	Double focus on small groups/families, including the subgroups in the community
Focus on treatment	Focus on prevention/promoting health
Orders provide the framework for nursing activities	Provides care based on the health assessment and needs for care
Main medical authority is the physician/healthcare provider	Nurse has medical autonomy
Communicates findings to the physician/healthcare provider	Soley responsible for the care and makes independent decisions and referrals
Delivers health services in a hospital setting	Delivers health services in the community (e.g., schools, health centers, shelters, senior centers)
Environment is more controlled and contained	Environment is not contained or controlled
Often only has contact while in hospital	Can develop long-term relationships

Source: Adapted from Mona, 2016.

Community health nursing involves advocacy and policy development to eliminate healthcare disparities. The most significant distinction between the two disciplines lies in their respective focuses. Public health is concerned with the scientific process of preventing infectious diseases. In contrast, community health is affected by the factors that influence a population's physical and mental health (Mona, 2016).

Population-Based

With the passage of the Patient Protection and Affordable Care Act in 2011, the emphasis on care shifted from an individual/client focus to health promotion and prevention for groups of people (Ariosto et al., 2018). *Population health* is defined as the health outcomes of a group of individuals, including the distribution of such outcomes within the group (Ariosto et al., 2018). These groups are often geographic populations such as nations or communities. Still, they can also be other groups such as employees, ethnic groups, disabled persons, prisoners, or any other defined group (Institute for Healthcare Improvement, 2023; Table 1.5).

TABLE 1.5 Comparison of Community Health, Public Health, and Population-Based Nursing

Topics	Community Health	Public Health	Population-Based
Focus on care	Focused on a specific area/ community/area	Focused on a large group of people	Analysis and design of interventions and management of large groups of citizens focused on improving their health status
Characteristics	Protecting the health of a specific area Advocacy and policy development to eliminate healthcare disparities	Promote health and prevent disease for entire population groups Provide healthcare to people and communities who are unable to seek assistance	Act of enhancing the well-being of a group sharing geographic, socioeconomic, or clinical criteria
Purpose	Overall factors that influence a population's physical and mental health	Protecting the health of all Scientific process-es of preventing infectious diseases and surveillance	Health outcomes of a group of individuals, including the distribution of such outcomes within the group

Source: Adapted from Bresnick, 2017.

TABLE 1.6 Recommendations for Future Population-Based Nursing Education

- Tackle the impact of SDOH on improving health
- Reduce health inequalities
- Consider adequate community resources
- Provide learning opportunities to build engagement
- Assess process and outcomes of population-/community-based interventions
- Improve population-based healthcare policies
- Enhance knowledge about big data/informatics and population health knowledge
- Develop new systems and tools that engage and empower patients to improve quality of care, outcomes, and wellness activities

Source: Ariosto et al., 2018.

More nursing curriculums are addressing population-based nursing to prepare future nurses to address the issues that face the world today. Future nurses must be taught about nursing outside of the acute care setting, as these are the populations whom they will see (Ariosto et al., 2018; Table 1.6).

Notable differences exist between community, public health, and population-based nursing, but some areas are the same. Future nurses must understand that population-based nursing addresses social factors contributing to health outcomes. Population-based health assists these groups in attaining and maintaining health with an increased focus on shared accountability for the upstream environment, social, and community factors contributing to chronic disease and cost (Ariosto et al., 2018).

Community Health Needs Assessment and Windshield Survey

Performing a windshield survey and a CHNA is critical to providing adequate care to a population and community. There are many tools and databases that can facilitate obtaining the information needed. Gathering observational data through a windshield survey and getting resident data through a systematic review and analysis will allow for a proper assessment of needs (CDC, 2018; Guin, 2020).

One way to assess community needs is through a windshield survey, which is conducted using a car and traveling through a specific area to determine what is seen (Guin, 2020). For example, reporting food availability, housing structures, sidewalks, parks, and healthcare facilities are ways to identify available resources (Table 1.7).

A CHNA can help understand the community dynamics and allow stakeholders and residents to make determinations (Guin, 2020). One way to assess the

TABLE 1.7 Example of Components of a Windshield Survey

- Environmental/street condition status (e.g., remodeling, building, abandoned buildings, debris, abandoned vehicles, garbage cans, air or noise pollution, potholes, signs, construction, vehicles parked on the side of the street, bus stops, etc.)
- Health services (e.g., from physicians, nurses, dentists, hospitals, dental clinics, etc.)
- Commercial and industrial space (e.g., types of stores, groceries, restaurants, gas stations, prices, quality, selection, atmosphere; types of industry, location, condition, etc.)
- Community agencies/churches/synagogues (e.g., social service agency/police/fire/rescue, number and condition of churches or places of worship, etc.)
- Residential/recreational space (e.g., single- or multiple-family housing, condition of homes, windows, doors, vacant homes, yard area, sidewalk conditions, bars, movie theaters, parks, recreation centers, etc.)

Source: Adapted from Guin, 2020.

community's needs is to assign a census tract to investigate detailed data that could identify a strength or need for improvement. A higher rate of lower-census income compared with those of the county and state could demonstrate problems with paying rent or for healthcare.

Intervention Wheel

In 1998, the Minnesota Department of Health Section of Public Health Nursing introduced the Public Health Intervention Model (Minnesota Department of Health, 2019). The Public Health Intervention Wheel (PHI) is a population-based practice model for public health nursing practice. The PHI wheel encompasses three levels of practice (community, systems, individual/family) and 17 public health interventions, organized in a color-coded pattern (Shafer et al., 2022; Minnesota Department of Health, 2019; Figure 1.4).

The PHI wheel explains what public health nursing does (Shafer et al., 2022). It is a framework used in public health nursing education (Shafer et al., 2022). Even though the PHI wheel was developed in the United States, the framework is also used in other countries (Shafer et al., 2022). For example, in 2013, England adopted the PHI wheel in its Public Health Outcomes Framework for its public health nursing and midwifery practices (Public Health England, 2013; Shafer et al., 2022).

The PHI wheel describes the scope of practice, which is similar across practice settings. The PHI wheel notes are practiced at three levels: individual/family, community, and systems. The PHI wheel displays what a PHN does and presents it as a specialty nursing practice. These interventions are not exclusive to public health nursing, as they are also used by other public health disciplines, except for delegated functions (Minnesota Department of Health, 2019).

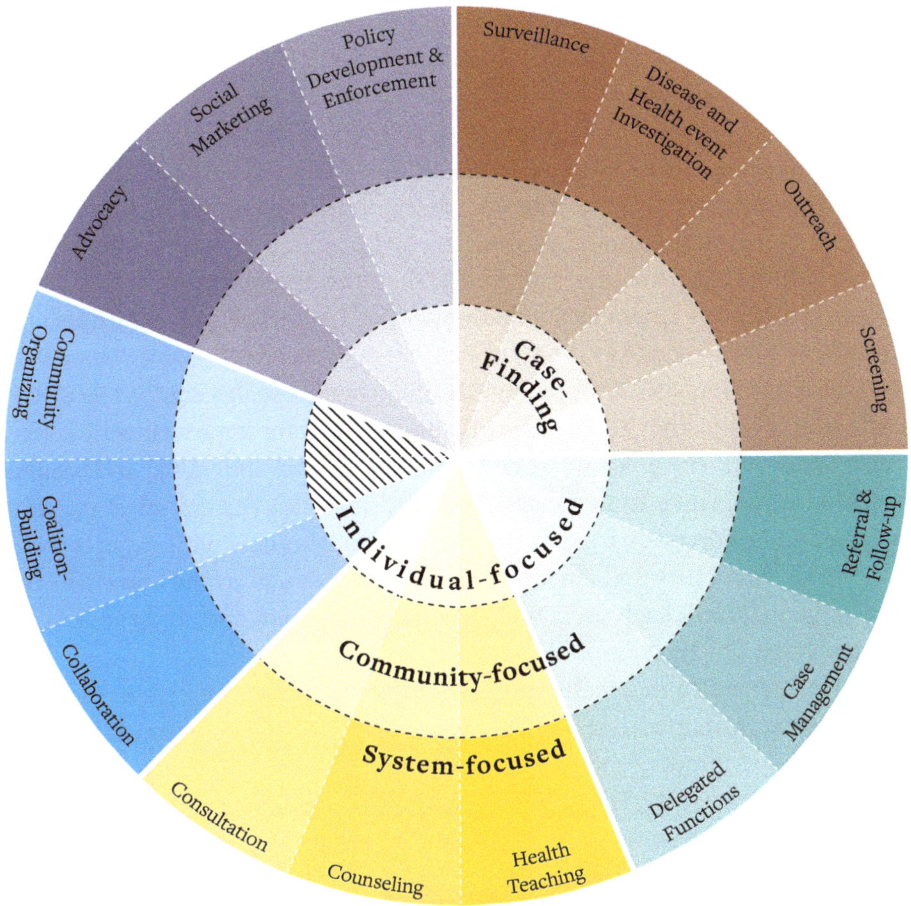

FIGURE 1.4 Minnesota Department of Health Intervention Wheel (Revised 2019)

Healthy People 2030

U.S. Surgeon General Julius Richmond (1979) compiled the landmark report titled *Healthy People: The Surgeon General's Report on Health Promotion and Disease Prevention*. Richmond identified that although there have been some positive gains and awareness in lifestyles and impact on healthy habits, the focus was on treatment and disability rather than on prevention (Richmond, 1979, p. 5). With the introduction of prevention, Richmond (1979) presented that the emphasis should work on the fact that prevention will save people's lives, improve their quality of life, and save money (pp. 10–11).

HP was initiated in 1990. HP 1990 was developed and set measurable 10-year objectives for individuals and nations to improve their health. The goals focused on decreasing deaths and increasing positive outcomes for independence among individuals. The objectives are reassessed and reevaluated every 10 years for progress, with new areas changed based on evidence (Department of Health and Human Services [DHHS], 2021).

HP 2030 noted similar topics, but the emphasis was on the information obtained over the past four decades (ODPHP, n.d.b.). The inclusion of the SDOH concepts plays a significant role in HP 2030 objectives and goals. Examples include reducing health disparities; increasing the lifespan; accessing preventive services; preventing disabilities, injuries, and premature deaths; and increasing education that promotes safe physical environments, healthy behaviors, mental healthcare, vulnerable population access, and inclusion in health services (DHHS, 2021).

Additional emphasis has been placed on increased health equity, the SDOH, health literacy, and an individual's well-being. Significant improvement has been seen by reviewing the progress made in each decade, but individual and national efforts must continue to improve. Collaborating with the community, state, national, and international organizations, HP collaborates with experts in the fields. It identifies new and emerging health issues to add to the objectives that need to be included, such as COVID-19, the opioid epidemic, and the usage of e-cigarettes (ODPHP, n.d.b.).

Since the health and well-being of all people and communities is one of the founding principles of HP 2030, nurses will need to promote this aspect to benefit all. Achieving such benefits requires eliminating health disparities, achieving health equity, attaining health literacy, and strengthening the physical, social, and economic environments (i.e., addressing SDOH; Pronk et al.,

BOX 1.5 ACTIVE LEARNING REFLECTION ACTIVITY

HP 2030 Framework

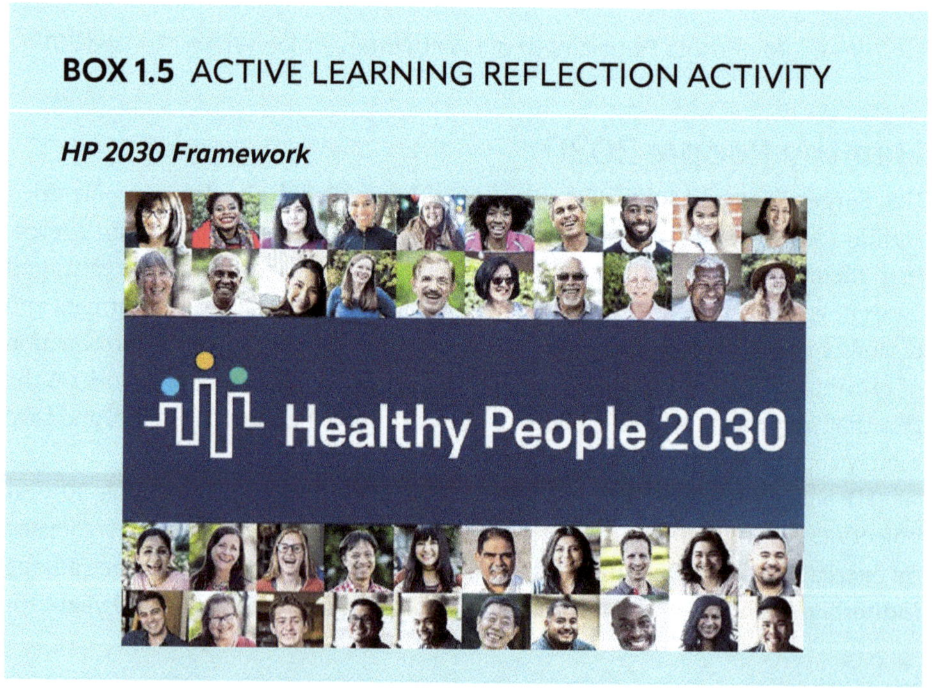

Go to the following site and watch the video on the HP 2030 framework: https://health.gov/healthypeople/about/healthy-people-2030-framework.

1. List the five critical areas of the framework.
2. Discuss in detail the definition and specific application of one of the essential areas of the framework.
3. Based on population-based nursing, discuss how your key area in question 2 could be applied to an adolescent population.

AACN *Essentials* (2021): Domains: #1; #2; #3; #4; #5; #9

- Competencies: 1.1; 1.2; 2.3; 2.4; 2.5; 3.1; 4.2; 5.1; 9.3
- Subcompetencies: 1.1b; 1.2c; 2.3c; 2.4b; 2.4c; 2.5c; 3.1a; 3.1c; 3.1e; 3.1f; 4.2c; 4.2d; 5.1a; 5.1c; 9.3g

Spheres of Care: Wellness/Disease prevention; Chronic disease management

Concepts: Evidence-based practice; Clinical judgment; SDOH, Compassionate care

Source: ODPHP, n.d.b.

2021). Promoting health and well-being requires private, public, and not-for-profit entities at all levels (national, state, tribal, and community; Pronk et al., 2021; Box 1.5).

Chapter Highlights

- Discussion about the differences between community health, public health, and population-based nursing
- Multiple active learning reflection activities to clarify community health, public health, population-based nursing, Lillian Wald, and HP
- Discussion regarding the history of public health
- Active learning strategies/reflection related to HP 2030
- Active learning strategies related to the PHI wheel
- Multiple active learning reflection activities
- Case studies related to HP 2030, the windshield survey, and the CHNA

Active Learning Exercises

INTERVENTION WHEEL ACTIVE LEARNING STRATEGY (ADDRESSING APPLICATION OF THE INTERVENTION WHEEL)

1. Visit the following link regarding the Minnesota Department of Health intervention wheel: https://www.health.state.mn.us/communities/practice/research/phncouncil/docs/PHInterventions.pdf.
2. Define the term and its meaning. Give a community example of how it might be applied for the following levels (systems-focused, community-focused, and individual-focused).

Interventions	Definition	Systems-Focused	Community-Focused	Individual-Focused
Social marketing				
Surveillance				
Community organizing				
Case management				
Outreach				

AACN *Essentials* (2021): Domains: #1; #2; #3; #4; #9

- Competencies: 1.3; 2.3; 3.1; 3.3; 3.4; 4.2; 9.3
- Subcompetencies: 1.3a; 1.3c; 2.3f; 3.1c; 3.1e; 3.1h; 3.3a; 3.3b; 3.4b; 3.4c; 4.2c; 9.3g

Spheres of Care: Wellness/Disease prevention; Chronic disease management

Concepts: Evidence-based practice; Clinical judgment; SDOH

Source: Minnesota Department of Health, 2019.

Case Studies

Case Study #1: Application to HP 2030

A community health fair is being held at the local mall, focusing on HP 2030 initiatives. You are part of the planning committee. The target population is older adults (older than age 65). Using the HP 2030 website and the following URL, specifically for older adults, investigate various ways in which the upcoming initiatives can be illustrated: https://health.gov/healthypeople/objectives-and-data/browse-objectives/older-adults.

1. Identify at least four suggested targets that were at baseline. What does *baseline* mean?
2. Identify whether any targets have exceeded or improved their goal.
3. Identify whether any targets have little or no detectable changes.
4. Identify three developmental areas. What do they mean?
5. Identify two areas that are getting worse.
6. How can this community health fair assist in developing initiatives to make changes?
7. Based on what you gathered from the targets, which three areas would you want to be integrated into the community health fair?

AACN *Essentials* (2021): Domains: #1; #2; #3; #4; #7; #8; #9

- Competencies: 1.1; 1.3; 2.7; 2.8; 3.1; 3.2; 3.3; 4.2; 7.1; 7.3; 8.2; 8.3; 9.1
- Subcompetencies: 1.1b; 1.3a; 1.3c; 2.7c; 2.8a; 2.8b; 2.8c; 2.8d; 3.1a; 3.1b; 3.1c; 3.1d; 3.1f; 3.1h; 3.2a; 3.2b; 3.3b; 4.2c; 4.2d; 4.2e; 7.1c; 7.3b; 8.2c; 8.2e; 8.3c; 9.1a; 9.1c

Spheres of Care: Wellness/Disease prevention

Concepts: Evidence-based practice; Compassionate care; SDOH; Ethics, Clinical judgment

Source: ODPHP, n.d.c.

Case Study #2: Application: Performing a Windshield Survey/Analysis of Findings

Below is a summary of an example of a windshield survey performed on an assigned census tract. Please read the information and analyze the census tract's physical environment.

Environmental Status

The census tract is mainly rural. There are 10 natural recreational parks with several trees and open spaces. These parks are located in the wealthy section of the census tract. In addition, this census tract has a significant area with a river running through it. The public green spaces are well maintained. The parks look clean and free of clutter. There are few public places with overgrown weeds. Some dense tree branches obstruct daylight and visibility. There are no sidewalks in the entire census tract. There is one main road that has a lot of noise.

Health Services

No medical facilities are found during the windshield survey. The closest hospital is 21 miles away, and the nearest pharmacy is 13 miles away, with no delivery services. The closest dental facility is approximately 22 miles away, and the physician's group is more than 17 miles away.

Commercial and Industrial Spaces

One small convenience store has no fresh fruit or vegetables but many alcoholic products. One gas station is located on the main road. No public transportation is available in the census tract. Agriculture is a significant industry in this census tract. There are four different companies growing crops within the perimeter.

Community Agencies

A fire department is located in the census tract. There are several churches noted, along with one community center.

Residential Space

There are multiple ranches and medium-sized farms in this census tract. The houses observed are single-family homes with large lawns and well-maintained gardens. A small neighborhood of mobile homes look to be in good condition.

1. What is one strength noted in the windshield survey? Please provide evidence-based support for this identified strength.
2. What needs for improvement are noted in the windshield survey? Please provide evidence-based support for these identified needs.

AACN *Essentials* (2021): Domains: #3 #4; #5; #8; #9

- Competencies: 3.1; 3.3; 4.2; 5.2; 5.3; 8.2; 9.3; 9.6
- Subcompetencies: 3.1b; 3.1c; 3.3b; 4.2c; 5.2a; 5.2c; 5.3a; 8.2c; 9.3g; 9.6a

Spheres of Care: Wellness/Disease prevention; Chronic disease management

Concepts: SDOH; Evidence-based practice

Sources: Based on instructor requirements developed for community nursing course; Guin, 2020.

Case Study #3: Population-Based Nursing Using Community Assessment (Application of a CHNA)

Nursing students have been assigned a clinical rotation at Spruce Canyon, which is a community located in an urban section of town.

Characteristics of the Spruce Canyon area include the following:

- Average mean age: 33.5 years
- Total residents: 3,410 (64% Hispanic, 18% Black, 13% White)
- Median income: 25,410 per year
- 32% use food stamps
- 70% of the residents ages 19–64 have no health insurance
- Spruce Canyon has a highly active community center that provides many services to its residents. Residents can receive help and application assistance with health insurance, food stamps, and employment. The director wants to start a food bank and community garden. The director of the community center wants to know about other types of needs and assistance that the residents of Spruce Canyon need. The instructor challenges the nursing students to develop a 10-question survey to assist the director in determining the community's needs and most significant problems.

1. Name at least five questions you would want to ask to assist the director.
2. Which three priority health education classes would you suggest?
3. Which three outside community resources might benefit the residents?
4. How might you help develop food bank and community garden plans? Develop two ways to do this.

AACN *Essentials* (2021): Domains: #3; #4; #5; #7; #8

- Competencies: 3.1; 3.2; 3.3; 3.5; 4.2; 5.1; 7.2, 8.2; 8.3
- Subcompetencies: 3.1a; 3.1b; 3.1c; 3.1f; 3.2a; 3.2b; 3.2c; 3.3a; 3.3b; 3.5c; 3.5d; 4.2c; 5.1a; 5.1f; 7.2b; 8.2c; 8.3a; 8.3c

Spheres of Care: Wellness/Disease prevention

Concepts: Evidence-based practice; Clinical judgment; SDOH

Sources: Based on instructor requirements developed for community nursing course; CDC, 2024.

NCLEX Questions

1. Which statement is the most prominent feature of public health nursing?
   a. Involves providing home care to sick people not confined in the hospital.
   b. Services are provided free of charge to people within the catchment area.
   c. Function as part of a team providing public health nursing services.
   d. Focuses on preventive, not curative services.
2. A PHN identifies the healthcare needs of the community members. Which is the nurse's most efficient initial approach to meet these needs?
   a. Involve community leaders to work within the political arena to obtain program funding.
   b. Draft research grants to explore the community's health needs in more detail.
   c. Design educational programs that address the identified community needs.
   d. Make residents aware of the resources in the community.

References

American Association of Colleges of Nursing. (2021). *The essentials: Core competencies for professional nursing education.* https://www.aacnnursing.org/Essentials

American Association of History of Nursing. (2018). *Lillian D. Wald.* https://www.aahn.org/wald

American Nursing Association. (n.d.). *Public health nursing.* https://www.nursingworld.org/practice-policy/workforce/public-health-nursing/

American Public Health Association. (2021a). *10 essential public health services.* https://www.apha.org/What-is-Public-Health/10-Essential-Public-Health-Services

American Public Health Association. (2021b). *What is public health?* https://www.apha.org/What-is-Public-Health

American Public Health Association. (2021c). *What is public health? Episode #1 of "That's Public Health."* YouTube, December 21, 2021. https://www.youtube.com/watch?v=ig2cnOLFBR4

Ariosto, D., Harper, E., Wilson, M., Hull, S., Nahm, E., & Sylvia, M. (2018). Population health: A nursing action plan. *Journal of American Medical Informatics Association, 1*(1), 7–10. 10.1093/jamiaopen/ooy003

Association of Public Health Nursing. (2022). *What is a public health nurse?* https://www.phnurse.org/what-is-a-phn-

Bates, R., & Memel, J. G. (2021). Florence Nightingale and responsibility for healthcare in the home. *European Journal for the History of Medicine and Health, 79,* 227–252. https://brill.com/view/journals/ehmh/79/2/article-p227_002.xml?language=en

Bresnick, J. (2017). *How do population health, public health, community health differ?* https://healthitanalytics.com/news/how-do-population-health-public-health-community-health-differ

Centers for Disease Control and Prevention. (2018). *Community health assessment and health improvement planning.* https://www.cdc.gov/publichealthgateway/cha/index.html

Centers for Disease Control and Prevention. (2022). *Community health assessments and health improvement plans.* https://www.cdc.gov/publichealthgateway/cha/plan.html

Centers for Disease Control and Prevention. (2023). *Public health professions gateway: 10 essential public health services*. https://www.cdc.gov/publichealthgateway/publichealthservices/essentialhealthservices.hml

Centers for Disease Control and Prevention. (2024). *Community planning for health assessment: CHA & CHIP*. https://www.cdc.gov/public-health-gateway/php/public-health-strategy/public-health-strategies-for-community-health-assessment-health-improvement-planning.html

Conway, P., Rosenblit, A., & Theisen, S. (2022). The future of home and community care. *The New England Journal of Medicine Catalyst*, 1–11. https://catalyst.nejm.org/doi/pdf/10.1056/CAT.22.0141

Council of Public Health Nursing Organizations. (2020). Public health nurses: The first line of prevention. YouTube, December 4, 2020. https://www.youtube.com/watch?v=X2uoIyrA8vc

Council of Public Health Nursing Organizations. (2023). *Looking back and ahead: CPHNO in historical perspective*. https://www.cphno.org/about/#:~:text=Since%20the%20organization's%20formation%20in,Health%20Nursing%20Organizations%20(QC).

CT.gov. (1999). *Hospitals today*. https://portal.ct.gov/-/media/OHS/ohca/HospitalStudy/HospTodaypdf.pdf?la=en

Department of Health and Human Services. (2021). *History of Healthy People*. Office of Health Promotion and Disease Prevention. https://health.gov/our-work/national-health-initiatives/healthy-people/about-healthy-people/history-healthy-people

Goodwin.edu. (2022). *What are the 3 core functions of public health?* https://www.goodwin.edu/enews/core-functions-public-health/

Guin, N. B. (2020). Windshield and walking surveys in community health nursing. *International Journal of Science and Research*, *9*(11), 523–525. https://www.ijsr.net/archive/v9i11/SR201022161001.pdf

Henry Street Settlement. (2023). *Baptism by fire* [video]. https://www.henrystreet.org/

Hirshon, J. M., Risko, N., Calvello, E. J. B., de Ramirez, S. S., Narayan, M., Theodosis, C., & O'Neill, J. Acute Care Research Collaborative at the University of Maryland Global Health Initiative. (2013). Health systems and services: The role of acute care. *Bulletin of the World Health Organization*, *91*(5), 386–388. https://doi.org/10.2471/blt.12.112664

Indeed. (2022). *Acute care nurse job description: Top duties and qualifications*. https://www.indeed.com/hire/job-description/acute-care-nurse?hl=en&co=US

Institute for Healthcare Improvement. (2023). *Population health*. https://www.ihi.org/Topics/Population-Health/Pages/default.aspx

Karen Teeley. (2016). *What is community/public health nursing?* YouTube, September 15, 2016. https://www.youtube.com/watch?v=pdTvSHAcQ1s

Kent, J. (2018). *Population health nurses require changes in education, practices*. https://healthitanalytics.com/news/population-health-nurses-require-changes-in-education-practices

Maraccini, A. M., Galiatsatos, P., Harper, M., & Slonim, A. D. (2017). Creating clarity: Distinguishing between community and population health. *American Journal of Accountable Care*, *5*(2), 32–37. https://www.ajmc.com/view/creating-clarity-distinguishing-between-community-and-population-health

Matthews, J. H., Whitehead, P. B., Ward, C., Kyner, M., & Crowder, T. (2020). Florence Nightingale: Visionary for the role of clinical nurse specialist. *Online Journal of Issues in Nursing*, *25*(2), Manuscript 1. https://doi.org/10.3912/OJIN.Vol25No02Man01

McDonald, L. (2020). Florence Nightingale's public health agenda. *Perspective in Public Health*, *140*(3), 137–138. https://doi.org/10.1177/1757913920916501

Minnesota Department of Health. (2019). *Public health interventions: Application for nursing practice* (2nd ed.). www.health.state.mn.us/communities/practice/research/phncouncil/docs/PHInterventions.pdf

Mona, M. (2016). *Major difference between hospital nurse and community nurse*. Nursing Exercise, May 2, 2016. http://nursingexercise.com/hospital-nurse-community-nurse/

National Academy of Medicine. (2021). *The Future of Nursing 2020–2030: Charting a Path to Health Equity*. National Academies Press. https://nam.edu/publications/the-future-of-nursing-2020-2030/

Nursing-Theory.org. (2023). *Lillian Wald*. https://nursing-theory.org/famous-nurses/Lillian-Wald.php

Office of Disease Prevention and Health Promotion. (n.d.a.). *Building a healthier future for all*. Healthy People 2030. https://health.gov/healthypeople

Office of Disease Prevention and Health Promotion. (n.d.b.). *Healthy People 2030 framework*. Healthy People 2030. https://health.gov/healthypeople/about/healthy-people-2030-framework

Office of Disease Prevention and Health Promotion. (n.d.c.). *Older adults*. Healthy People 2030. https://health.gov/healthypeople/objectives-and-data/browse-objectives/older-adults

Pronk, N., Kleinman, D. V., Goekler, S. F., Ochiai, E., Blakey, C., & Brewer, K. H. (2021). Promoting health and well-being in Healthy People 2030. *Journal of Public Health Management and Practice, 27*(Suppl 6), S242–S248. https://doi.org/10.1097/phh.0000000000001254

Public Health England. (2013). *Nursing and midwifery contribution to public health: Improving health and wellbeing*. https://www.gov.uk/government/publications/nursing-and-midwifery-contribution-to-public-health

Public Health Nursing. (n.d.). *Role of the public health nurse*. https://publichealthnursing.weebly.com/community-vs-public-health-nursing.html

Richmond, J. (1979). *Healthy People: The surgeon general's report on health promotion and disease prevention*. U.S. Department of Health, Education and Welfare. https://profiles.nlm.nih.gov/spotlight/nn/catalog/nlm:nlmuid-101584932X92-doc

Shafer, M. A., Strohschein, S., & Glavin, K. (2022). Twenty years with the public health intervention wheel: Evidence for practice. *Public Health Nursing, 39*(1), 195–201. https://doi.org/10.1111/phn.12941

Valentine-Maher, S. K., Van Dyk, E. J., Aktan, N. M., & Bliss, J. B. (2021). Teaching population health and community-based care across diverse clinical experiences: Integration of conceptual pillars and constructivist learning. *Journal of Nursing Education, 53*(3), S11–S18. https://doi.org/10.3928/01484834-20140217-01

Walker, A. (2024). *Nursing ranked as the most trusting profession for the 22nd year in a row*. Nurse.org, January 23, 2024. https://nurse.org/articles/nursing-ranked-most-honest-profession/

World Health Organization. (2016). *Transitions of care: Technical series on safer primary care*. apps.who.int/iris/bitstream/handle/10665/252272/9789241511599-eng.pdf

Credits

Fig. 1.1: American Association of Colleges of Nursing (AACN), "The Essentials Four Sphere of Care," https://www.aacnnursing.org/Essentials. Copyright © 2021 by American Association of Colleges of Nursing (AACN).

Fig. 1.2: Jon Mark Hirshon, et al., "Health Systems and Services: The Role of Acute Care," *Bulletin of the World Health Organization*, vol. 91, no. 5. Copyright © 2013 by World Health Organization (WHO).

Fig. 1.3: Adapted from Public Health Accreditation Board, "The Essential Public Health Core Services (2020 Version)," https://phaboard.org/center-for-innovation/public-health-frameworks/the-10-essential-public-health-services/. Copyright © 2020 by Public Health Accreditation Board.

Fig. 1.4: Minnesota Department of Health, "Public Health Intervention Wheel," https://www.health.state.mn.us/communities/practice/research/phncouncil/wheel.html. Copyright © by Minnesota Department of Health. Reprinted with permission.

IMG 1.1: U.S. Department of Health and Human Services, "Healthy People 2030 Logo," https://health.gov/healthypeople/about/healthy-people-2030-framework, 2023.

CHAPTER 2

Social Determinants of Health Culture, Ethnicity, Health Equity, Health Disparities, and Vulnerable Populations

"It is absolutely imperative that every human being's freedom and human rights are respected, all over the world."

—Jóhanna Sigurðardóttir, former prime minister of Iceland

Learning Outcomes

After reading this chapter, students should be able to:

1. Describe the social determinants of health (SDOH)
2. Understand the health beliefs of culture, race, and ethnic groups
3. Apply the SDOH to the community and healthcare access
4. Understand health disparities and health equality and inequalities
5. Identify various vulnerable populations
6. Use case studies and active learning activities to promote the SDOH, health disparities, and health equity

Keywords and Concepts

Culture; ethnicity; health disparities; health equality/inequality; health disparities; race; social determinants of health (SDOH); vulnerable populations

Definitions of the Keywords

Culture: Specific beliefs, values, customs, thoughts, behaviors, rituals, manners, and religions that specific groups practice (National Center for Cultural Competence [NCCC], n.d.)

Ethnicity: A large group of individuals with a shared culture and traditions, language, and history (Cambridge Dictionary, n.d.a.)

Health disparities: Disease conditions that occur at higher levels in specific populations than in others (Centers for Disease Control and Prevention [CDC], 2022b)

Health equality/inequalities: Differences between various social populations and financial levels for individuals and societies (World Health Organization [WHO], 2018)

Race: Individuals who are divided into other groups based on physical characteristics such as skin color and eye shape (Cambridge Dictionary, n.d.b.)

SDOH: The health risks and outcomes that develop from where an individual lives, is educated, is employed, and interacts socially (CDC, 2021)

Vulnerable populations: Groups and communities at a higher risk for poor health due to the barriers they experience to social, economic, political, and environmental resources and illness and disability limitations (National Collaborating Centre for Determinants of Health, 2022)

Introduction

Over the past three decades, the understanding of health and its determinants has changed (Gottlieb et al., 2019). Social factors related to where a person lives as well as their education level and income can affect health consequences. In recent years, social risks have become more critical to understanding positive health outcomes of the individual, family, community, and population (Gottlieb et al., 2019).

The American Academy of Colleges of Nursing (AACN; 2021) noted the importance of the SDOH in nursing education. The new AACN document designated SDOH as a concept integrated within the ACCN essentials (2021). Concepts such as the SDOH serve as core components in understanding multiple situations within the nursing practice (AACN, 2021).

Health outcomes depend on many variables. The difference between the SDOH and health disparities must be clearly understood. Health disparities research has focused on the understanding that populations with higher social disadvantages experience worse health outcomes. Scientific evidence notes that the SDOH affects population health and health disparities, but the pathways and mechanisms of how this occurs have yet to be established (Palmer et al., 2019).

An individual's educational levels reflect a person's understanding of what could lead to appropriate or inappropriate health and life decisions. Those individuals who are considered to be in vulnerable populations can be forgotten or not included (McEnroe-Petitte, 2020). Overall, understanding the value of the SDOH areas related to health inequities, health disparities, vulnerable populations, and cultural/ethnic groups is vital to how health must be seen and promoted for all individuals and their communities (CDC, 2022d). This chapter will discuss determinants of health and associated factors, such as health literacy, health equality, culture, and health disparities.

Background of the Concepts

Determining SDOHs allows healthcare professionals to focus on the specific needs of various populations. By examining each of the determinants, a better understanding can be achieved, along with developing plans, interventions, and evaluations for each determinant. The SDOH include the following areas: education access and quality, healthcare and quality, neighborhood and built environment, social and community context, and economic stability (CDC, 2022d). Without the definitions and understanding of each determinant characteristic, effective community care cannot be provided, and the population's needs cannot be fulfilled (Artiga & Hinton, 2018).

Social Determinants of Health

The SDOH are essential to individuals of all ages. The areas where a person may live, be employed, worship, be educated, and play shape various policies, laws, programs, cultures, and communities are critical for health outcomes (Office of Disease Prevention and Health Promotion [ODPHP], n.d.i.). By reviewing the qualities of the SDOH, individuals can see their impacts on a person's health, well-being, and quality of life (ODPHP, n.d.i.).

Healthcare workers focus on the categories of SDOH to provide individuals and communities with the essential resources they need to understand and access. For example, sometimes people do not receive recommended healthcare services, such as cancer screenings and immunizations, because they do not have a primary care provider or knowledge of access to healthcare resources (Furr-Holden et al., 2020). They may lack safe housing, and their access to education, jobs, nutritious foods, and healthy air and water may be affected (ODPHP, n.d.i.).

Enhancing the SDOH initiative in Healthy People (HP) 2030 is geared toward reducing health inequities using upstream approaches (Shah, 2021). Upstream approaches should be at the macro level for systemwide changes to occur. An example of an upstream macro approach that affects health could be addressing income through living-wage policy changes or healthcare for all (Shah, 2021).

Definition of SDOH

HP 2030 enhanced its goals related to the SDOH. The goals promote social, physical, and economic environments, encouraging attaining total health and well-being potential (ODPHP, n.d.i.). Many objectives in HP 2030 enhance the upstream approach to improve health and are related to the SDOH. Some examples of the SDOH are safe housing/neighborhoods, racism, discrimination, education, income, access to nutritious foods, polluted air, and literacy/language skills (ODPHP, n.d.i.).

SDOH are grouped into five domains, which are education access and quality, healthcare access and quality, neighborhood and built environment, social and community context, and economic stability (Figure 2.1). These domains encompass many aspects of the environment that affect a person's quality of life and well-being (ODPHP, n.d.i.).

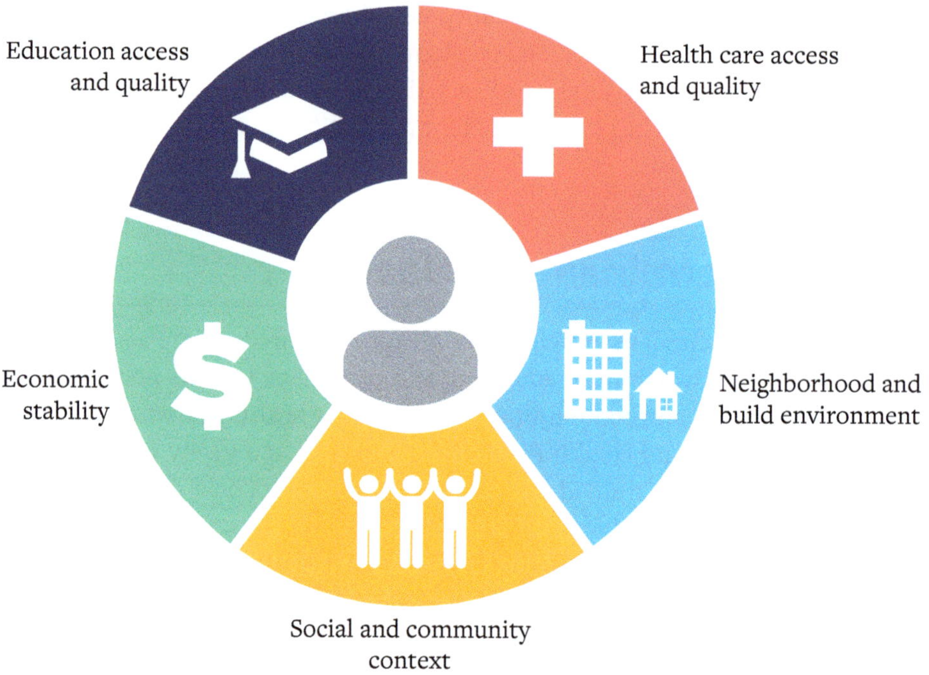

FIGURE 2.1 Social Determinants of Health: Five Domains

Education Access and Quality

Education is an important area to understand when discussing SDOH. With proper education, employment may be available to all and positively affect income. Stryzhak (2020) noted that higher levels of education are associated with higher income levels, which help people live happier lives.

Unfortunately, education at all levels is not open to all individuals around the globe. The United Nations (UN) Sustainable Developmental Goals (SDGs; 2022d) related to quality education revealed that the COVID-19 pandemic profoundly affected education. Those most affected by school disruptions due to COVID-19 were girls, children from disadvantaged backgrounds, those living in rural areas, children with disabilities, and children of ethnic minorities (UN, 2022d).

Many school systems around the United States have math and reading scores that do not meet proficiency levels for proper education and adequate future incomes. More developmental and research objectives have been added to HP 2030 to provide baseline information on how problematic eighth-grade reading and math scores are (ODPHP, n.d.c.). Ongoing data for fourth-grade math skills at or above the proficiency level rose from 40.2% in 2017 to 41.1% in 2019 but are still below the goal of 43% (ODPHP, n.d.c.). However, data for fourth-grade reading skills at or above proficiency decreased from 36.6% in 2017 to 35.3% in 2019, noting a worsening problem below the goal of 41.5% (ODPHP, n.d.c.).

Healthcare Access and Quality

The Agency for Healthcare Research and Quality (AHRQ, 2021) evaluates health and quality, offering reports on the U.S. population and disparities in racial and socioeconomic groups. The report identifies six specific areas for quality: patient safety, person-centered care, care coordination, effective treatment, healthy living, and care affordability (AHRQ, 2021). Although the overall trend in access to care has improved, significant disparities by race, ethnicity, household income, and location of residence persist for access to health insurance and access to dental insurance, including inequalities by race, ethnicity, household income, location of residence, and insurance type (AHRQ, 2021).

The WHO (2020) views healthcare quality as encompassing services that allow for increases in positive health outcomes for individuals and populations. A resounding theme is the need for quality healthcare for all without financial hardship. One of the key themes is primary care access, which is difficult due to a shortage of these services (WHO, 2020).

HP 2030 (ODPHP, n.d.d.) noted that about 10% of the U.S. population do not have health insurance. Those with health insurance are more likely to have primary care providers, thus requiring primary and early secondary prevention (screenings). The distance to a provider, cost, and lack of transportation are reasons for getting quality healthcare (ODPHP, n.d.d.). In the United States, the number of those older than age 35 who received all the recommended high-priority preventive services in 2015 was 8.5%, and in 2018, that number dropped to 6.9% (ODPHP, n.d.d.). The target for this objective is 11.5% of the population (ODPHP, n.d.d.).

Neighborhood and Built Environment

Creating neighborhoods and environments that promote health and safety is a goal of HP 2030 (ODPHP, n.d.g.). Unfortunately, many individuals in the United

States live, work, play, and learn in unsafe situations. Racial/ethical minorities and low-income individuals are more prone to dangerous conditions due to high violence and hazardous air and water (ODPHP, n.d.g.).

HP 2030 objectives for neighborhood and built environment entail many different avenues. Developmental objectives related to increasing respiratory issues, such as chronic obstructive pulmonary disease and asthma, are now in place to monitor for the future. In 2018, there were 9.4 asthma deaths per 100,000, but in 2020, this rate increased to 11.3 asthma deaths per 100,000 (ODPHP, n.d.g.). The goal for asthma deaths is 8.9 per 100,000 (ODPHP, n.d.g.).

One of the UN's SDGs is managing water and sanitation for all (UN, 2022c). More than 730 million people live in areas with high and critical levels of water stress. At the current rate, by 2030, 1.6 billion individuals will lack proper water, 2.8 billion will lack adequate sanitation, and 1.9 billion will lack good hygiene facilities (UN, 2022c).

Pinter-Wollman et al. (2018) identify three specific themes related to the environment that promote health. The first is to look at the physical environment and how interventions can increase physical activity to assist with obesity and obesity-associated conditions, such as diabetes, heart disease, and cancer. Their second theme supports proper nutritional habits related to obesity, and the final theme identifies mental health, housing, and urban design. Housing locations, whether urban or rural, can influence the development of depression and anxiety (Pinter-Wollman et al., 2018).

Social and Community Context

HP 2030's social and community context goal involves the importance of relationships with family, friends, coworkers, and community members (ODPHP, n.d.h.). Positive relationships and adequate social support can improve health and well-being (ODPHP, n.d.h.). By developing interventions to increase love and respect, social relationships can be used to help with critical issues while improving the health and well-being of all.

Social support is essential to the early years of development. In 2016–2017, only 68.5% ages 6 to 17 had parents who reported that they and their child could share ideas and talk about things that mattered, whereas in 2018–2019, this number worsened, dropping to 65.3% (ODPHP, n.d.h.). The target goal for improving communication between parents and children is 73% (ODPHP, n.d.h.).

The Rural Health Information Hub (RHIhub) has developed programs with interventions focusing on SDOH issues that affect the rural community (RHIhub, 2022b). Specifically, programs related to social and community contexts have been developed. The importance of where people live, the creation of relationships between neighbors and their community, and civic connections could be crucial to improving health outcomes. The programs have developed interventions focused on civic participation, discrimination, incarceration and crime, social cohesiveness and connectedness, and community capacity (RHIhub, 2022b).

Economic Stability

The UN (2022a) is determined to end poverty worldwide. SDG #1 noted a decrease in poverty from 10.1% to 8.6% from 2015 to 2018. However, the COVID-19 pandemic raised the rate from 8.3% in 2019 to 9.2% in 2020. The changes in inflation and the war in Ukraine have also been factors in reversing a steady decline in poverty for almost 30 years (UN, 2022b).

HP 2030 (ODPHP, n.d.b.) states that one in 10 U.S. individuals lives in poverty. The United States has high housing costs, food insecurity, and problems with attaining affordable healthcare. Individuals with a steady income are more likely to be healthier and less likely to live in poverty (ODPHP, n.d.b.). People with disabilities, injuries, or other disabling diseases are more inclined to suffer from economic issues (ODPHP, n.d.b.).

Rising housing costs are causing more individuals to spend more of their income on this factor. HP 2030 has now added an objective to monitor and provide interventions to keep the percentage of income going to housing down. Baseline numbers were 34.6% in 2017, and families used 30% of their income for housing (ODPHP, n.d.b.). The goal is 25.5% (ODPHP, n.d.b.). Specific characteristics and an example of the HP 2030 objective for all five SDOH areas are noted in Table 2.1.

TABLE 2.1 Five Categories With Characteristics and an Example of an HP 2030 SDOH Objective

Type of SDOH	Characteristics	Objective Example From HP 2030
Education Access and Quality	• Educational opbportunities at all levels • Reading/math proficiency skills • Graduation rates	Increase the proportion of high school students who graduate in four years—AH-08
Healthcare and Quality	• Food insecurity/hunger/healthy food options • Access to healthcare • Health insurance • Transportation issues • Primary/secondary prevention (immunizations/screenings)	Increase the proportion of people with a substance use disorder who received treatment in the past year—SU-01
Neighborhood and Built Environment	• Inaccessibility of food and for nutritious choices • Access to adequate housing, water, utilities, and clean/toxin-free air • Crime rates/violence • Park access • Internet access • School safety • Fluoride access in water • Hearing loss due to environment • Mass transportation access • Tobacco usage/work/home	Increase the proportion of adults with broadband Internet—HC/HIT-05

Social and Community Context	• Social inclusion/exclusion • Racial segregation/discrimination • Culture and social norms • Use of information technology for health • Communication with parents/ community • Health literacy	Increase the proportion of children and adolescents who communicate positively with their parents—EMC-01
Economic Stability	• Income levels/unemployment • Amount of housing cost • Disabilities that restrict working • Work-related injuries • Affording food	Reduce the proportion of adults with arthritis whose arthritis limits their work—A-03

Source: Adapted from ODPHP, n.d.i.

Culture/Ethnicity/Race

Understanding the effects of culture, race, and ethnicity will become even more critical as the United States becomes more diversified. Culturally competent nurses will be essential in providing positive health outcomes. Nurses must invest in cultural awareness of the population and community and provide cultural sensitivity regarding various races and ethnicities (Young & Guo, 2020).

Transcultural nursing has become even more imperative in nursing education as immigration and globalization occur (Albougami et al., 2016). Many transcultural models have been developed that could assist in understanding the practices and beliefs of particular populations. Understanding different cultures could lead to better healthcare delivery, effective disease management, and an improvement in the overall health of these individuals and populations (Albougami et al., 2016; Leininger, 2002). Comparing culturally competent models could provide a more thorough assessment of transcultural nursing (Table 2.2).

Culture

Culture is critical at many levels. Nurses must know other cultures' varying perceptions and acceptance of healthcare practices (Albougami et al., 2016). In 2008, the AACN developed a cultural competency toolkit for nursing students (AACN, 2008). Further clarification of the importance of culture is noted in the revised AACN essentials that were released (AACN, 2021; Table 2.3).

Cultural competence, which is learned over time, requires personal reflection and experiences (Young & Guo, 2020). Understanding cultural differences better through realistic education and training can increase the efficacy of nursing practice for diverse populations (Young & Guo, 2020). The new essentials designated diversity, equity, and inclusion (DEI) as a concept, with the understanding that cultural competency is critical for nursing students to understand and apply (AACN, 2021). Assessment of necessary skills, attitudes, and awareness needed for effective cultural care is essential for all nurses in the future.

TABLE 2.2 Models of Culturally Competent Care Comparison

Name of Model	Specific Characteristics	Application Example
Leininger sunrise model/transcultural nursing theory/ cultural care theory (2002; Nursing Theory, 2020)	Culturally specific care Culturally congruent care	On admission and ongoing, performs a holistic assessment of beliefs, including health, relationships, religion, language, sexual orientation, and appearance
Giger and Davidhizar's transcultural assessment model (2008)	Six dimensions common to every culture: communication, space, social organization, time, environmental control, and biological variation	Time is subdivided into whether the group is clock-oriented, like most Westerners, or socially oriented. The clock-oriented group is fixated on time itself, and individuals with this orientation seek to keep appointments to avoid being seen as impolite or offensive.
Purnell model for cultural competence (2002)	Involves 12 domains: overview or heritage, communication, family roles and organization, workforce issues, biocultural ecology, high-risk behaviors, nutrition, pregnancy, death rituals, spirituality, healthcare practices, and healthcare professionals	Depending on their place of origin, individuals or groups are accustomed to specific foods and draw meaning from the foods they eat. Food consumption associated with particular traditions may affect health. Some ethnic groups suffer from certain nutritional limitations and deficiencies.

Source: Adapted from Albougami et al., 2016.

TABLE 2.3 Vital Cultural Competencies for Undergraduate Nursing Students

These five competencies identify the key elements considered essential for baccalaureate nursing graduates to provide culturally competent care. These competencies provide a framework for integrating suggested content and learning experiences into existing curricula.

- Competency 1: Apply knowledge of social and cultural factors that affect nursing and health care across multiple contexts.
- Competency 2: Use relevant data sources and the best evidence in providing culturally competent care.
- Competency 3: Promote achievement of safe and quality outcomes of care for diverse populations.
- Competency 4: Advocate for social justice, including a commitment to the health of vulnerable populations and the elimination of health disparities.
- Competency 5: Participate in continuous cultural competence development.

Source: AACN, 2008.

Race and Ethnicity Defined

- **Race** is a socially defined category, based on real or perceived biological differences between groups of people.
- **Ethnicity** is a socially defined category based on common language, religion, nationality, history, or another cultural factor.

FIGURE 2.2 *Race* Versus *Ethnicity* Defined

Race/Ethnicity

Many people do not know the difference between race and ethnicity and often use the terms interchangeably. *Race* is about characteristics provided by parents, meaning something inherited. *Ethnicity* is a cultural expression associated with something learned (Morin, 2022; Figure 2.2). Proper language about race and ethnicity is critical for effective communication (Table 2.4).

TABLE 2.4 Preferred Terms for Races and Cultures

Instead of This	Try This
• Referring to people by their race/ethnicity (for example, *Blacks*, *Hispanics*, *Latinos*, *Whites*, *American Indians*, etc.) • Referring to people as *colored people*, *colored Indian* (regarding American Indians) • Native American (for federal publications) • Eskimo • Oriental • Afro-American • Negro • Caucasian • The [racial/ethnic] community (for example, "the Black community") • Non-White (used with or without specifying non-Hispanic or Latino)	**Racial groups:** • American Indian or Alaska Native persons/communities/populations • Asian persons • Black or African American persons; Black persons • Native Hawaiian persons • Pacific Islander persons • White persons • People who identify with more than one race, people of more than one race, persons of multiple races **Ethnic groups:** • Hispanic or Latino persons • Non-Hispanic persons When describing a combination of racial/ethnic groups (for example, three or more subgroups), use "people from some racial and ethnic groups" or "people from racial and ethnic minority groups."

Source: Adapted from CDC, 2022c.

The racial and ethnical makeup has changed in the United States. From 2010 to 2021, the non-Hispanic population decreased from 63.8% to 59.3%. In contrast, the Hispanic/Latino population increased from 16.4% to 18.9% (USA Facts, 2021). The Hispanic/Latino population is rising at a higher rate than the African American population and is now more prominent (USA Facts, 2021; Figure 2.3).

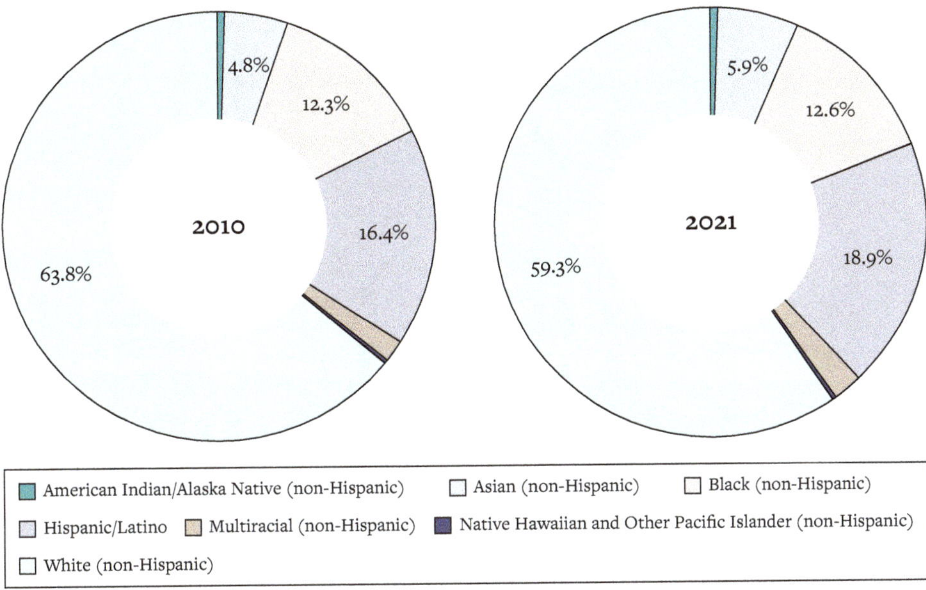

FIGURE 2.3 Racial and Ethical Changes From 2010 to 2021

Health Equality/Equity/Inequalities/Inequities

CDC (2022b) defines *health equity* as the state in which all individuals have a fair and equal opportunity to achieve their highest level of health. Many societal factors will need to change to achieve health equity. Changes in policy and social factors at the macro level will be the key to reducing health inequity (CDC, 2022b).

In 2021, the CDC expanded on the priority of health equity concerning the SDOH. CDC developed a framework containing six pillars to address healthy equity and SDOH. These pillars are data and surveillance, evaluation and evidence building, partnerships and collaboration, community engagement, infrastructure and capacity, and policy and law (CDC, 2021; Figure 2.4). The National Center for Chronic Disease Prevention and Health Promotion (NCCDPHP) is the primary agency leading the process of the six pillars. These pillars are CDC agencywide processes to improve and promote cross-cutting efforts to address SDOH and health equity issues and help leadership decide where to invest SDOH resources (CDC, 2021; Table 2.5).

Health equity is a priority at the global level. Within the SDOH department at the WHO is the Equity and Health (EQH) unit. The EQH unit addresses the SDOH and equity. Much like the CDC, it provides strategic leadership in developing evidence, norms, and standards that strengthen the case for investment; building national capacities; and fostering global advocacy (WHO, n.d.). The health-related targets of the UN SDG agenda noted the need for equity for all to ensure healthy lives (SDG #3; Hosseinpoor et al., 2018) and

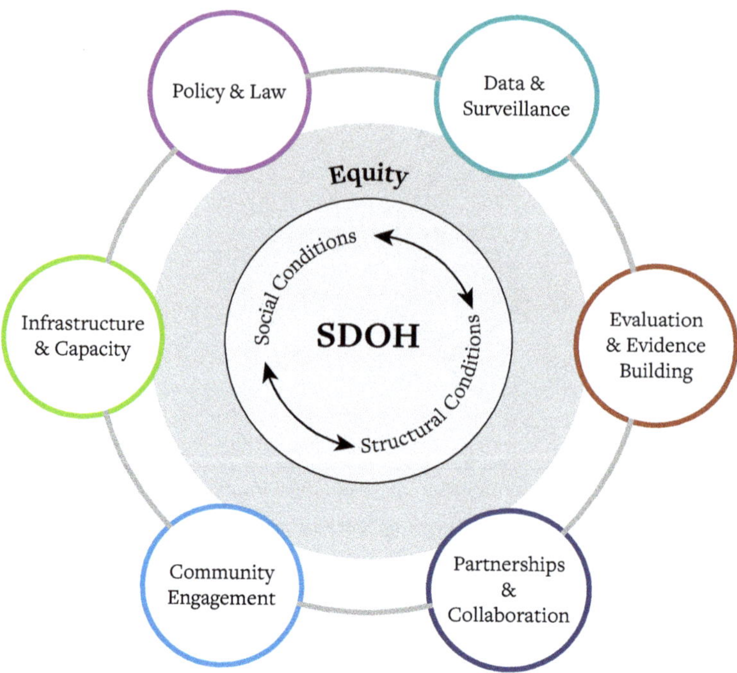

FIGURE 2.4 CDC Framework of Six Pillars to Address the SDOH and Health Equity

TABLE 2.5 CDC Framework of Six Pillars to Address the SDOH and Health Equity With Definitions and Characteristics

Pillar	Definition/Characteristic
Data and surveillance	Standardization, collection, analysis, and dissemination of data across the agency
Evaluation and evidence-building	Advance evaluation and build evidence for strategies to reduce disparities and promote health equity
Partnerships and collaboration	Establish criteria, steps, and procedures for partnerships, collaborations, and relationships that result in improved health outcomes
Community engagement	Foster meaningful, sustained community engagement across all phases of CDC intervention planning and implementation
Infrastructure and capacity	Strengthen and sustain infrastructures such as workforce, training, and access to financial resources required to reduce health disparities
Policy and law	Identify evidence, tools, and resources to enhance communication about policies with policymakers and other stakeholders

Source: Adapted from CDC, 2021.

gender equality (SDG #5; UN, 2022b). The key to understanding how to address, monitor, and solve health equality issues is understanding the population subgroups (Hosseinpoor et al., 2018; Box 2.1).

BOX 2.1 APPLICATION OF HEALTH EQUITY ACTIVE LEARNING EXERCISE (EVIDENCE-BASED)

Watch the following video regarding health equity released by the American Public Health Association (APHA): https://www.youtube.com/watch?v=Arpzx6TJuQI.

Reflect on the video by answering the following question:

1. Based on the video, think about/research three specific interventions/programs using health equity in the community. Provide evidence-based literature to support these.

AACN *Essentials* (2021): Domains: #1, #3; #4; #6; #9

- Competencies: 1.2; 3.1; 3.3; 4.2; 6.4; 9.2; 9.3
- Subcompetencies: 1.2c; 3.1c; 3.1h; 3.3a; 3.3b; 4.2c; 6.4d; 9.2d; 9.3g

Spheres of Care: Wellness/Disease prevention, Chronic disease management

Concepts: Evidence-based practice; Diversity, equity, inclusion (DEI), SDOH

Sources: APHA, 2021; CDC, 2021.

Application to SDOH and HP 2030

The NCCDPHP has strengthened efforts to address the SDOH and health equity in the past few years. In 2020, it identified five areas related to the HP 2030 SDOH that complemented existing work and were related to chronic disease outcomes (Hacker & Houry, 2022). These areas are noted in Table 2.6.

TABLE 2.6 CDC/NCCDPHP Application to HP 2030 Goals

- **Social connectedness**, which is the degree to which individuals have quality relationships to create a sense of belonging and support
- **Community-clinical linkages**, which connect individuals to the services that they need
- **Tobacco-free policy**, which includes population-based preventive measures to reduce tobacco use and tobacco-related morbidity and mortality
- **The built environment**, which refers to human-made surroundings and can consist of issues related to housing and transportation
- **Food and nutrition security, which** exists when people consistently have physical, social, and economic access to food to meet dietary needs for a productive and healthy life

Source: Hacker & Houry, 2022.

The WHO (2022) addressed COVID-19 and stated that it was a significant threat to the world regarding contracting and preventing the disease. Social factors such as limitations to healthcare and vaccinations were noted. Age, transportation, access to healthcare, and lack of vaccine equity contributed to the rates of COVID-19 (WHO, 2022).

Additional concerns with COVID-19 led to health inequities that developed for other reasons. The effects on specific populations include older adults, individuals with chronic conditions, and those without appropriate economic resources. COVID-19 caused numerous disruptions in many areas of healthcare (WHO, 2022). Due to the vast numbers requiring hospitalizations and care, many preventative and elective care/surgeries were postponed. These actions caused many conditions to go undetected and allowed the development of diseases. As the WHO (2022) looks deeper into the effects of COVID-19, the need to review the beginning, middle, and current status of COVID-19 will be essential to improve the quality of care that the pandemic presented (WHO, 2022). Despite the countries' income, COVID-19 was a significant condition and threat to the public, leading to many health inequalities (Okonkwo et al., 2021).

Health Disparities

Despite attempting to provide health equity to all, specific populations experience health disparities (CDC, 2020). Understanding the impact of health disparities is critical to delivering optimal healthcare. Certain SDOH factors could be just one of the variables affecting particular populations with higher issues and diseases. Understanding of disparity revolves around sex, race or ethnic background, level of education, amount of income, presence of any disability, living location, and sexual orientation (CDC, 2020; ODPHP, 2022).

A specific example of health disparity issues in the COVID-19 pandemic was the death rate. Non-Hispanic persons accounted for more than two-thirds of U.S. deaths, and the non-Hispanic Native American and Black populations died disproportionately at higher rates (USA Facts, 2022). Non-Hispanic persons comprise only 60% of the U.S. population (USA Facts, 2022; Figure 2.5).

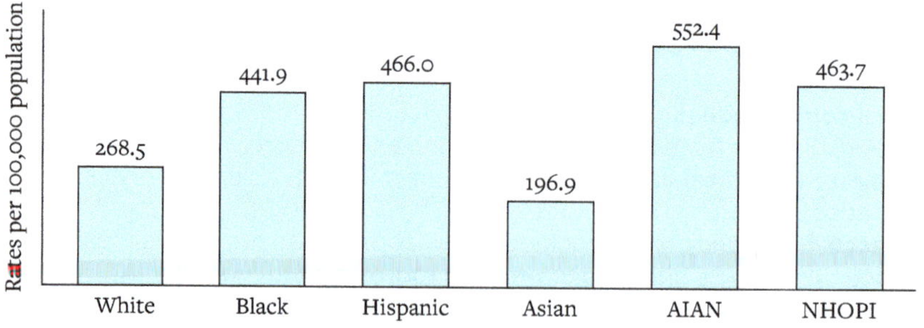

FIGURE 2.5 Cumulative COVID-19 Age-Adjusted Mortality Rates and Ethnicity 2020–2022. (AIAN) refers to American Indian or Alaska Native; (NHOPI) refers to Native Hawaiian or Other Pacific Islander.

Definition

Health disparities are differences in the incidence, prevalence, and mortality of a disease and the related adverse health conditions among specific population groups. These groups may be characterized by gender, age, race or ethnicity, social class, disability, geographic location, or sexual orientation (CDC, 2020). The occurrence of tuberculosis (TB), viral hepatitis, human immunodeficiency virus (HIV), and sexually transmitted diseases (STDs) at higher levels in specific populations is referred to as a *health disparity* (CDC, 2020). Higher conditions can occur by gender and sexual orientation (CDC, 2020). SDOH factors such as income, built environment, and education are also linked to health disparities (CDC, 2020; Table 2.7).

TABLE 2.7 Specific Population Health Disparities Examples in the United States

Population	Specific Examples of Health Disparities and Rates
African American	HIV: African American/Black people's death rates were higher (16.3 per 100,000) compared with those of any other racial/ethnic group (2.5 per 100,000 for White people).
Hispanic	STDs: The rate of reported chlamydia cases among Hispanic people was 392.6 cases per 100,000 population, which was 1.9 times the rate among White individuals.
Asian	TB: The rate in Asian people was 17 cases per 100,000, which is 31 times higher than the rate of TB disease in non-Hispanic persons (0.5 cases per 100,000 population).

Application to Health Disparities and Inequalities and HP 2030

Race or ethnicity, sex, sexual orientation, age, disability, socioeconomic status, and geographic location all can contribute to an individual's ability to achieve good health (ODPHP, n.d.e.). It is essential to recognize the impact of SDOH outcomes on specific populations as there has been an increased concentration on developing new programs and policies/procedures. Steps to making positive changes to the environment where individuals live, decrease health disparities, and make significant improvements for all people are critical (ODPHP, n.d.e.). Environmental conditions influence health and well-being outcomes, functioning, and quality-of-life outcomes and risks and are primarily responsible for health inequities (Gómez et al., 2021).

HP 2030 (ODPHP, 2022) strives to improve the health of all groups. The disparities in access and availability of medical facilities and services are significant. Horvath (2022) discusses findings that stress socioeconomic factors in minority communities are required to travel more distances for healthcare than in White neighborhoods. The reasons relate to poor socioeconomic factors, including monies, insurance coverage, educational levels, racism, and marginalized communities (Horvath, 2022). Differences in distances to medical facilities are also common in rural communities. Services such as those given with obstetric care, emergency services, and intensive care units are often a considerable distance for this population (Horvath, 2022).

The AHRQ reports yearly on healthcare quality and disparity. SDOH factors may substantially influence the population's health and well-being more than services delivered by practitioners and healthcare delivery organizations (AHRQ, 2022). Even though the percentage of people with health insurance coverage has significantly increased in the past decade, non-Hispanic American Indian, Alaska Native, and Hispanic groups are considerably less likely to be insured (AHRQ, 2022).

Vulnerable Populations

Certain factors, such as sex, age, and income, can influence an individual's health risk for certain diseases and risk of being seriously affected by public

TABLE 2.8 Five Most Vulnerable Populations in Healthcare

Type	Issue
Chronically ill and disabled	These populations report twice the number of poor-health days than the general population.
Low-income and homeless	Low-income individuals have more chronic illnesses. *Homeless* means the lack of a safe place to live, which equates to a higher number of adverse-related outcomes.
Certain geographical communities	Rural populations have worse health than that of the general population. Native Americans have a lower life expectancy and lack of access to care.
Lesbian, gay, bisexual, transgender, and queer or questioning (LGBTQ+) population	Black transgender women have higher rates of HIV. This population lacks safe housing and healthcare providers who are culturally educated about the LGBTQ+ population.
Older adults and children	Older adults don't receive the preventive care recommended for them. There are negative effects of climate change on children (such as air and water pollution, which leads to more respiratory problems such as asthma).

Source: Adapted from Joszt, 2018.

health emergencies. The same is valid for population groups (CDC, 2022a). CDC (2022a) tracks the social vulnerability of U.S. communities based on how they prepare and respond to hazardous events. Poverty, lack of access to transportation, and proper housing may weaken a community's ability to properly prevent significant population loss and rebuild due to its social vulnerability (CDC, 2022a).

Definition

Significant disparities exist in healthcare for vulnerable populations in the United States. Several groups are considered vulnerable populations, including racial and ethnic minorities, the economically disadvantaged, and those with chronic health conditions. For vulnerable populations, their health and healthcare issues may be exacerbated by social factors such as more significant risk factors, worse access to care, and increased morbidity and mortality (Joszt, 2018; Table 2.8; Box 2.2).

BOX 2.2 VULNERABLE POPULATIONS ACTIVE LEARNING ACTIVITY (ADDRESSING THE SDOH, HEALTH EQUITY, AND HEALTH DISPARITIES)

Visit the following link: https://www.ruralhealthinfo.org/toolkits/sdoh.

Complete all aspects of "Module 1: Introduction to social determinants of health for rural populations."

Answer the following questions:

1. Discuss two health equity/health disparity issues with rural populations.
2. Using the five categories of the SDOH, specifically address unique issues in rural communities for each category.
3. Name two population considerations specific to rural communities.

AACN *Essentials* (2021): Domains: #1; #2; #3; #4; #6; #7; #9

- Competencies: 1.2; 2.1; 3.1; 3.3; 3.4; 4.2; 6.1; 7.2; 9.2; 9.3
- Subcompetencies: 1.2c; 2.1c; 3.1a; 3.1b; 3.1c; 3.1d; 3.1e; 3.1h; 3.1i; 3.3a; 3.3b; 3.4b; 4.2c; 6.1d; 7.2b; 9.2d; 9.3a; 9.3g

Spheres of Care: Wellness/Disease prevention; Chronic disease management

Concepts: Evidence-based; Clinical judgment; DEI; Ethics; SDOH

Source: Adapted from RHIhub, 2022.

Application to the SDOH and HP 2030

HP 2030 continues to focus on vulnerable groups to better understand and provide specific interventions. Objectives are divided into five topics: population, health behaviors, health conditions, health settings, and SDOH. Particular populations, such as LGBTQ, children, older adults, and people with disabilities, are specifically identified in the population section (ODPHP, n.d.a.).

LBGTQ-specific objectives have been expanded with HP 2030. Data have now expanded to include bullying of transgender students; adolescent illicit drug use for transgender, gay, lesbian, and bisexual students; suicide thoughts in transgender, gay, lesbian, and bisexual adolescent students; and the need for improvement to the public health structure at the local and state levels on addressing sexual orientation and gender identity (ODPHP, n.d.f.).

RHIhub (2022a) contains an SDOH toolkit for rural communities, which includes evidence-based and promising models and resources to support organizations implementing programs to address the SDOH in rural communities across the United States. Other evidence-based toolkits are regarding care coordination, community health workers, health promotion and disease prevention, telehealth, health networks and coalition, service integration, and rural transportation (RHIhub, 2022a; Box 2.3).

BOX 2.3 SDOH ACTIVE LEARNING ACTIVITY (USING HP 2030)

1. Use the following URL to access the SDOH categories: https://health.gov/healthypeople/objectives-and-data/browse-objectives#social-deterMinants-of-health.
2. List two objectives noted in each category. Focus on ones not in development or research but with established data.
3. Discuss one of the objectives in detail for each category. (Note the baseline and target statistics along with the summary of the detailed objective.)
4. Discuss how each objective might be used in a community by giving a specific example for each noted with evidence-based resources.

SDOH Assignment Category	
Economic Stability	
Education Access and Quality	
Healthcare Access and Quality	
Neighborhood and Built Community	
Social and Community Context	

AACN *Essentials* (2021): Domains: #1; #3; #4; #8; #9

- Competencies: 1.2; 3.1; 3.3; 3.4; 4.2; 4.3; 8.1; 8.2; 9.3; 9.6
- Subcompetencies: 1.2c; 3.1a; 3.1b; 3.1c; 3.3a; 3.3b; 3.4b; 4.2c; 4.3d; 8.1c; 8.1d; 8,1e; 8.2c; 8.2d; 9.3a; 9.3g; 9.6a; 9.6c

Spheres of Care: Wellness/Disease prevention; Chronic disease management

Concepts: DEI; Ethics; Evidence-based practice; SDOH

Source: Adapted from ODPHP, n.d.i.

Chapter Highlights

- Discussion with examples of the SDOH
- Discussion with examples of culture, health equity, health disparities, and vulnerable populations
- Application/active learning exercise related to health equity
- Active learning exercises related to SDOH
- Active learning exercise related to vulnerable populations (rural)
- Case studies related to the SDOH, culture, health equality, and health disparities

Active Learning Exercises

Application to Intervention Wheel: Referral and Follow-Up Intervention: Vulnerable Population of Interest (Homeless)

Use the following link: www.health.state.mn.us/communities/practice/research/phncouncil/docs/PHInterventions.pdf.

Go to the "Referral and Follow-Up Intervention" (Green Wedge). Note the practice-level example regarding "Adults Experiencing Homelessness."

Read the "Referral and Follow-Up Intervention" definition, including the information at the systems, community, and individual/family levels. Answer the following questions:

1. Briefly discuss the overall statistics for homelessness in the United States.
2. Discuss three specific issues noted regarding homelessness.
3. Discuss what was done at the systems level.

4. Discuss what was done at the community level.
5. Discuss what was done at the individual/family level.
6. Apply one level to resources/referral opportunities for people experiencing homelessness in your community.

AACN *Essentials* (2021): Domains: #1; #2; #3; #4; #6; #7; #8; #9

- Competencies: 1.2; 2.1; 3.1; 3.2; 3.4; 4.2; 6.1; 7.2; 8.4; 9.2; 9.3; 9.6
- Subcompetencies: 1.2c; 1.2e; 2.1a; 2.1b; 3.1b; 3.1c; 3.1e; 3.1g; 3.1h; 3.1i; 3.2a; 3.3b; 3.2c; 3.4b; 3.4c; 4.2c; 6.1d; 7.2b; 8.4b; 8.4d; 9.2b; 9.2d; 9.3g; 9.6a; 9.6c

Spheres of Care: Wellness/Disease prevention; Chronic disease management; Regenerative/restorative care

Concepts: Communication; Compassionate care; DEI; Ethics; SDOH; Clinical Judgment

Source: Adapted from Minnesota Department of Health, 2019.

Case Studies

Case Study #1: SDOH Application

Susie Jones is a single, unmarried Caucasian mother. She lives in Section 8, a lower-income community in an urban town. She is 25 and has three children ages 7, 5, and 2. Susie receives minimal child support for her three children, who all have different fathers, none of who are involved with their children. She is unable to work because of the cost of daycare. Susie did not graduate high school due to her first pregnancy. Susie has not seen a healthcare provider since the birth of her last child and is currently dating Tommy Hoffman.

1. Apply two SDOH categories to the scenario, providing rationale and evidence-based resources.
2. What are two priority interventions regarding assisting Suzie? Provide rationales and evidence-based resources to support the answer.
3. What other questions/assessments are needed from Susie? Provide rationales and evidence-based resources to support the response.

AACN *Essentials* (2021): Domains: #1; #2; #3; #4; #5

- Competencies: 1.3; 2.3; 2.9; 3.3; 3.5; 4.1; 5.1
- Subcompetencies: 1.3b; 1.3c; 2.3c; 2.9a; 3.3b; 3.5c; 4.1b; 5.1a; 5.1f

Spheres of Care: Wellness/Disease prevention

Concepts: Clinical judgment; Evidence-based practice; SDOH

Source: Created by authors.

Case Study #2: SDOH Application With Cultural and Ethnicity Factors

Manuel Rodriguez is a 49-year-old mechanic who lives next door to Susie Jones. He works at a mechanic shop located across town. Manuel needs a driver's license and a car to get to work. A bus stop is close to his house but often runs late. Manuel is divorced and has no children. English is not Manuel's first language. Manuel learned his trade in Puerto Rico about 10 years ago before coming to the country. He can read only at a third-grade level.

1. Apply two SDOH categories to the scenario, providing rationale and evidence-based resources.
2. What two cultural and/or ethnic factors should be considered in this scenario? Provide a rationale and evidence-based resources to support the response.
3. What other questions/assessments are needed from Manuel? Provide a rationale and evidence-based resources to support the response.

AACN *Essentials* (2021): Domains: #2; #3; #6; #7; #8; #9; #10

- Competencies: 2.2; 2.6; 2.8; 3.2; 6.1; 7.2; 8.2; 8.3; 9.2; 9.3; 9.6; 10.2
- Subcompetencies: 2.2b; 2.2e; 2.6b; 2.8c; 3.2c; 6.1b; 7.2b; 8.2d; 8.3c; 9.2d; 9.3g; 9.6c; 10.2f

Spheres of Care: Wellness/Disease prevention

Concepts: Communication; DEI; Evidence-based practice; SDOH; Ethics

Source: Created by authors.

Case Study #3: SDOH Application With Health Disparities and Health Inequality Factors

Joseph, age 35, and Destiny Johnson, age 32, are an African American couple who live in the same community as Susie and Manuel (from case study #2). They have been married for 13 years. They have four children who are ages 14, 12, 7, and 3. Joseph works at a local fast-food restaurant where he was just turned down for a managerial promotion despite being the most qualified applicant. Joseph's health insurance premiums are too much for the family to afford any insurance. Destiny recently noticed a lump in her right breast but didn't know how the family could afford healthcare regarding the issue. Damian is age 3, is not talking yet, and is often seen flapping his hands. None of the children see a pediatrician or have a regular healthcare provider.

1. Apply two SDOH categories to the scenario, providing a rationale and evidence-based resources to support the response.
2. What two health disparities and/or health inequality factors should be considered in this scenario? Provide a rationale and evidence-based resources to support the response.

3. What other questions/assessments are needed from the Johnson family? Provide a rationale and evidence-based resources to support the response.

AACN *Essentials* (2021): Domains: #2; #3; #7; #9

- Competencies: 2.2; 2.5; 2.8; 2.9; 3.3; 7.1; 7.2; 9.2; 9.3
- Subcompetencies: 2.2e; 2.5c; 2,5e; 2.8a; 2.8b; 2.9e; 3.3a; 3.3b; 7.1d; 7.2b; 9.2d; 9.2e; 9.3a; 9.3g

Spheres of Care: Wellness/Disease prevention; Chronic disease management; Regenerative/restorative care

Concepts: Evidence-based practice; DEI; SDOH; Clinical judgment

Source: Created by authors.

NCLEX Questions

1. Under which SDOH category should food insecurity be addressed?
   a. Healthcare access
   b. Economic stability
   c. Social and community context
   d. Education

2. A nurse works in a community clinic with a large population of Hispanic people. If implemented by the nurse, which strategy would decrease health disparities for the Hispanic population?
   a. Improve public transportation to the clinic.
   b. Update supplies and equipment at the clinic.
   c. Obtain low-cost medication for the clinic clients.
   d. Teach clinic staff about Hispanic health beliefs.

References

Agency for Healthcare Research and Quality. (2021). *2021 National Healthcare Quality and Disparities Report.* https://www.ahrq.gov/sites/default/files/wysiwyg/research/findings/nhqrdr/2021qdr.pdf

Agency for Healthcare Research and Quality. (2022). *2022 National Healthcare Quality and Disparities Report.* https://www.ahrq.gov/sites/default/files/wysiwyg/research/findings/nhqrdr/2022qdr-final-es.pdf

Albougami, A., Pounds, K., & Alotaibi, J. (2016). Comparison of four cultural competence models in transcultural nursing: A discussion paper. *International Archives of Nursing and Health Care, 2*(4), 1–5. http://clinmedjournals.org/articles/ianhc/international-archives-of-nursing-and-health-care-ianhc-2-053.php?jid=ianhc

American Association of Colleges of Nursing. (2008). *Tool kit of resources for culturally competent education for baccalaureate nurses*. https://www.aacnnursing.org/Portals/42/AcademicNursing/CurriculumGuidelines/Cultural-Competency-Bacc-Tool-Kit.pdf

American Association of Colleges of Nursing. (2021). *AACN essentials*. https://www.aacnnursing.org/AACN-Essentials

American Public Health Association. (2021). *Health equity*. YouTube. https://www.youtube.com/watch?v=Arpzx6TJuQI

Artiga, S., & Hinton, E. (2018). *Issue brief beyond health care: The role of social determinants in promoting health and health equity*. Kaiser Family Foundation. https://www.kff.org/racial-equity-and-health-policy/issue-brief/beyond-health-care-the-role-of-social-determinants-in-promoting-health-and-health-equity/

Cambridge Dictionary. (n.d.a.). *Ethnicity*. https://dictionary.cambridge.org/us/dictionary/english/ethnicity

Cambridge Dictionary. (n.d.b.). *Race*. https://dictionary.cambridge.org/us/dictionary/english/race

Centers for Disease Control and Prevention. (2020). *Defining health disparities*. https://www.cdc.gov/nchhstp/healthdisparities/default.htm

Centers for Disease Control and Prevention. (2021). *What is CDC doing to address social determinants of health?* https://www.cdc.gov/about/sdoh/cdc-doing-sdoh.html

Centers for Disease Control and Prevention. (2022a). *CDC/ATSDR SVI fact sheet*. https://www.atsdr.cdc.gov/placeandhealth/svi/fact_sheet/fact_sheet.html

Centers for Disease Control and Prevention. (2022b). *Health equity*. https://www.cdc.gov/healthequity/whatis/index.html#:~:text=Health%20equity%20is%20the%20state,health%20and%20health%20care%3B%20and

Centers for Disease Control and Prevention. (2022c). *Preferred terms for select population groups and communities*. https://www.cdc.gov/health-communication/php/toolkit/preferred-terms.html?CDC_AAref_Val=https://www.cdc.gov/healthcommunication/Preferred_Terms.html

Centers for Disease Control and Prevention. (2022d). *Social determinants of health*. https://www.cdc.gov/publichealthgateway/sdoh/index.html

Furr-Holden, D., Carter-Pokras, O., Kimmel, M., & Mouton, C. (2020). Access to care during a global health crisis. *Health Equity*, *4*(1), 150–157. https://doi.org/10.1089/heq.2020.29001.rtl2

Giger, J., & Davidhizar, R. (2008). *Transcultural nursing: Assessment and intervention* (5th ed). Mosby.

Gómez, C., Kleinman, D., Pronk, N., Wrenn Gordon, G., Ochiai, E., Blakey, C., Johnson, A., & Brewer, K. (2021). Addressing health equity and social determinants of health through Healthy People 2030. *Journal of Public Health Management and Practice*, *27*(Suppl 6), S249–S257. https://doi.org/10.1097/phh.0000000000001297

Gottlieb, L., Fichtenberg, C., Alderwick, H., & Adler, N. (2019). Social determinants of health: What's a healthcare system to do? *Journal of Healthcare Management*, *64*(4), 243–257. https://doi.org/10.1097/jhm-d-18-00160

Hacker, K., & Houry, D. (2022). Social needs and social determinants: The role of the Centers for Disease Control and Prevention and public health. *Public Health Report*, *137*(6), 1049–1052. https://doi.org/10.1177/00333549221120244

Hill, L., & Ariga, S. (2022). *COVID-19 cases and deaths by race/ethnicity: Current data and changes over time*. Kaiser Family Foundation. https://www.kff.org/coronavirus-covid-19/issue-brief/covid-19-cases-and-deaths-by-race-ethnicity-current-data-and-changes-over-time/

Horvath, L. (2022). *Health equity: Inequitable access to healthcare's racist roots*. RTI Health Advance. https://healthcare.rti.org/insights/health-equity-racism-and-proximity-to-hospitals?gclid=Cj

0KCQjw39uYBhCLARIsAD_SzMSnNzUtEPt2QT2U7nm1b6XuMXoR-ZzgDqnOGlitVD7qj-UV9ha5JcsaAnfmEALw_wcB

Hosseinpoor, A., Bergen, N., Schlotheubera, A., & Grove, J. (2018). Measuring health inequalities in the context of sustainable development goals. *Bulletin World Health Organization, 96*, 654–659. http://dx.doi.org/10.2471/BLT.18.210401

Joszt, L. (2018). 5 vulnerable populations in healthcare. *American Journal of Managed Care*. July 20, 2018. https://www.ajmc.com/view/5-vulnerable-populations-in-healthcare

Leininger, M. (2002). Culture care theory: A major contribution to advance transcultural nursing knowledge and practices. *Journal of Transcultural Nursing, 13*(3), 189–192. https://doi.org/10.1177/10459602013003005

McEnroe-Petitte, D. M. (2020). Caring for patients who are homeless. *Nursing, 50*(3), 24–30. https://doi.org/10.1097/01.nurse.0000654600.98061.61

Minnesota Department of Health. (2019). *Public health interventions: Applications for public health nursing practice* (2nd ed.). www.health.state.mn.us/communities/practice/research/phncouncil/docs/PHInterventions.pdf

Morin, A. (2022). *Differences between race vs. ethnicity: How the US Census Bureau identifies ethnicity and race*. Verywell Mind. https://www.verywellmind.com/difference-between-race-and-ethnicity-5074205

National Center for Cultural Competence. (n.d.). *Bridging the cultural divide in healthcare settings: The essential role of cultural broker programs*. https://nccc.georgetown.edu/culturalbroker/

National Collaborating Centre for Determinants of Health. (2022). *Vulnerable populations*. https://nccdh.ca/glossary/entry/vulnerable-populations

Nursing Theory. (2020). *Leininger's culture care theory*. https://nursing-theory.org/theories-and-models/leininger-culture-care-theory.php

Office of Disease Prevention and Health Promotion. (n.d.a.). *Browse objectives*. Healthy People 2030. https://health.gov/healthypeople/objectives-and-data/browse-objectives

Office of Disease Prevention and Health Promotion. (n.d.b.). *Economic stability*. Healthy People 2030. https://health.gov/healthypeople/objectives-and-data/browse-objectives/economic-stability

Office of Disease Prevention and Health Promotion. (n.d.c.). *Education access and quality*. Healthy People 2030. https://health.gov/healthypeople/objectives-and-data/browse-objectives/education-access-and-quality

Office of Disease Prevention and Health Promotion. (n.d.d.). *Healthcare access and quality*. Healthy People 2030. https://health.gov/healthypeople/objectives-and-data/browse-objectives/health-care-access-and-quality

Office of Disease Prevention and Health Promotion. (n.d.e.). *Healthy People partners and SDOH*. Healthy People 2030. https://health.gov/healthypeople/priority-areas/social-determinants-health/healthy-people-partners-and-sdoh

Office of Disease Prevention and Health Promotion. (n.d.f.). *LGBT*. Healthy People 2030. https://health.gov/healthypeople/objectives-and-data/browse-objectives/lgbt

Office of Disease Prevention and Health Promotion. (n.d.g.). *Neighborhood and built environment*. Healthy People 2030. https://health.gov/healthypeople/objectives-and-data/browse-objectives/neighborhood-and-built-environment

Office of Disease Prevention and Health Promotion. (n.d.h.). *Social and community context*. Healthy People 2030. https://health.gov/healthypeople/objectives-and-data/browse-objectives/social-and-community-context

Office of Disease Prevention and Health Promotion. (n.d.i.). *Social determinants of health*. Healthy People 2030. https://health.gov/healthypeople/objectives-and-data/social-determinants-health

Office of Disease Prevention and Health Promotion. (2022). *Disparities.* Healthy People 2030. https://health.gov/healthypeople/priority-areas/health-equity-healthy-people-2030

Okonkwo, N. E., Aguwa, U. T., Jang, M., Barre, I. A., Page, K. R., Sullivan, P. S., Beyrer, C., & Baral, S. (2021). COVID-19 and the US response: Accelerating health equities. *BMJ Evidence-Based Medicine, 26*(4), 176–179. http://dx.doi.org/10.1136/bmjebm-2020-111426

Palmer, R., Ismond, D., Rodriquez, E., & Kaufman, J. (2019). Social determinants of health: Future directions for health disparities research. *American Journal of Public Health, 109,* S1–S2. https://ajph.aphapublications.org/doi/10.2105/AJPH.2019.304964

Pinter-Wollman, N., Jelic, A., & Wells, N. (2018). The impact of the built environment on health behaviours and disease transmission in social systems. *Philosophical Transactions Royal Society B, 373,* 20170245. http://dx.doi.org/10.1098/rstb.2017.0245

Purnell, L. (2002). The Purnell model for cultural competence. *Journal of Transcultural Nursing, 13,* 193–196. https://doi.org/10.1177/10459602013003006

Rural Health Information Hub. (2022a). *Module 1: Introduction to social determinants of health.* https://www.ruralhealthinfo.org/toolkits/sdoh/1/introduction

Rural Health Information Hub. (2022b). *Programs that focus on improving social and community context.* https://www.ruralhealthinfo.org/toolkits/sdoh/2/social-and-community-context

Shah, H. (2021). *Addressing the social determinants of health upstream.* Loma Linda University Health. https://ihpl.llu.edu/blog/addressing-social-determinants-health-upstream

Stryzhak, O. (2020). The relationship between education, income, economic freedom and happiness. *SHS Webs of Conferences, 75,* 03004. https://www.shs-conferences.org/articles/shsconf/pdf/2020/03/shsconf_ichtml_2020_004.pdf

United Nations. (2022a). *Goal 1: No poverty.* https://www.un.org/sustainabledevelopment/poverty/

United Nations. (2022b). *Goal 5: Gender equality.* https://www.un.org/sustainabledevelopment/gender-equality/

United Nations. (2022c). *Goal 6: Ensure availability and sustainability management of water and sanitation for all.* https://sdgs.un.org/goals/goal6

United Nations. (2022d). *Quality education.* United Nations Sustainable Goals. https://www.un.org/sustainabledevelopment/education/

USA Facts. (2021). *Our changing population: United States.* https://usafacts.org/data/topics/people-society/population-and-demographics/our-changing-population?gclid=CjwKCAjw-L-ZBhB4EiwA76YzOZXXdJGnL9Pi4jfvwET_SgG1ydwDrx6GkaaU9IjRdXZ3-DX4enAe5xoCFRsQAvD_BwE

USA Facts. (2022). *COVID-19 death data shows racial disparities during the pandemic.* https://usafacts.org/articles/covid-19-death-data-shows-racial-disparities-during-the-pandemic/?utm_source=google&utm_medium=cpc&utm_campaign=ND-COVID&gclid=Cj0KCQiAsoycBhC6ARIsAPPbeLuKHJGP8jgFHiikcX6Vk2HHOifKtb7q3i5qtW2ECSx0_mmK9rMBecsaAt1SEALw_wcB

Wonsor, R. (n.d.). *Lesson 9: Race and ethnicity.* Introduction to Sociology. https://slideplayer.com/slide/6596093/

World Health Organization. (n.d.). *Equity and health.* https://www.who.int/teams/social-determinants-of-health/equity-and-health

World Health Organization. (2018). *Health inequities and their causes.* https://www.who.int/news-room/facts-in-pictures/detail/health-inequities-and-their-causes

World Health Organization. (2020). *Quality health services.* https://www.who.int/news-room/fact-sheets/detail/quality-health-services

World Health Organization. (2021). *About social determinants of health. What are social determinants of health?* https://www.cdc.gov/socialdeterminants/about.html

World Health Organization. (2022). *World Health Statistics 2022: Monitoring health for the SDGs.* https://apps.who.int/iris/bitstream/handle/10665/356584/9789240051140-eng.pdf

Young, S., & Guo, K. L. (2020). Cultural diversity training: The necessity of cultural competence for health care provider and in nursing practice. *The Health Care Manager, 39*(2), 100–108. https://doi.org/10.1097/hcm.0000000000000294

Credits

Fig. 2.1: U.S. Department of Health and Human Services, "Social Determinants of Health," https://health.gov/healthypeople/priority-areas/social-determinants-health, 2023.

Fig. 2.2: Robert Wonser, https://slideplayer.com/slide/6596093/. Copyright © by Robert Wonser.

Fig. 2.3: USA Facts, "Racial and Ethical Changes from 2010-2021," https://usafacts.org/data/topics/people-society/population-and-demographics/our-changing-population?gclid=CjwKCAjw-L-ZBhB4EiwA76YzOZXXdJGnL9Pi4jfvwET_SgG1ydwDrx6GkaaU9IjRdXZ3-DX4e-nAe5xoCFRsQAvD_BwE. Copyright © 2021 by USAFacts Institute.

Fig. 2.4: Centers for Disease Control and Prevention, "CDC Framework of Six Pillars to Address SDOH/Health Equity," https://www.cdc.gov/about/priorities/social-determinants-of-health-at-cdc.html?CDC_AAref_Val=https://www.cdc.gov/about/sdoh/cdc-doing-sdoh.html, 2021.

Fig. 2.5: Kaiser Family Foundation, "COVID-19 Age-Adjusted Mortality Rates by Race/Ethnicity 2020-2022," https://www.kff.org/coronavirus-covid-19/issue-brief/covid-19-cases-and-deaths-by-race-ethnicity-current-data-and-changes-over-time/. Copyright © 2022 by Kaiser Family Foundation.

CHAPTER 3

Levels of Prevention

"Prevention is a whole less costly than treatment.
And maybe more effective."

—Debra Adair

Learning Outcomes

After reading this chapter, students should be able to:

1. Understand the definitions of the levels of prevention
2. Compare and contrast the levels of prevention
3. Compare and contrast the upstream, midstream, and downstream approaches
4. Apply the levels of prevention using active learning exercises
5. Use case studies to enhance learning related to levels of prevention

Keywords and Concepts

Downstream approach, midstream approach, primary prevention, primordial prevention, quaternary prevention, secondary prevention, tertiary prevention, upstream approach

Definitions of the Keywords

Downstream approach: Refers to managing chronic diseases and focuses on individual response (Merck, 2018)

Midstream approach: Refers to modifying individual behavior (Merck, 2018). Intermediary determinant changes generally occur at the micro policy level (Lewis & Holland-Penny, 2022)

Primary prevention: Refers to actions or interventions initiated before the disease or problem manifests itself (World Health Organization [WHO], 2022)

Primordial prevention: Consists of risk factor reduction targeted toward an entire population (Kisling & Das, 2023)

Quaternary prevention: An action taken to protect individuals from medical interventions that are more harmful than helpful (Kisling & Das, 2023)

Secondary prevention: Refers to early detection through screening and/or early treatments to improve positive health outcomes (WHO, 2022)

Tertiary prevention: Refers to the reduction of the effects of long-term complications through effective rehabilitation practices (Institute for Work and Health [IWH], 2015; Kisling & Das, 2023)

Upstream approach: Interventions and strategies that focus on improving and supporting health at the macro level to help individuals achieve optimal health through policies and research on the social determinants of ill health (Ingleby, 2019; National Collaborating Centre for Determinants of Health [NCCDH], 2014)

Introduction

The focus within healthcare in many parts of the globe is treatment rather than preventive services. Nowhere is this truer than in the United States. The cost of U.S. healthcare is tremendous and continues to rise yearly. Healthcare use and costs are much higher for chronic conditions than for those who are healthy (Buttorff et al., 2017).

U.S. healthcare spending grew 9.7% in 2020, reaching $4.1 trillion, or $12,530 per person (Centers for Medicare & Medicaid Services [CMS], 2022). As a share of the nation's gross domestic product, health spending accounted for 19.7% (CMS, 2022). This amount of spending is higher than in other advanced countries (Emanuel et al., 2021).

Ninety percent of the $4.1 trillion spent annually on healthcare is attributed to chronic diseases and mental health issues (Centers for Disease Control and Prevention [CDC], 2022a; CMS, 2022). Chronic conditions and mental health are essential as older individuals are also affected by diabetes, hypertension, end-stage renal disease, asthma, and obesity. Holman (2020) suggests that at least 50% of the population in the United States has some form of chronic illness and expresses the view that this is an epidemic. The expenses to assist with effective interventions of chronic disease are costly, leading to 86% of expenses. Holman (2020) notes that current medical professionals have not approached the continuing prevalence and, therefore, have not made plans to deal with the increase in chronic illness.

Holman (2020) discusses looking at chronic illness and focusing on effective education and research. A review of various methods to improve client outcomes is needed. Clients who are more adherent to an effective plan of care could lower healthcare costs and have positive effects on controlling chronic conditions. Initially, preventive prevention is preferred, but this is often not the case. If the chronic condition is already present, the focus should be on secondary and tertiary care related to early treatment and preventing complications. Healthcare professionals should always focus on primary and secondary prevention early in the care of clients (Holman, 2020).

If primary prevention is the preferred method of health promotion and disease prevention, why is its use still so low in the United States? Levine et al. (2019) note four major levers or influencers of preventive care in healthcare organizations and industries. The most prominent theme is financial and economic considerations. Healthcare sectors must still be profitable to sustain their business. Decisions regarding how to invest resources, which health benefits to cover, and how to bill for clinical services are essential components of that formula. The second theme is inconsistent metrics and reporting that is outcome-focused. The third theme is that healthcare payers must expand their outreach and increase preventive services using influence and incentives. The last theme is the need to transition to a value-based from a volume-based reimbursement model.

This chapter focuses on understanding and applying levels of prevention and proper approaches for more effective health outcomes. Including active learning strategies along with relevant case studies and reflections will help further development of the concepts.

Background of the Concepts

Focusing on levels of prevention and various approaches allows healthcare providers to effectively include various methods to reduce the risks or threats to health. With the multitude of information and recommending bodies, it is often challenging for healthcare professionals to remain current on changing evidence-based practices (Kisling & Das, 2023).

Primordial, Primary, Secondary, Tertiary, and Quaternary Prevention

Understanding definitions and applying the levels of prevention are vital to providing effective client interventions at the community and population-based levels. The main levels of prevention are primary, secondary, and tertiary (Figure 3.1). However, recent changes include the primordial and quaternary levels of prevention. Each area specifically addresses the need for strategies to further assist in managing individuals, families, communities, and populations.

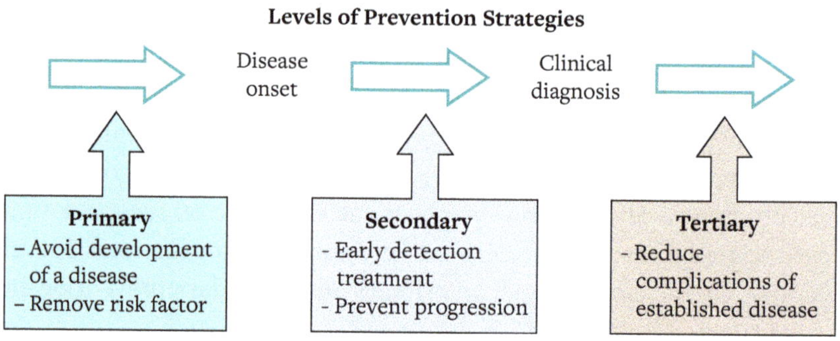

Levels of Prevention Strategies

Disease onset

Clinical diagnosis

Primary
- Avoid development of a disease
- Remove risk factor

Secondary
- Early detection treatment
- Prevent progression

Tertiary
- Reduce complications of established disease

FIGURE 3.1 Definitions of Main Levels of Prevention (Visual Interpretation)

Primordial Prevention

Development of the primordial level helps rectify prevention at a more systemic level. Recently, there has been a shift of preventive strategies earlier in the lifeline stages to prevent risk factor establishment in a population or even before the risk profile has been established (Hussain, 2021). Using more primordial prevention interventions could reduce the burden of the effectiveness of later complications from chronic diseases (Hussain, 2021).

One example of an application to using primordial prevention is associated with the human papillomavirus (HPV) vaccine. This vaccine was developed in 2006 to combat the growing problem of cervical cancer in women (CDC, 2021a). The first focus of the HPV vaccine was regarded only for female use. In 2011, the HPV vaccine was recommended for men (Meites et al., 2019). Even though this vaccine has been marketed for mostly female use, further systemic education should occur for males. The HPV vaccine is not required for entering school in all states, but what would happen if this recommendation changed? Could implementing a mandatory HPV vaccination for entrance into middle school reduce the possible risk factor for men to succumb to head and neck cancer in the future?

Primordial prevention is not widely used in public health practices. As chronic conditions remain the primary cause of death in developed countries, the focus may need to shift to ways to reduce risk factors earlier in life. Nurses should take an active role in policy development at a systemic level. See the application of primordial prevention (Box 3.1).

BOX 3.1 APPLICATION OF PRIMORDIAL PREVENTION LEARNING EXERCISE (EVIDENCE-BASED EXERCISE)

Using the CDC website for HPV vaccinations https://www.cdc.gov/vaccines/by-disease/index.html:

1. Provide two possible systemic solutions for better action for promoting the HPV vaccine for men. Use evidence-based interventions with statistical backup to determine how there might be a case for mandatory vaccinations.
2. In three states (Hawaii, Virginia, and Rhode Island) as well as Puerto Rico and Washington, D.C., the HPV vaccine is required for school admission (National Conference of State Legislators, 2022). Is there evidence of lower cases of HPV, including oral and neck cancer, in these areas?

American Association of Colleges of Nursing (AACN) *Essentials* (2021): Domains: #2; #3; #5; #6; #8; #9

- Competencies: 2.5; 2.8; 3.1; 3.3; 3.4; 3.5; 5.1; 6.4; 8.2; 8.3; 9.4
- Subcompetencies: 2.5d; 2.8c; 3.1b; 3.1c; 3.1d; 3.1i; 3.3a; 3.4b; 3.5d; 5.1a; 5.1d; 6.4d; 8.2c; 8.3e; 9.4a

Spheres of Care: Wellness/Disease prevention

Concepts: Communication; Evidence-based practice

Sources: CDC, 2021b; National Conference of State Legislators, 2022.

Primary Prevention

Primary prevention is often seen as the first level of prevention. Intervening before the disease or problem could lower the situation's incidence. Effective primary prevention strategies include altering risky behaviors, banning harmful substances, educating on proper oral hygiene, and preparing for emergency disasters (WHO, 2022).

Another effective form of primary prevention is vaccinations (WHO, 2022). However, there are some vaccines available that are currently underused. For instance, the HPV vaccination rate in the United States was only 48% for adolescents ages 13 through 15 who received recommended vaccine doses through 2018 (Office of Disease Prevention and Health Promotion [ODPHP], n.d.a.). The Healthy People 2030 goal is to reach 80% of this target population (ODPHP, n.d.a.). The HPV vaccination is most effective when administered before the onset of sexual activity (Meites et al., 2019; Quinlan, 2021).

Unfortunately, although head, neck, and oral cancers are decreasing, HPV-caused oral and neck cancer is rising in men (CDC, 2019; Farris & McEnroe-Petitte, 2013). HPV is the most transmitted sexually transmitted infection in the United States (Quinlan, 2021). In June 2020, the U.S. Food and Drug Administration (FDA) approved adding the prevention of HPV-associated head and neck cancers as an indication to the label of the Gardasil HPV vaccine (Quinlan, 2021).

The CDC (2019) notes that the rate of oral squamous cell carcinoma (HPV-associated) for men is 9.1 per 100,000, age-adjusted for all races and ethnicities. Rates are higher in the southern, Midwest, and northern states, whereas western states have the least number of cases. In 2019, 17,899 new cases of HPV-associated oral squamous cell carcinoma were diagnosed. These new cases were in men older than age 40 who did not have access to the HPV vaccine, as it is not available for those older than age 26 and was not accessible for men until 2011. Could increasing HPV vaccination rates change these numbers in the future if men are vaccinated as adolescents?

So, why is vaccination hesitancy such an issue, especially with the HPV vaccine? Lavelle et al. (2019) found several factors that influence the vaccination rate for parents, adolescents, and adults. For all three groups, vaccine effectiveness was the most influential factor. Others were the recommendation of primary care providers (PCPs) and out-of-pocket cost of the vaccine. Interestingly, the risk of illness, vaccine side effect risks, vaccination locations, and time for vaccination were not essential factors in the decision to get vaccinated. Factors that could provide more vaccine uptake by adolescents include strong PCP recommendations that mention the vaccine's effectiveness and healthcare policies to lower the cost of the vaccinations. Nurses must invest in strong advocacy for policies and practical education that could increase HPV and vaccination rates. Educating that the efficacy rate of the HPV vaccine is greater than 93% could be a factor in rising rates, as could educating clients that most sexually related cancers, including HPV-associated oral cancer, are spread through sexual activity (Quinlan, 2021).

Many problems could be addressed with enhanced primary prevention. Heart disease is the deadliest chronic disease, especially in the United States (CDC, 2022b). The key to the future could be to invest in more primary prevention strategies to reduce the number of cases. Arnett et al. (2019) note several primary prevention guidelines for cardiovascular disease that could reduce the incidence of these issues (Table 3.1; Box 3.2).

TABLE 3.1 Primary Prevention Guidelines for Cardiovascular Disease (2019)

- Evaluate SDOH factors for all clients for educational/resource needs (e.g., health literacy, psychological stressors, financial issues, sleep health, and self-efficacy).
- Promote a healthy lifestyle throughout the lifespan during each encounter.
- Consume a healthy diet that emphasizes the intake of vegetables, fruits, nuts, whole grains, lean vegetables or animal protein, and fish and minimizes the intake of trans fats, red meat/processed red meats, refined carbohydrates, and sweetened beverages.
- Adults should engage in at least 150 minutes of accumulated moderate-intensity physical activity or 75 minutes per week of vigorous-intensity physical activity.
- Clients should be assessed during every healthcare visit for tobacco use, and those who use tobacco should be assisted and strongly advised to quit.
- Aspirin should be used infrequently in routine primary prevention because of the lack of net benefit.

Source: Arnett et al., 2019.

BOX 3.2 PRIMARY PREVENTION ACTIVE LEARNING EXERCISE (USING THE HEALTHY PEOPLE 2030 SITE)

1. Proceed to the following website on Healthy People 2030 using the following URL: https://odphp.health.gov/healthypeople/tools-action/browse-evidence-based-resources/violence-prevention-primary-prevention-interventions-reduce-perpetration-intimate-partner-violence-and-sexual-violence-among-youth
2. Click on the tab labeled "Read more about this resource."
3. Under "Snapshot," list the three primary strategies under "Intervention."
4. Using evidence-based resources, give a specific example for each primary strategy.

Extra resource: https://www.thecommunityguide.org/media/pdf/OnePager-Violence-IPV-SV.pdf

AACN *Essentials* (2021): Domains: #1; #2; #3; #4; #5; #9

- Competencies: 1.1; 2.1; 2.5; 2.8; 3.1; 3.3; 4.2; 5.1; 5.2; 9.3; 9.4
- Subcompetencies: 1.1a; 1.1b; 2.1a; 2.1b; 2.5d; 2.8e; 3.1b; 3.1c; 3.1i; 3.3b; 4.2c; 5.1c; 5.1f; 5.2c; 9.3a; 9.3g; 9.4a

Spheres of Care: Wellness/Disease prevention

Concepts: Compassionate care; Evidence-based practice; Clinical judgment

Sources: ODPHP, n.d.c.; Community Preventive Services Task Force, 2018.

Secondary Prevention

Secondary prevention strategies focus on screenings and early treatment (Kisling & Das, 2023). The healthcare professional should assess and identify problems early and when there is the possibility of detection of the disease. During the screening process, the opportunity to educate individuals on the primary development of various conditions and the need to participate in activities to prevent an actual condition from presenting or exacerbating is prime. Delaying the recognition of conditions could be detrimental. Through education, clients can begin to practice healthy activities and prevent further compromising their health (Kisling & Das, 2023).

Secondary prevention is also vital concerning HPV. Early screening and treatment could affect the overall prognosis of the problem. Screening for HPV infection effectively identifies precancerous lesions and allows for early interventions that can prevent the development of cancer (Quinlan, 2021). The five-year relative survival rate for those with localized HPV-associated oral disease at diagnosis is 83%, compared with only 36% in clients whose cancer has metastasized (American

Dental Association [ADA], 2019). There is insufficient evidence to recommend for or against oral cancer screening in asymptomatic individuals (American Academy of Family Physicians, 2020; Quinlan, 2021). The ADA recommends that dentists routinely perform visual and tactile examinations for oral and oropharyngeal carcinoma in all clients (ADA, 2019; Quinlan, 2021). Unlike HPV-associated cervical cancer, there are no FDA-approved HPV tests for men or the oropharynx (Quinlan, 2021).

Early diagnosis and treatment are another vital consideration for HPV-associated oropharyngeal cancers (OPCs). One of the most significant issues is that asymptomatic HPV-associated OPCs are hard to diagnose (Mirghani et al., 2017). Signs and symptoms of early precursors to HPV-associated OPCs are white or red oral lesions that do not resolve after two weeks. Further indications of HPV-associated OPCs include a lump or thickening in the oral soft tissues, soreness or feeling that something is caught in the throat, difficulty chewing or swallowing, ear pain, difficulty moving the jaw or tongue, hoarseness, numbness of the tongue or areas of the mouth, and swelling of the jaw (ADA, 2019). Clients at risk must be educated about these issues and receive an oral examination immediately.

The Power of Prevention

Preventive Screening Schedule

PLUS
See your doctor annually for a physical exam, blood pressure test, medication review, exercise review, fall-prevention tips, and BMI measurement.

Screening	Procedure	Frequency	Age
Breast cancer+	Mammogram	Every 2 years	40–74
Colorectal cancer	Colonoscopy Flexible sigmoidoscopy Cologuard® Fecal occult blood test (FOBT)	Every 10 years Every 5 years Every 3 years Annually	45-75 45-75 45-75 45-75
Diabetes eye disease*	Check for eye damage from diabetes	Annually if diabetic retinopathy is present; if not, every 2 years	18–75
Diabetes kidney disease*	Check for kidney damage from diabetes	Annually	18–75
Diabetes A1C*	Have A1C levels checked for controlled blood sugar	Annually, or more often as doctor-directed	18–75
Flu	Flu Shot	Annually prior to flu season	All
Osteoporosis+	Check bone mass	At least once	65+
Osteoporosis after a fracture+	Check bone mass	Within 6 months of fracture	65–85
Urinary incontinence	Talk to your doctor	When experiencing leaking urine	All

+For women *For individuals with diabetes

FIGURE 3.2 Examples of Secondary Prevention Screenings

There are many screening opportunities for prominent issues and diseases. Blood pressure screening, colon screening, Pap smears, mammograms, and lab tests can identify problems and lead to early treatment (Kisling & Das, 2023). Specific age-related screenings must be taught and acknowledged during client encounters (Figure 3.2).

Men are less likely to seek a healthcare provider than are women (Cleveland Clinic, 2018). Cleveland Clinic (2018) notes that 40% of men visit a healthcare provider only when there is a severe health issue and do not prefer routine check-ups. Men fear a diagnosis, and about 21% noted anxiety and nervousness about finding out that there was something wrong. The pressure on men to conceal problems is intense, leading to a state of denial that could delay screening and treatment (Cleveland Clinic, 2018; Davis et al., 2012).

Tertiary Prevention

Tertiary prevention focuses on what occurs in the presence of the disease process and the complications (IWH, 2015; Kisling & Das, 2023). During this time, interventions are initiated to treat the specific condition and reduce the potential complications. Forms of tertiary prevention are commonly used in rehabilitation efforts, such as occupational and physical therapy in burn clients, cardiac rehabilitation in post-myocardial infarction clients, stroke rehabilitation, and chronic obstructive pulmonary disease management (Kisling & Das, 2023).

Even at the tertiary level, HPV-associated OPCs can be controlled if they are treated early. This condition is often seen as a disease of inequality due to the inability to vaccinate those in resource-limited areas, especially in Africa, Asia, and Latin America. Involvement with the WHO has provided a unique opportunity to assist with making significant changes and lifting barriers to HPV (Alfaro et al., 2021).

Opioid abuse has risen significantly among college students. During this time, students tend to be introduced to various substances, issues with college life, and related stresses that contribute to the addition of alcohol and other highly addictive drug usage (Lipari & Jean-Francois, 2016). Combining these substances adds to legal situations, individual and family disruptions, and medical conditions such as hepatitis B and C. Comprehensive educational instructions have been implemented to rectify the problem. Educational actions include using naloxone hydrochloride (Narcan), providing necessary resources for users, and offering treatment and relapse avoidance strategies to cope with individual situations (Daniels-Witt et al., 2017). Although indicated for college students, the actions taken can also be used for other age groups when these problems occur rapidly (Table 3.2).

TABLE 3.2 Tertiary Level of Prevention: Strategies to Address Opiate Abuse Among American College Students

Develop a group on campus using guidelines from Narcotics Anonymous.	Mock simulations, including practicing overdose emergencies
Supply the campus counseling services with individuals who are certified drug counselors.	Lists of local drug providers to be used as a referral database
Install a 24-hour helpline that is separate from the campus police access.	All university-wide areas to have Narcan available, including the campus police, campus pharmacies, and resident hall directors
Initiate a campus withdrawal policy by which students affected by opiate usage can complete courses through distance learning methods.	Education of campus police, faculty, staff, and students on how to administer Narcan and provide care and training for overdose prevention

Source: Daniels-Witt et al., 2017.

Quaternary Prevention

Martins et al. (2018) discuss the concept of quaternary prevention. The quaternary level of prevention was first associated with clients who had an illness without a disease, including identifying clients at risk of overmedication and protection from invasive medical interventions. The definition of *quaternary prevention* has recently encompassed the idea that healthcare providers should protect clients from medical interventions that cause more harm than good.

All healthcare providers should understand this form of prevention and incorporate it when developing plans of care and considering protection from any harmful interventions. These negative actions can include overmedication, overtreatment, and other potentially harmful activities (Martins et al., 2018). Further, quaternary prevention can affect all other prevention levels (Martins et al., 2018; Figure 3.3).

Quaternary Prevention –

Action taken to avoid medical interventions that are more harmful than beneficial to the client.

The overall goal is reducing overdiagnosis, overtreatment, and iatrogenic harm.

Example 1: The use of a "watchful waiting" strategy (watch and follow-up) when a young healthy client without any cardiovascular risk or symptom worries about his cholesterol level.

Example 2: The appropriate use of antibiotics in upper respiratory tract infections when the cause may be viral and not bacterial.

FIGURE 3.3 Quaternary Prevention With Examples

Upstream, Midstream, and Downstream Approaches

Including the upstream, midstream, and downstream concepts is vital to understanding the importance of applying these approaches to individual, family, community, and population-based care. The development of upstream, midstream, and downstream approaches to healthcare prevention are viable methods to note inequities in care made available to individuals in society. *Upstream* care looks at the wide variety of resources at the macro level in economic and societal aspects that support equitable usage, including social status, race/ethnicity, and income (NCCDH, 2014). An example of the upstream approach is to provide easy access and availability for chronic disease management to those with low incomes. The Bay Area Regional Health Inequalities Initiative report (2020) identified that higher-income individuals living in the Bay Area would live longer than those with a lower income.

BOX 3.3 UPSTREAM AND DOWNSTREAM PARABLE REFLECTION

Watch the following video: https://www.youtube.com/watch?v=qarQXqKbmLg (change the subtitle to English under "Settings").

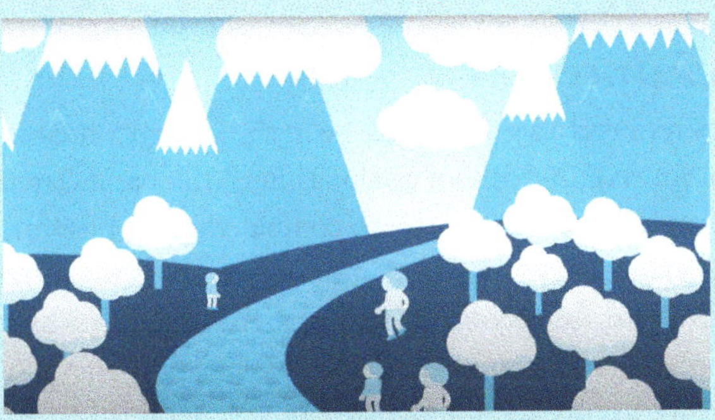

https://salud-america.org/the-upstream-downstream-parable-for-health-equity/

1. **Reflection:** Based on the video, think about three specific ways these approaches could be used in population-based nursing for heart disease.

AACN *Essentials* (2021): Domains: #1; #2; #3; #4; #5; #9; #10

- Competencies: 1.1;1.2; 1.3; 2.4; 3.1; 3.3; 4.2; 5.1; 9.1; 9.2; 9.3; 10.2
- Subcompetencies: 1.1a; 1.1b; 1.2a; 1.3a; 1.3b; 1.3c; 2.4b; 2.4c; 3.1c; 3.1e; 3.3a; 3.3b; 4.2a; 4.2b; 4.2c; 5.1a; 5.1b; 5.1f; 9.1a; 9.2d; 9.3g; 10.2d; 10.2f

Spheres of Care: Wellness/Disease prevention; Chronic disease management

Concepts: Clinical judgment; Evidence-based practice; SDOH; Diversion, equity, and inclusion (DEI)

Sources: Merck, 2018; Upstream, 2013.

Midstream care modifies a person's behaviors (Merck, 2018) and is noted to be at the meso level. This level includes high school completion, availability of affordable housing, and food security (NCCDH, 2014). *Downstream* care focuses on the individual or micro perspective on managing chronic disease conditions, providing equitable access to care, and responding to individuals who need immediate assistance with food, clothing, and shelter (NCCDH, 2014; Merck, 2018). Using primary, secondary, and tertiary levels of prevention to assess the individual needs, whether upstream, midstream, or downstream, should be implemented within an effective plan.

In 1979, J. B. McKinlay introduced the upstream concept at an American Heart Association presentation using an interesting analogy (1979). This classic public health parable told the story of a witness who saw a person caught in a river current. The witness saved the person but noted that more people were floating down the river. After rescuing many people, the witness investigated why this continued to happen upstream. The story illustrates the ongoing struggle between public health protection mandates to respond to emergencies (help people caught in the current) and prevention and promotion mandates (i.e., stop people from falling into the river; Butterfield, 2017; NCCDH, 2014; Box 3.3).

Upstream Approach

Vaccine hesitancy remains a significant issue in the United States as more states now allow exemptions for required school vaccinations. Miller and Carroll (2021) discuss the need for a comprehensive approach to combat vaccine hesitancy. The upstream approach should include evidence-based initiatives at the state, provider, and practice levels. Many cultural and socioeconomic factors drive vaccine hesitancy. Unfortunately, the COVID-19 vaccination has only exemplified vaccine hesitancy and increased health disparities in vaccine access and uptake (Miller & Carroll, 2021; Table 3.3).

TABLE 3.3 Upstream (Macro-Level) Approaches to Vaccine Hesitancy

Population-Level Interventions
• Create school-mandated vaccinations/policies at the state and local levels • Eliminate nonmedical exemptions • Provide better access/targeting to underserved populations
Practice-Level Interventions
• Maintain registry for unimmunized clients • Create unimmunized client policies, such as mandating regular well visits, eliminating walk-in visits, requiring clients and accompanying caregivers to wear masks, avoiding the waiting room when sick, and using a refusal-to-vaccinate form
Provider-Level Interventions
• Build rapport and trust with underimmunized and unimmunized clients/parents • Use motivational interviewing • Be culturally competent and apply SDOH factors • Continue education with each visit on appropriate vaccines and their importance

Source: Miller & Carroll, 2021.

Butterfield (2017) used an expanded nursing approach utilizing the upstream concept. The Butterfield Upstream Model for Population Health (BUMP Health) further expands on the need for a broader approach to the upstream approach. The BUMP Health framework emphasizes addressing the determinants of health and health inequality that influence health outcomes, focusing specifically on specific populations. A determination of the factors that would have the most significant impact is a specific point of the BUMP framework, much as in the essential components of public health.

So, what would be an upstream approach to HPV-associated OPCs? In HPV-associated OPCs, it would be to diminish the causes of causes (NCCDH, 2014). Since men can develop HPV-associated OPCs later in life, illustrating the need for HPV vaccination (primary prevention/upstream approach) for younger males is critical. Nurses play a crucial role in educating and advocating for oral cancer prevention by encouraging HPV vaccination (Da Rosa et al., 2021).

Midstream Approach

The midstream approach is not used as often as the upstream and downstream approaches but has grown in popularity. This approach is geared toward the meso level, or the subpopulation. The meso level considers cultures and social factors at the regional level that could influence behavioral health promotion changes (Waithaka et al., 2018). Adjusting health issue messages to the subpopulations could be helpful in improving health outcomes.

Social marketing to subpopulations could be an excellent midstream approach. Effective social marketing is concerned with the customer's immediate social environment. Midstream social marketing programs have the potential to shift focus away from the two traditional domains and attempt to understand the behavior in context as well as the structural barriers to change (Fletcher-Brown, 2021).

A midstream approach with HPV-associated OPCs may be an avenue that could be used to improve understanding of the issue. Fletcher-Brown (2021) used a social marketing midstream approach to facilitate a better understanding of how to improve breast cancer behavior in India. The approach used community health nurses and key stakeholders to develop healthcare resources for vulnerable populations through appropriate social media campaigns and mobile health technology. Approaching the target population for HPV-associated OPCs with a proper social media campaign (midstream approach) could entice effective primary and early secondary prevention interventions (Box 3.4).

BOX 3.4 HPV VACCINE (USING THE CDC SITE)

1. Proceed to the following link at the CDC website: https://www.cdc.gov/hpv/vaccines/reasons-to-get.html?CDC_AAref_Val=https://www.cdc.gov/hpv/parents/vaccine/six-reasons.html.
2. You are preparing a required health promotion presentation for your community health class assignment for a group of middle school students. Your assignment is regarding primary prevention and the HPV vaccine.
3. Using this website and other information, develop a short conversation/outline to present to the group. What three priority items will you offer to encourage the administration of the HPV vaccine?

AACN *Essentials* (2021): Domains: #1; #2; #3; #5; #6; #8; #9

- Competencies: 1.1;1.3; 2.2; 2.8; 3.1; 3.3; 5.1; 6.1; 8.5; 9.3; 9.4
- Subcompetencies: 1.1a; 1.1b; 1.3a; 1.3c; 2.2b; 2.8a; 2.8d; 3.1e; 3.1h; 3.3a; 3.3b; 5.1c; 6.1e; 8.5b; 9.3a; 9.4a

Spheres of Care: Wellness/Disease prevention

Concepts: Communication; Evidence-based practice; Clinical judgment

Source: CDC, 2021c.

Downstream Approach

The downstream approach provides access to care for all individuals regardless of their level as well as services for various health and social needs (NCCDH, 2014). The individual identifies and implements behavioral changes while they make decisions. One example of obesity is noted in a person's choices, such as working on eating healthier, losing weight, and obtaining their goals (Rutter et al., 2017). There is a need for motivation, encouragement, and further communication with individuals presenting education and intense health information to make significant lifestyle changes. The downstream environment can negatively affect the progression of weight loss instead of obesity stigma, economic status, income, and ability/cost to exercise (Rutter et al., 2017).

Williams and Fullagar (2018) present the term *lifestyle drift* (p. 1), stating that the upstream approach focuses on health inequalities, and the downstream approach regards an individual's behavior and ability to make changes. These authors describe a "citizen shift" (p. 15) in which there is a means to services but no responsibility to ensure that individuals find them valuable. For example, when looking at exercise and physical activity, services are developed in a public setting with access for large groups of individuals of various economic levels and ethnicities in small and large cities. Social marketing has promoted these settings, but some do not use nor have the means to afford them (Williams & Fullagar, 2018).

Shifting responsibility and an individual's perceptions of exercise may be a promising approach. The culture then blames the shift and relates this to the individual, the director of the exercise setting, and then those who continue to be sedentary and do not want to exercise. This low participation sheds light on the residents of the area and their overall health status (Powell et al., 2017). The ability to adopt policy changes, review individual and social motivational aspects, and, overall, move the downstream approach to upstream approaches must be developed and encouraged for all members of society (Williams & Fullagar, 2018).

Despite low HPV vaccination rates, most interventions still use a downstream approach (Miller & Carroll, 2021). The stigma of the COVID-19 vaccine has further affected the individual's perception of the importance of primary prevention vaccines (Miller & Carroll, 2021). Unless there is further investigation into the specific behaviors of individuals and overall vulnerable populations associated with SDOH interventions, the downstream approach will still be a factor in ongoing issues with HPV vaccination rates and further HPV-associated OPCs in the future (Miller & Carroll, 2021; Table 3.4).

TABLE 3.4 Examples of Upstream, Midstream, and Downstream Approaches to SDOH

SDOH Categories	Upstream/ Macro	Midstream/Meso	Downstream/ Individual
Education access and quality	Federal policies to increase reading and writing scores	Support adult high school completion programs locally	Address the small number of children who participate in early education
Healthcare and quality	Federal cigarette tax increase for tobacco products	Increase the number of community organizations providing preventive services	Expand mobile services to individuals with no public or personal transportation
Economic stability	Advocacy for living-wage policies and progressive taxation	Make jobs available for low-income veterans and unhoused individuals	Address income level to ensure that chronic disease prevention programs are accessible to individuals
Social and community context	Policy improvements for the juvenile justice system	Assurance of food security to children in a particular community	Increase the number of individuals who use I.T. to track correct healthcare data
Neighborhood and built environment	Enhancement of residential areas by adding parks, walkways, and green spaces	Increase broadband Internet in areas with low rates	Clean up inhabitable residences with infestations

Sources: ODPHP, n.d.b.; NCCDH, 2014.

Frank (2022) revisits the idea of using an older public health conceptual framework, which was created by epidemiologist Geoffrey Rose. Rose's framework notes using primordial, primary, secondary, and tertiary prevention rather than upstream and downstream approaches.

An example of Rose's framework approach can be seen regarding the obesity epidemic (Frank, 2022). In Rose's framework, emphasis on primordial prevention using a more upstream approach could be the catalyst to shedding some light on the ever-growing obesity issue. Addressing many causes could be the ultimate way to manage obesity at the population level (Figure 3.4). This proposal may also provide a way to oversee many other diseases, problems, and issues at this level.

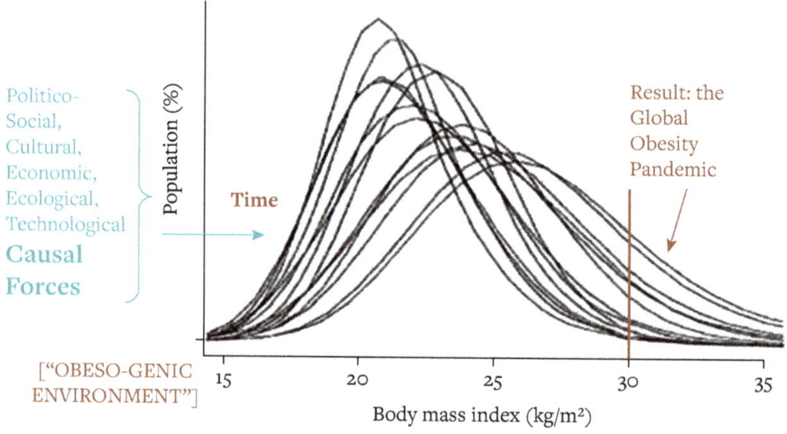

FIGURE 3.4 Rose's Population Strategy as Applied to Obesity

Chapter Highlights

- Discussion with examples of levels of prevention
- Discussion with examples of upstream, midstream, and downstream approaches
- Application of upstream, midstream, and downstream approaches to SDOH
- Application of HPV (vaccinations and OPCs) with levels of prevention and different approaches
- Active learning exercises/reflections related to levels of prevention
- Case studies related to HPV and the levels of prevention

Active Learning Exercises

Application to Intervention Wheel: Primary Prevention (Using the Intervention Wheel)

Use the following document to assist in completing the assignment: www.health.state.mn.us/communities/practice/research/phncouncil/docs/PHInterventions.pdf.

1. Using the Minnesota Department of Health document, develop a social marketing/public service primary prevention announcement on cyberbullying at the system, community, and individual levels.

AACN *Essentials* (2021): Domains: #1; #3; #4; #8; #10

- Competencies: 1.1; 1.3; 3.3; 3.5; 4.1; 8.1; 10.1
- Subcompetencies: 1.1a; 1.1b; 1.3a;1.3b; 1.3c; 3.3a; 3.3b; 3.5b; 3.5d; 4.1g; 8.1b; 8.1d; 8.1e; 10.1a

Spheres of Care: Wellness/Disease prevention

Concepts: Communication; Evidence-based practice; Clinical judgment

Source: Minnesota Department of Health, 2019.

Case Studies

Case Study #1: Primary Prevention HPV

A mother arrives at the pediatric clinic with her 11-year-old son, Jason. He is there for a sports physical and an update on mandatory school vaccines. According to the CDC immunization schedule, Jason is due for the tetanus, diphtheria, & acellular pertussis (Tdap) and meningococcal vaccine. Also listed on the schedule is the human papillomavirus (HPV) vaccine. His mother acknowledges the Tdap and meningococcal vaccine but is hesitant about the HPV vaccine.

1. What evidence-based information can be offered to Jason and his mother about the facts of the HPV virus, prevention of cancers, mandatory state legislation rules regarding vaccines, schedule of immunizations, cost, vaccine safety, side effects, contraindications, and benefits?
2. If Jason lived in Florida, what vaccine requirements are mandated by his state legislation for HPV?
3. What three specific primary prevention strategies could be used for HPV?
4. In the article by McQuillan et al. (2017), what are the findings related to cultural aspects of the prevalence and prevention of HPV? How can these assist healthcare providers in increasing the number of those receiving the vaccine?

5. With HPV, children and teens are not of the age to consent, and the responsibility is given to the adult. What are some ethical concerns that should be taken into consideration when deciding what is best for the child?
6. Present a plan to increase your community's education and vaccination rates and compare and contrast this plan with a country outside the United States. What roadblocks may be encountered, and how can we overcome them?

Use the article by McQuillan et al. (2017) to assist with the case study.

AACN *Essentials* (2021): Domains: #1; #2; #3; #5; #7; #8; #9; #10

- Competencies: 1.1; 2.7; 2.8; 3.1; 3.2; 3.4; 5.1; 7.3; 8.1; 8.3; 9.1; 9.3; 9.4; 10.1
- Subcompetencies: 1.1b; 2.7a; 2.8a; 2.8e; 3.1b; 3.1d; 3.1e; 3.2a; 3.4c; 5.1f; 7.3b; 7.3c; 8.1b; 8.3c; 8.3e; 9.1a; 9.3a; 9.4a; 10.1a

Spheres of Care: Wellness/Disease prevention

Concepts: Communication; Evidence-based practice; Ethics; Health policy; SDOH

Source: McQuillan et al., 2017.

Case Study #2: Secondary Prevention HPV

Joe is a 45-year-old White man with a negative history of smoking and alcohol usage. He noticed a pea-size nodule on the left side of his neck. It quickly grew and doubled in size and was painful to the touch. Joe sought care from his healthcare provider. An ultrasound, a computed tomography (CT) scan of the neck, an abdominal CT scan, and a chest X-ray were ordered. The abdominal scan was negative, so a neck biopsy to identify the growth was performed. The biopsy produced a diagnosis of stage 3 squamous cell adenocarcinoma. The primary source of cancer could not be determined, but the tonsils were suspected.

1. Could his condition have been prevented, and how would this have been accomplished?
2. What areas identify Joe's signs and symptoms related to the development of HPV? List several other presentations that would help with the diagnosis of this condition.
3. In reviewing the CDC website on HPV statistics, what information can be gained to further identify the prevalence of HPV in women, but with an emphasis on the male population?

After diagnosis, Joe began chemotherapy using an implanted port. His medications included three separate chemotherapeutic agents along with steroids and antiemetics. During the treatments, which lasted 21 days, he developed several side effects, such as constipation, diarrhea, nausea, and hypotension. Thirty-nine radiation treatments were given for three weeks but soon stopped due to side effects. Joe became weak during this time, his throat was irritated, and he had difficulty eating. He lost a total of 60 pounds over two months. However, with follow-up testing, remission was determined.

1. What education would be offered to Joe during his chemotherapy and radiation treatments to assist him and his caregivers through this time?
2. As a multidisciplinary team member, which other professionals should be included, and what would their roles be in helping Joe with his quality of life while he was being cared for in the home setting?

AACN *Essentials* (2021): Domains: #2; #3; #6; #9

- Competencies: 2.1; 2.4; 2.8; 3.3; 6.3; 9.2
- Subcompetencies: 2.1a; 2.1b; 2.4d; 2.8c; 2.8d; 3.3b; 6.3a; 9.2b; 9.2c; 9.2g

Spheres of Care: Chronic disease care; Regenerative/restorative care; Hospice/palliative/supportive care

Concepts: Communication; Compassionate care; Evidence-based practice

Sources: CDC, 2024; adapted from Farris & McEnroe-Petitte, 2013.

Case Study #3: Tertiary Prevention for HPV

Approximately six months later, Joe (refer to case study #2) began developing pain in his shoulders and hips. A positron emission tomography scan was done, with spots noted throughout his bones and chest. Chemotherapy and radiation were restarted with no change in his symptoms. Side effects from the radiation were affecting his salivary glands, causing dry mouth and burns. The pain in his shoulder and hip worsened. Eating was difficult again, and the weight loss continued. After a discussion with his healthcare provider, he decided to use palliative care treatment. Hospice care was initiated soon, as Joe chose not to continue with any curative treatments. He passed away a few days later at his home.

1. Based on the case study, what is the difference in care during palliative and hospice?
2. What tertiary prevention support was given to Joe and his family?
3. What tertiary prevention interventions could be given to Joe and his family?
4. What support will Joe's family have after his death?

AACN *Essentials* (2021): Domains: #1; #2; #3; #6; #9

- Competencies: 1.3; 2.1; 2.4; 2.8; 3.3; 6.3; 9.2
- Subcompetencies: 1.3b; 1.3c; 1.3c; 2.1a; 2.1b; 2.4d; 2.8c; 2.8d; 3.3b; 6.3a; 9.2b; 9.2c; 9.2g

Spheres of Care: Chronic disease care; Regenerative/restorative care; Hospice/palliative/supportive care

Concepts: Communication; Compassionate care; Evidence-based practice; Clinical judgment

Source: Adapted from Farris & McEnroe-Petitte, 2013.

NCLEX Questions

1. The nurse is participating in a local mall health fair, giving senior citizens influenza vaccinations. What level of prevention is the nurse practicing?
   a. Primary prevention
   b. Secondary prevention
   c. Tertiary prevention
   d. Quaternary prevention
2. A client experienced a myocardial infarction four weeks ago and is currently participating in daily cardiac rehabilitation sessions at the local fitness center. At what level of prevention is the client participating?
   a. Primary prevention
   b. Secondary prevention
   c. Tertiary prevention
   d. Quaternary prevention

References

Alfaro, K., Maza, M., Cremer, M., Masch, R., & Soler, M. (2021). Removing global barriers to cervical cancer prevention and moving towards elimination. *Nature Reviews Cancer, 21*, 607–608. https://doi.org/10.1038/s41568-021-00396-4

American Academy of Family Physicians. (2020). *Clinical preventive service recommendation. Oral cancer.* https://www.aafp.org/patient-care/clinical-recommendations/all/oral-cancer.html

American Association of Colleges of Nursing. (2021). *The essentials: Core competencies for professional nursing education.* https://www.aacnnursing.org/Essentials

American Dental Association. (2019). *ADA expands policy on oral cancer detection to include oropharyngeal cancer.* https://www.ada.org/resources/research/science-and-research-institute/oral-health-topics/cancer-head-and-neck

Arnett, D. K., Blumenthal, R. S., Albert, M. A., Buroker, A. B., Goldberger, Z. D., Hahn, E. J., Himmelfarb, C. D., Khera, A., Lloyd-Jones, D., McEvoy, J. W., Michos, E. D., Miedema, M. D., Muñoz, D., Smith, Jr., S. C., Virani, S. S., Williams, Sr., K. A., Yeboah, J., & Ziaeian, B. (2019). 2019 ACC/AHA guideline on the primary prevention of cardiovascular disease: A report of the American College of Cardiology/American Heart Association Task Force on Clinical Practice. *Circulation, 140*, e596–e646. https://doi.org/10.1161/CIR.0000000000000678

Bay Area Regional Health. (2020). *Bay Area Regional Health Inequalities Initiative* (*BARH11*). http://www.phi.org/wp-content/uploads/migration/uploads/application/files/qwsx208hrfk-pqlrljyczf7vuanmc3vhjf59sg28mdm2efsl2xk.pdf

BlueCross BlueShield Minnesota. (2022). *The power of prevention*. https://blog.bluecrossmn.com/2022-report-to-the-community/

Brodersen, J., Schwartz, L., & Woloshin, S. (2014). Overdiagnosis: How cancer screening can turn indolent pathology into illness. *APMIS Journal of Pathology, Microbiology, and Immunology, 122*(8), 683–689. https://doi.org/10.1111/apm.12278

Butterfield, P. G. (2017). Thinking upstream: A 25-year retrospective and conceptual model aimed at reducing health inequities. *Advances in Nursing Science, 40*(1), 2–11. https://doi.org/10.1097/ans.0000000000000161

Buttorff, C., Ruder, T., & Bauman, M. (2017). *Multiple chronic conditions in the United States*. RAND Corporation. http://www.rand.org/t/TL221

Centers for Disease Control and Prevention. (2019). *Cancers caused by associated risk factors: HPV-associated cancers*. https://gis.cdc.gov/Cancer/USCS/#/RiskFactors/

Centers for Disease Control and Prevention. (2021a). *HPV infection*. https://www.cdc.gov/vaccines/vpd/hpv/public/index.html

Centers for Disease Control and Prevention. (2021b). *Human papillomavirus (HPV) vaccination & cancer prevention*. https://www.cdc.gov/vaccines/vpd/hpv/index.html

Centers for Disease Control and Prevention. (2021c). *Human papillomavirus (HPV): Reasons to get vaccinated*. https://www.cdc.gov/hpv/vaccines/reasons-to-get.html?CDC_AAref_Val=https://www.cdc.gov/hpv/parents/vaccine/six-reasons.html

Centers for Disease Control and Prevention. (2022a). *Health and economic costs of chronic diseases*. https://www.cdc.gov/chronicdisease/about/costs/index.htm

Centers for Disease Control and Prevention. (2022b). *Heart disease*. https://www.cdc.gov/heartdisease/index.htm

Centers for Disease Control and Prevention. (2024). *HPV stats*. https://www.cdc.gov/cervical-cancer/statistics/index.html

Centers for Medicare & Medicaid Services. (2022). *National health expenditure data: Historical*. https://www.cms.gov/Research-Statistics-Data-and-Systems/Statistics-Trends-and-Reports/NationalHealthExpendData/NationalHealthAccountsHistorical

Cleveland Clinic. (2018). *Cleveland Clinic 2018 MENtion It Survey*. https://newsroom.clevelandclinic.org/wp-content/uploads/sites/4/2018/08/Cleveland-Clinic-MENtion-It-Survey-Results-2018.pdf

Community Preventive Services Task Force. (2018). *The community guide: Violence prevention: Primary prevention interventions to reduce perpetration of intimate partner violence and sexual violence among youth*. https://www.thecommunityguide.org/media/pdf/OnePager-Violence-IPV-SV.pdf

Daniels-Witt, Q., Thompson, A., Glassman, T., Federman, S., & Bott, K. (2017). The case for implementing the levels of prevention model: Opiate abuse on American college campuses. *Journal of American College Health, 65*(7), 518–524. https://doi.org/10.1080/07448481.2017.1341900

Da Rosa, P., Koenecke, L., Gudgeon, L., Keller, W., & Gu, W. (2021). Role of nurses in the prevention and early detection of oral cavity and pharynx cancers. *Online Journal of Rural Nursing and Health Care, 21*(2), 152–167. https://doi.org/10.14574/ojrnhc.v21i2.692

Davis, J., Buchanan, K., Katz, R., & Green, B. L. (2012). Gender differences in cancer screening beliefs, behaviors, and willingness to participate: Implications for health promotion. *American Journal of Men's Health, 6*(3), 211–217. https://doi.org/10.1177/1557988311425853

Emanuel, E., Gudbranson, E., Van Parys, J., Gortz, M., Helgeland, J., & Skinner, J. (2021). Comparing health outcomes of privileged U.S. citizens with those of average residents of other developed countries. *JAMA Internal Medicine, 181*(3), 339–344. https://jamanetwork.com/journals/jamainternalmedicine/fullarticle/2774561

Farris, C., & McEnroe-Petitte, D. (2013). Head, neck, and oral cancer update. *Home Healthcare Nurse, 31*(6), 322–328. https://doi.org/10.1097/nhh.0b013e3182932f01

Fletcher-Brown, J. (2021). *Innovating social marketing to affect cancer healthcare resources for vulnerable consumers in an emerging country context: A midstream approach* (JFB UP717123) [doctoral thesis, University of Portsmouth]. https://researchportal.port.ac.uk/en/studentTheses/innovating-social-marketing-to-affect-cancer-healthcare-resources

Frank, J. (2022). Controlling the obesity pandemic: Geoffrey Rose revisited. *Canadian Journal of Public Health, 113*, 736–742. https://doi.org/10.17269/s41997-022-00636-6

Frank, J., Jepson, R., & Williams, A. (2016). *Disease prevention: A critical toolkit.* Oxford University Press.

Holman, H. R. (2020). Commentary: The relation of the chronic disease epidemic to the health care crisis. *American College of Rheumatology, 2*(3), 167–173. https://doi.org/10.1002/acr2.11114

Hussain, M. (2021). Primordial prevention: The missing link in neurological care. *Journal of Family Medicine and Primary Care, 10*(1), 31–34. https://doi.org/10.4103/jfmpc.jfmpc_1806_20

Ingleby, D. (2019). Moving upstream: Changing policy scripts on migrant and ethnic minority health. *Health Policy, 123*(9), 809–817. https://doi.org/10.1016/j.healthpol.2019.07.015

Institute for Work and Health. (2015). *Primary, secondary, and tertiary prevention.* "What researchers mean by ..." series. https://www.iwh.on.ca/what-researchers-mean-by/primary-secondary-and-tertiary-Prevention

Kisling, L., & Das, J. (2023). *Prevention strategies.* StatPearls Publishing. https://www.ncbi.nlm.nih.gov/books/NBK537222/

Lavelle, T., Messonnier, M., Stokley, S., Kim, D., Ramakrishnan, A., Gebremariam, A., Simon, N., Rose, A., & Prosser, L. (2019). Use of a choice survey to identify adult, adolescent and parent preferences for vaccination in the United States. *Journal of Patient-Reported Outcomes, 3*(51), 1–12. https://doi.org/10.1186/s41687-019-0135-0

Levine, S., Malone, E., Lekiachvili, A., & Briss, P. (2019). Healthcare industry insights: Why the use of preventive services is still low. *Preventing Chronic Disease, 16*, E30. https://doi.org/10.5888/pcd16.180625

Lewis, J., & Holland-Penny, J. (2022). *Psychoactive substance use and social policy.* University of Windsor. https://ecampusontario.pressbooks.pub/psychoactivesubstancesvls1/

Lipari, R. N., & Jean-Francois, B. (2016). *A day in the life of college students aged 18 to 22: Substance use facts.* The CBHSQ Report. Center for Behavioral Health Statistics and Quality, Substance Abuse and Mental Health Services Administration. https://www.samhsa.gov/data/sites/default/files/report_2361/ShortReport-2361.html

Martins, C., Godycki-Cwirkob, M., Bruno, H., & Brodersen, J. (2018). Quaternary prevention: Reviewing the concept quaternary prevention aims to protect patients from medical harm. *European Journal of General Practice, 24*(1), 106–111. https://doi.org/10.1080/13814788.2017.1422177

McKinlay, J. B. (1979). A case for refocusing upstream: The political economy of illness. In: E. G. Jaco (Ed.), *Patients, physicians, and illness* (3rd ed.; pp. 9–25). Free Press.

McQuillan, G., Kruszon-Moran, D., Markowitz, L. E., Unger, E. R., & Paulose-Ram, R. (2017). *Prevalence of HPV in adults aged 18–69: United States, 2011–2014.* NCHS data brief, 280. National Center for Health Statistics. https://www.cdc.gov/nchs/data/databriefs/db280.pdf

Meites, E., Szilagyi, P., Chesson, H., Unger, E., Romero, J., & Markowitz, L. (2019). Human papillomavirus vaccination for adults: Updated recommendations of the Advisory Committee on Immunization Practices. *Mortality and Morbidity Weekly Report, 68*(32), 698–702. https://www.cdc.gov/mmwr/volumes/68/wr/mm6832a3.htm

Merck, A. (2018). *The upstream-downstream parable for health equity.* Salud America!, October 8, 2018. https://salud-america.org/the-upstream-downstream-parable-for-health-equity/

Miller, J. M., & Carroll, R. S. (2021). An informed approach to vaccine hesitancy and uptake in children. *Delaware Journal of Public Health*, 8(1), 60–64. https://doi.org/10.32481/djph.2022.03.009

Minnesota Department of Health. (2019). *Public health interventions: Application for nursing practice* (2nd ed.). www.health.state.mn.us/communities/practice/research/phncouncil/docs/PHInterventions.pdf

Mirghani, H., Jung, A. & Fakhry, C. (2017). Primary, secondary and tertiary prevention of human papillomavirus-driven head and neck cancers. *European Journal of Cancer,* 78, 105–115. http://dx.doi.org/10.1016/j.ejca.2017.03.021

National Collaborating Centre for Determinants of Health. (2014). *Let's talk: Moving upstream.* "Let's Talk" series. St. Francis Xavier University. https://nccdh.ca/images/uploads/Moving_Upstream_Final_En.pdf

National Conference of State Legislators. (2022). *HPV vaccine: State legislation and regulation.* https://www.ncsl.org/research/health/hpv-vaccine-state-legislation-and-statutes.aspx#:~:te

Office of Disease Prevention and Health Promotion. (n.d.a.). *Increase the proportion of adolescents who get recommended doses of the HPV vaccine—IID-08.* Healthy People 2030. Office of the Assistant Secretary for Health. https://health.gov/healthypeople/objectives-and-data/browse-objectives/vaccination increase-proportion-adolescents-who-get-recommended-doses-hpv-vaccine-iid-08

Office of Disease Prevention and Health Promotion. (n.d.b.). *Social determinants of health.* Healthy People 2030. Office of the Assistant Secretary for Health. https://health.gov/healthypeople/priority-areas/social-determinants-health

Office of Disease Prevention and Health Promotion. (n.d.c.). *Violence prevention: Primary prevention interventions to reduce perpetration of intimate partner violence and sexual violence among youth.* Healthy People 2030. Office of the Assistant Secretary for Health. https://health.gov/healthypeople/tools-action/browse-evidence-based-resources/violence-Prevention-primary-prevention-interventions-reduce-perpetration-intimate-partner-violence-and-sexual-violence-among-youth

Powell, K., Thurston, M., & Bloyce, D. (2017). Theorising lifestyle drift in health promotion: explaining community and voluntary sector engagement practices in disadvantaged areas. *Critical Public Health, 27*(5), 554–565. https://doi.org/10.1080/09581596.2017.1356909

Primary Care Online Resources and Education. (n.d.). *Preventive services.* https://edblogs.columbia.edu/pcore/prevention/prevention-preventive-services/

Quinlan, J. (2021). *Human papillomavirus: Screening, testing, and prevention.* https://www.aafp.org/pubs/afp/issues/2021/0800/p152.html

Rose, G. (2008). *The strategy of preventive medicine* (2nd ed.). Oxford University Press.

Rutter, H., Bes-Rastrollo, M., de Henauw, S., Lahti-Koski, M., Lehtinen-Jacks, S., Mullerova, D., Rasmussen, F., Rissanen, A., Visscher, T., & Lissner, L. (2017). Balancing upstream and downstream measures to tackle the obesity epidemic: A position statement from the European Association for the study of obesity. *Obesity Facts, 10,* 61–63. https://doi.org/10.1159/000455960

Upstream. (2013). *Introduction to upstream.* YouTube, September 25, 2013. https://www.youtube.com/watch?v=qarQXqKbmLg

Waithaka, D., Tsofa, B., & Barasa, E. (2018). Evaluating healthcare priority setting at the meso level: A thematic review of empirical literature. *Wellcome Open Research*, *3*(2), 1–18. https://wellcomeopenresearch.org/articles/3-2

Williams, O., & Fullagar, S. (2018). Lifestyle drift and the phenomenon of 'citizen shift' in contemporary U.K. health policy. *Sociology of Health & Illness*, *41*(5), 20–35. https://doi.org/10.1111/1467-9566.12783

World Health Organization. (2022). *About us*. http://www.emro.who.int/about-who/public-health-functions/health-promotion-disease-prevention.html

Credits

Fig. 3.1: Primary Care Online Resources and Education, "Definitions of Main Levels of Prevention," https://edblogs.columbia.edu/pcore/prevention/prevention-preventive-services/. Copyright © by The Trustees of Columbia University.

Fig. 3.2: Blue Cross Blue Shield Minnesota, "Examples of Secondary Prevention Screenings," https://blog.bluecrossmn.com/longevity/power-of-prevention/. Copyright © 2018 by Blue Cross Blue Shield Association.

Fig. 3.3: Adapted from Carlos Martins, Maciek Godycki-Cwirko, Bruno Heleno and John Brodersen, "Quaternary prevention: an evidence-based concept aiming to protect patients from medical harm," *British Journal of General Practice*, vol. 69, no. 689. Copyright © 2019 by Royal College of General Practitioners.

IMG 3.1: Upstream, Screenshot from "The Upstream-Downstream Parable for Health Equity," https://www.youtube.com/watch?v=qarQXqKbmLg. Copyright © 2014 by Upstream.

Fig. 3.4: Adapted from copyright © 2016 by John W. Frank (CC BY 4.0) at https://link.springer.com/article/10.17269/s41997-022-00636-6.

CHAPTER 4

Health Promotion and Disease Prevention

"Everything hinges on education. Without it, you can't advocate for proper health care, for housing, for a civil rights bill that ensures your rights."

—Susan L. Taylor

Learning Outcomes

After reading this chapter, students should be able to:

1. Understand the definitions of *health promotion* and *disease prevention*
2. Apply the concepts of health promotion and disease prevention
3. Apply the three levels of the learning domain
4. Differentiate between the learning styles
5. Understand the issue of health literacy
6. Apply the stages of change
7. Apply at least two health belief/health promotion models
8. Create SMART (*specific*, *measurable*, *achievable*, *realistic*, and *timely*) objectives
9. Understand the teach-back method

Keywords and Concepts

Affective learning domain; auditory/aural learning style; cognitive learning domain; disease prevention; health literacy; health promotion; kinesthetic/tactile learning style; psychomotor learning domain; read/write learning style; SMART objectives/goals; teach-back method; visual learning style

Definitions of the Keywords

Affective learning domain: Involves emotion/feeling toward learning (Centers for Disease Control and Prevention [CDC], n.d.)

Auditory/aural learning style: The idea that learning is enhanced by hearing and listening to, understanding, and remembering things that have been heard and storing information by sounds (EducationPlanner.org, n.d.)

Cognitive learning domain: Involves intellect through understanding and applying the information to learning (CDC, n.d.)

Disease prevention: Population-based and individual-based interventions emphasizing primary and early secondary levels to minimize disease and risk factors (World Health Organization [WHO], 2023)

Health promotion: Empowering individuals to control their health using health literacy and actions to increase healthier behaviors (WHO, 2023)

Health literacy: The information a person finds and uses to make appropriate decisions regarding health-related needs (CDC, 2022b)

Kinesthetic/tactile learning style: Requires manipulation or touching to enhance learning (EducationPlanner.org, n.d.)

Psychomotor learning domain: Involves physicality and how that develops from basic motor skills to intricate performance (CDC, n.d.)

Read/write learning style: Preference is information as words and reading materials (Visual, Aural, Reading, Kinesthetic [VARK], 2023a)

SMART goals/objectives: Used for goal setting; *SMART* is an acronym for *specific, measurable, achievable, realistic*, and *timely* (CDC, 2022a)

Teach-back method: Technique used by healthcare providers to ensure that explained medical information is communicated effectively (Agency for Healthcare Research and Quality [AHRQ], 2021)

Visual learning style: The idea that reading or viewing pictures enhances learning (EducationPlanner.org, n.d.)

Introduction

Individuals, families, communities, and populations must be educated about health risks and adverse outcomes that lead to preventable illnesses. Without understanding how to prevent issues, health conditions can become significant concerns down the road. A lack of knowledge about certain problems can cause specific populations to experience many issues that lead to chronic diseases (Zajacova & Lawrence, 2018).

The nurse's role is to foster the importance of health-promoting activities. Examples include healthy eating, physical exercise, stress management, adequate sleep, hygiene, and healthy personal relationships (Ross et al., 2017). However, understanding that health literacy is intricately linked to health promotion and disease prevention is critical in providing effective vital strategies and interventions (Ferreira et al., 2022).

This chapter will address health prevention and disease promotion for individuals, families, communities, and populations. The importance of education and interventions that persons should incorporate into their daily lives could foster better health outcomes. The chapter will discuss the concepts of health promotion, disease prevention, health literacy, different health promotion models, SMART goals/objectives, and the teach-back method.

Background of the Concepts

Various health promotion and disease prevention aspects determine success in meeting practical well-being. Social factors and issues with health equity can influence many populations who cannot obtain services to promote and maintain health, manage diseases, and reduce disabilities and premature deaths (CDC, 2023a; Office of Disease Prevention and Health Promotion [ODPHP], n.d.a.). Healthcare professionals (HCPs) must be able to assess all individuals for access usage and identify barriers to necessary services (Gallaway et al., 2022).

Evidence-based research has identified that national and international communities need more access to healthcare resources. Some individuals have health insurance but cannot pay for out-of-pocket costs and hence cannot access routine treatments, well-child visits, or immunizations. Those without health insurance may be employed but unable to pay for the insurance as income is used for other needs, such as food and housing (McEnroe-Petitte, 2020). Minority groups may also be included in this area. Researchers have found that many children, families, and adults report the lack of healthcare insurance, the lack of a routine personal doctor or healthcare provider, or high medical costs for diagnosed conditions and treatments, leading to no follow-up care or preventative needs. Other healthcare areas, such as eye and dental care, are additionally not used due to high costs and lack of access to care (Gallaway et al., 2022). Uninsured adults are less likely to receive preventive services for chronic conditions such as diabetes, cancer, and cardiovascular disease (CVD; ODPHP, n.d.a.).

Individuals who are less educated and who belong to culturally different groups have identified that healthcare is more challenging to access and more costly (Gallaway et al., 2022). Healthcare staffing shortages and insufficient healthcare provided have affected the availability of healthcare to meet the needs of vulnerable populations. Incorporating telehealth has assisted in areas that lack access and healthcare provider availability. Telehealth allows for resources in areas where healthcare is limited, especially rural settings (Gallaway et al., 2022). The stigma and bias present among the medical community, especially in dealing with conditions such as mental health, HIV/AIDS, gender and hormonal disorders, abortions, sexual orientation, race, and culture, can affect how the healthcare worker perceives the person. Language barriers will also affect the care processes as they cannot effectively understand what the person needs or is trying to communicate (Gallaway et al., 2022).

Additional barriers exist, such as the inability to access transportation, the inability to obtain needed equipment, and little to no availability of healthcare resources. Huot et al. (2019) discuss the issues leading to these barriers. These include the physical geography of the individuals, provider-related obstacles, culture and language problems, and systemic factors. The financial requirements, stress, and time away from family members were found to be an issue. The consideration for the harshness of winter weather was addressed as this affected care. The costs for travel and charges for deliveries of medical equipment were high. This research also found that staff shortages and frequent turnover limited available care. By analyzing individuals' environment and surroundings, the ability to meet and provide a more holistic method of healthcare delivery could be accomplished (Huot et al., 2019).

Health Promotion and Disease Prevention

Health promotion and disease prevention through population-based interventions, including action to address social determinants of health (SDOH) and health inequity, are vital to prevention success (WHO, 2023). Healthy People (HP) 2030's overall goals are health and well-being, with the program noting that all healthcare providers are responsible for promoting and assessing (Pronk et al., 2021).

Health Promotion/Disease Prevention Definitions

Health promotion, as defined by the WHO (2023), is the ability of individuals to empower themselves to take control of their health and health activities. Effective health promotion can be enhanced by health literacy and education, as healthy behaviors and actions can improve effective health promotion. The WHO (2023) has found that disease prevention is based on population and individual interventions that focus on the levels of primary and secondary actions to minimize diseases and recognize risk factors that may contribute to specific conditions. At the population level, they can eliminate health disparities, improve quality of life, and improve the availability of healthcare and related services. Health promotion and disease prevention can empower individuals to make healthier choices and reduce their risk of developing diseases and disabilities (CDC, 2023a).

Application of Health Promotion and Disease Prevention

Health promotion and disease prevention are part of an individual's knowledge and health literacy. Health promotion encourages individuals to have the power to understand and make decisions about their health and health practices (Ferreira et al., 2022). The need to increase the knowledge of an individual or group of people leads to assertive actions taken to provide the needed measures for facilitating learning and continuing education. The importance of including various topics to meet the specific needs of multiple groups is emphasized depending on individual needs. Meeting the needs of particular groups, such as women, children, and older adults, can be an appropriate approach (Nouri et al., 2019). The ability to educate individuals nationally and internationally requires adequate resources. Proper inclusion of relevant content will assist with increasing knowledge and developing skills for an individual's health and that of the community and populations around them (Nutbeam et al., 2018).

With health promotion, vitality includes coordinating between not just the health facilities but also the community partners. This can easily be accomplished through the development of specific programs conducive to all aspects of healthy living for all ages, such as promotion of successful social interaction and mental health; the inclusion of physical activities and healthy eating patterns; early identification, prevention, and continual monitoring of chronic disease appropriate follow-up and medication/treatment regimens; and inclusion of safety measures and accident prevention (Baixinho et al., 2019; Cardoso et al., 2017; Ferreira et al., 2022).

The 2010 Affordable Care Act (ACA) provided more emphasis on preventive care (Department of Health and Human Services [DHHS], 2022). Medicare introduced the Annual Wellness Visit under the ACA, which includes a comprehensive assessment of preventive services for the older adult, explicitly focusing on the cognitive and functional impairments that may be present (Chung et al., 2018). Medicare's coverage has made it possible to facilitate preventive visits that place the focus on older adults (Chung et al., 2018).

Research of older adults in California and their use of preventative care found that only half received such services as influenza and pneumococcal vaccinations, colonoscopy/sigmoidoscopy or fecal occult blood tests, and mammography for women. The continued lack of coverage with fee-for-service (FFS) payments is viewed as a barrier. Healthcare visits are routinely short and do not allow for an appropriate conversation to discuss acute and chronic conditions, education, counseling, and screening options (Chung et al., 2018). Most insurance plans now must cover necessary primary and secondary preventions. Unfortunately, preventive visit rates are low for those in the United States (Chung et al., 2018).

Chung et al. (2018) found that preventative measures were included primarily for women (59.8%), non-Hispanic White individuals (64.4%), and Medicare FFS beneficiaries (80.7%). The summary included the fact that only 32% attended a preventive visit. Visits tended to decline as individuals' ages and comorbidities increased. Disparities with the low use of preventive measures for Hispanics and African-American older adults continue (Chung et al., 2018).

The ODPHP provides information on the preventive services suggested for particular genders and ages. The link to *MyHealthfinder* allows individuals to access trusted information to help families and communities stay safe and healthy (ODPHP, 2023; Box 4.1).

BOX 4.1 ACTIVE LEARNING REFLECTION ON USING THE *MYHEALTHFINDER* TOOL

Go to https://health.gov/myhealthfinder and type in "male aged 70."

1. Note at least five areas identified on the website.
2. Click on "Colorectal Cancer Screening" and discuss some specific essential and action items noted. Name at least two for each.

American Association of Colleges of Nursing (AACN) *Essentials* (2021):
Domains: #2; #3; #5; #8

- Competencies: 2.3; 2.4; 3.1; 3.3; 5.1; 8.3
- Subcompetencies: 2.3e; 2.4d; 3.1b; 3.1c; 3.1f; 3.3b; 5.1d; 5.1f; 8.3a

Spheres of Care: Wellness/Disease prevention

Concepts: Evidence-based practice; SDOH

Source: ODPHP, 2023.

The Advisory Committee on Immunizations Practices (ACIP) recommends vaccinations through the CDC. In contrast, the Women's Preventive Services Initiative (WPSI) makes recommendations appropriate for women (WPSI, 2022). Additionally, various specialty organizations, such as the American College of Obstetrics and Gynecology and American Cancer Society, make prevention endorsements (CDC, 2023b).

The United States Preventive Services Task Force (USPSTF) is an independent, volunteer panel of disease prevention and evidence-based medical practices. This task force of national experts delivers recommendations about clinical preventive services to help improve people's health in this country. Specific primary and secondary prevention strategies are the priorities for this panel (USPSTF, n.d.b.; Box 4.2).

The ACA charges the USPSTF with making an annual report to Congress that identifies gaps in the evidence base for clinical preventive services and recommends priority areas that deserve further examination. The USPSTF hopes that by annually highlighting high-priority evidence gaps, as requested by Congress, it will assist public and private researchers and research funders in targeting their efforts, ensuring a collaborative approach to improving preventive health and healthcare for all Americans (USPSTF, n.d.c.).

BOX 4.2 ACTIVE LEARNING REFLECTION ON HEALTH PROMOTION/PREVENTION

Watch this video about the USPSTF's new guidelines for breast cancer screening: https://www.youtube.com/watch?v=r6olpv75gnM.

1. What level of prevention is screening?
2. Which specific ethnicity is more affected by breast cancer? How would you promote this health promotion activity to this target population (name two ways)?
3. How have the new guidelines changed from the 2016 guidelines? Name two ways.

AACN *Essentials* (2021): Domains: #2; #3; #4; #9

- Competencies: 2.3; 2.4; 2.7; 2.8; 2.9; 3.1; 3.2; 4.2; 9.1; 9.2
- Subcompetencies: 2.3a; 2.3b; 2.3e; 2.4d; 2.7a; 2.8c; 2.8e; 2.9a; 3.1a; 3.1b; 3.1i; 3.2c; 4.2c; 4.2d; 9.1c; 9.2d; 9.2g

Spheres of Care: Wellness/Disease prevention

Concepts: Diversity, equity, and inclusion (DEI); Evidence-based practice; SDOH

Source: USPSTF Info, 2024.

An example of recent evidence-based change in health promotion and disease prevention intervention was the administration of aspirin use in clients with CVD. For many years, the standard of practice was that low-dose aspirin should be used for those with CVD. In April 2022, the USPSTF recommended aspirin for adults ages 40 to 59 with an estimated 10% or greater 10-year CVD risk. However, the decision to initiate low-dose aspirin use for the primary prevention of CVD should be made during a discussion between the healthcare provider and the client. For other age groups, low-dose aspirin with CVD risk is no longer recommended (USPSTF, n.d.a.).

Learning Domains

Bloom and other researchers developed the taxonomy of learning domains (Hoque, 2016). The learning domains are a method to facilitate adult learning through cognitive, affective, and psychomotor techniques formulated from a specific aspect to a more complex process. These learning outcomes determine the learning strategies incorporated into lesson plans. Examples may include activities, assessments, and modes of presentations that are desirable to ensure learning has taken place (Hoque, 2016).

Cognitive Learning Domain

Cognitive learning encompasses understanding information and basic content recall. The latest understanding of Bloom's technology notes cognition is emphasized using

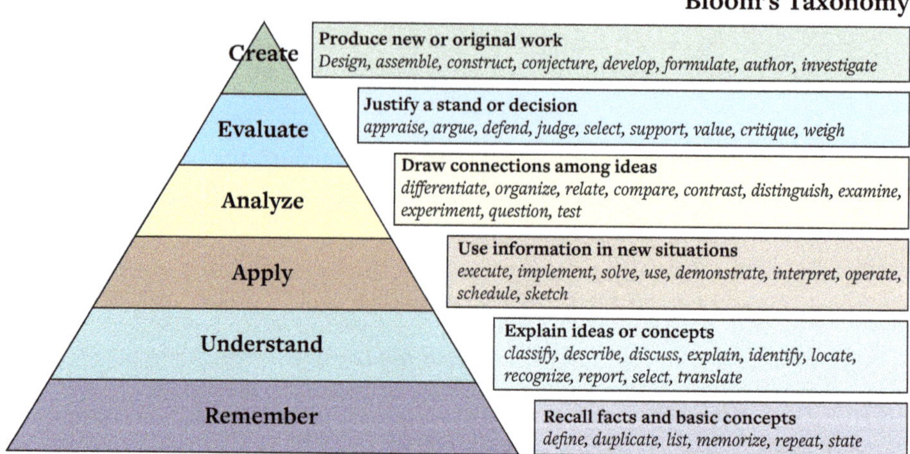

FIGURE 4.1 Bloom's Taxonomy (Updated) for Cognitive Domain Learning

the following areas: remember, understand, apply, analyze, evaluate, and create (Hoque, 2016). Remember that it is the lowest level, but an individual cannot achieve the highest level (create) without first using the lower levels. The cognitive domain contains learning skills chiefly related to the mental (thinking) process (Hoque, 2016; Figure 4.1).

Affective Learning Domain

Affective learning focuses on emotional processes such as attitudes, motivation, participation, values, and incorporation of lifelong learning. By doing so, individuals can listen, participate, be involved, advocate, and be willing to change behaviors and lifestyles. This domain includes dealing with things emotionally and is categorized into five subdomains: receiving, responding, valuing, organization, and characterization (Hoque, 2016; Figure 4.2).

Psychomotor Learning Domain

The psychomotor learning domain notes the ability to progress from a lower-order to a higher-order process while performing an activity that requires skill. The psychomotor domain is specific to discreet physical functions, reflex actions, and interpretive movements (Hoque, 2016). The form of learning occurs through recognition, recall, or memorization. Learning progression adds analysis, interpretations, and advanced insights (Figure 4.3).

Mallillin (2020) examined the different domains of learning and respondents' academic performance to identify the extent of the domains of learning and the students' academic performance regarding skills in learning, attitude toward studies, and educational achievements. Results noted that using various learning domains improved the students' academic performance and overall achievement (Mallillin, 2020; Box 4.3).

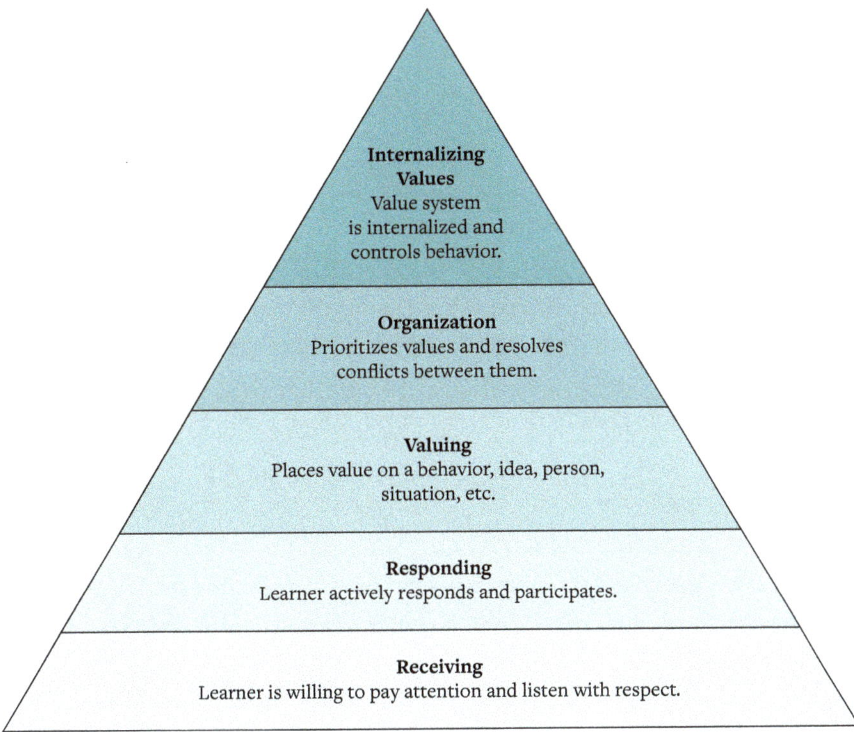

FIGURE 4.2 Subdomains of Affective Learning

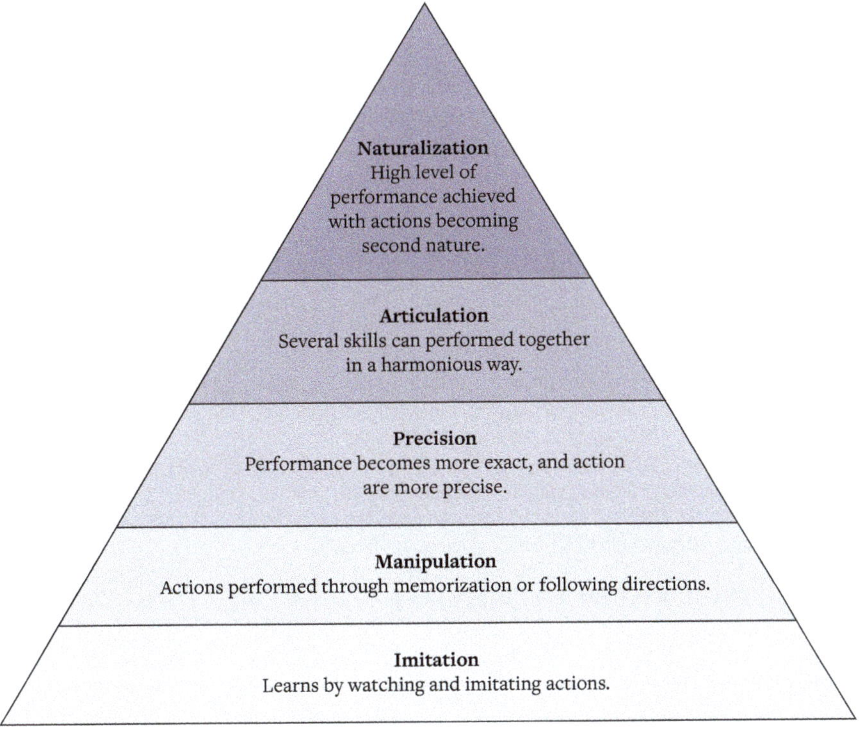

FIGURE 4.3 Subdomains of Psychomotor Learning

BOX 4.3 ACTIVE LEARNING REFLECTION ON LEARNING DOMAINS

Watch the following video about the three learning domains (click on the first video): https://www.cdc.gov/healthyschools/professional_development/e-learning/pd201/section_02.html

1. After watching the video, apply all the learning domains to an example of a new, younger adult client with diabetes who will now receive insulin. Provide a short synopsis of each learning domain as applied to the scenario.

AACN *Essentials* (2021): Domains: #1; #2; #6; #8; #9

- Competencies: 1.1; 1.3; 2.2; 2.3; 2.4; 2.5; 2.7; 6.1; 8.4; 9.2
- Subcompetencies:1.1b; 1.3c; 2.2b; 2.3a; 2.3b; 2.3d; 2.3e; 2.3g; 2.4b; 2.4c; 2.4d; 2.5a; 2.5b; 2.5c; 2.5d; 2.7a; 6.1e; 8.4b; 9.2b; 9.2c

Spheres of Care: Wellness/Disease prevention; Chronic disease management

Concepts: Communication; Compassionate care; Evidence-based practice; Clinical judgment

Source: Adapted from CDC, 2018.

Learning Styles (VARK)

A *learning style* describes an attribute or characteristic of learning (VARK, 2023a). Individuals may have one learning style preference or multiple modalities. Neil Fleming discovered four different learning styles: *v*isual, *a*uditory, *r*eading/writing, and *k*inesthetic (VARK; 2023a; Box 4.4).

BOX 4.4 ACTIVE LEARNING REFLECTION ON VARK LEARNING STYLES

Watch the following video on the four VARK learning styles: https://vark-learn.com/introduction-to-vark/. Reflect on what you learned.

1. Name the four learning styles and provide a specific example that an individual would use for each.

AACN *Essentials* (2021): Domains: #1; #2; #8

- Competencies: 1.3; 2.5; 8.1; 8.3
- Subcompetencies: 1.3a; 1.3b; 1.3c; 2.5d; 8.1c; 8.3a

Spheres of Care: Wellness/Disease prevention

Concepts: Evidence-based practice; Clinical judgment

Source: VARK, 2023a.

Visual Learning Style

Visual learning includes identifying images, tables, and graphics to analyze and understand the content. This style notes the depiction of information in maps, diagrams, charts, graphs, flow charts, and the symbolic arrows, circles, hierarchies, and other devices that people use to represent what could have been presented in words. It does not include still pictures or photographs of reality, movies, videos, or PowerPoint. It includes designs, white space, patterns, shapes, and various formats used to highlight and convey information noted in graphics (VARK, 2023a).

Auditory/Aural Learning Style

The auditory/aural learning style entails listening to voices and sounds while incorporating speech through lectures and group discussions. Learners with auditory learning as their primary preference report learning best from lectures, group discussions, radio, email, mobile phones, speaking, and talking. The auditory/aural preference includes talking aloud and to oneself (VARK, 2023a).

Reading/Writing Learning Style

The reading/writing learning style notes the use of reading and writing to enhance learning through note-taking, essay writing, and online or in-person presentations. Not surprisingly, many teachers and students prefer this style. Being able to write well and read widely are attributes that employers of graduates seek. People who choose this modality are often addicted to PowerPoint, the Internet, lists, diaries, dictionaries, and words (VARK, 2023a).

Kinesthetic/Tactile Learning Style

The kinesthetic/tactile method occurs when one learns using one's senses, examples, and case studies. People who prefer this mode are connected to reality through simulation, personal experiences, demonstrations, and videos. People with this preference learn from the experience of doing something and value their own experiences and, less so, the experiences of others (VARK, 2023a; Box 4.5).

BOX 4.5 ACTIVE LEARNING REFLECTION ACTIVITY USING THE VARK QUESTIONNAIRE

Take the VARK questionnaire using the following URL: https://vark-learn.com/the-vark-questionnaire/. Reflect on your results by identifying your learning style(s).

1. Discuss two ways you plan to use your identified learning style(s). Give specific applications.

AACN *Essentials* (2021): Domains: #1; #2; #3; #8; #9

- Competencies: 1.3; 2.2; 2.5; 3.5; 8.1; 8.3; 9.2
- Subcompetencies: 1.3b; 2.2e; 2.5d; 3.5d; 8.1c; 8.3a; 9.2g

Spheres of Care: Wellness/Disease prevention

Concepts: Communication; Evidence-based practice

Source: VARK, 2023b.

Providing different modes of relating information and material to others requires various learning styles. Those who do not have a standout learning style with one preference are defined as *multimodal* (VARK, 2023a). Providing knowledge in numerous avenues allows multimodal individuals to learn.

Stages of Change

Health promotion and disease prevention entail identifying problems and noting how one might make positive changes. One such model of change is the Transtheoretical or Change Model. Developed by Prochaska and DiClemente in the late 1970s, the Transtheoretical Model (TTM) focuses on individuals' decision-making and is a model of intentional change (Rural Health Information Hub [RHIhub], 2023b). The TTM operates on the assumption that people do not change behaviors quickly and decisively but undergo cyclical processes. Instead, change in behavior, especially habitual, occurs continuously through a cyclical process. The model portrays a straightforward method to assist individuals who want to change their behaviors. The details include separate stages: precontemplation, contemplation, preparation, action, maintenance, and termination. By reviewing these, an individual can determine whether they are ready to make changes to their behavior (RHIhub, 2023b; Table 4.1; Figure 4.4).

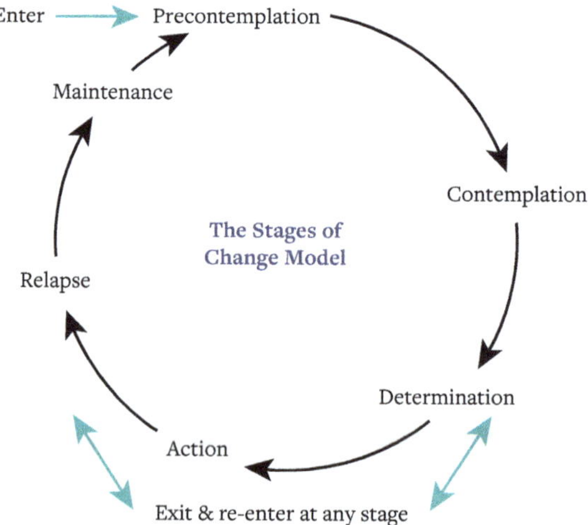

FIGURE 4.4 Visual Interpretation of the Transtheoretical or Change Model

TABLE 4.1 Details of Transtheoretical or Change Model (Using an Example of Nicotine Usage)

Stage	Definition/Example
Precontemplation	• There is no intention to act • Client will keep the same behavior (e.g., nicotine usage)
Preparation	• There are intentions to act and a plan to do so soon • Client understands the risks of nicotine usage but is not planning to quit at this time
Action	• Behavior has been changed for a short time • Client has stopped using nicotine for two weeks, experienced decreased shortness of breath, and tried nicotine patches but has now begun using nicotine through cigarette smoking again
Maintenance	• Behavior has been changed and continues to be maintained for the long term • Client has not used nicotine through cigarette smoking for several weeks through regular nicotine patches and gum use. Client has been able to increase activities without shortness of breath and notes how much better they feel
Termination	• There is no desire to return to prior negative behaviors • Client has developed a plan that does not include nicotine use

Source: Adapted from RHIhub, 2023b.

Health Promotion Models

Models can be beneficial in incorporating health promotion and disease prevention. Models allow for collecting concepts that relate to various ways individuals can produce an organized approach to dealing with issues. The following models will be discussed: the Health Belief Model (HBM), Pender's Health Promotion Model (HPM), and Orem's Self-Care Deficit Nursing Theory (SCDNT). Each model has specific vital elements and beliefs that individuals may utilize and relate to health practices and various health conditions, including their approaches and particular individual needs (RHIhub, 2023a).

Health Belief Model

The HBM focuses on completing behaviors relating to health promotion, such as screenings or measures that will assist an individual in preventing injury or adverse outcomes, such as wearing a seatbelt or other protective equipment. In an individual's use of the HBM, the following elements are noted: perceived susceptibility, severity, benefits, and barriers to behaviors (McLean et al., 2019).

The area of self-efficacy is also included, in which the action can and will be conducted despite the barrier. The inclusion of motivation allows the individual to use physical or verbal cues to effectively complete the required behavior (McLean et al., 2019; Table 4.2).

TABLE 4.2 Health Belief Model Key Elements

Modifying Factors	Individual Beliefs	Example
Perceived susceptibility	Perceived threat to sickness or disease	"Am I susceptible to getting the condition?"
Perceived severity	Belief of consequence	"Will I die from this disease?"
Perceived benefits	Potential positive benefits of action	"I will get a flu vaccine so I can be protected from the severity of the condition."
Cues to action	Perceived barriers to action, exposure to factors that prompt action	"Having chest pain means a healthcare professional must evaluate me."
Self-efficacy	Confidence in the ability to succeed	"With hypertension, I need to check my blood pressure every morning and record it."

Source: Boston University School of Public Health, 2022a.

There needs to be a process for the implementation of the HBM. Initially, a needs assessment, which looks at individuals and populations who are at risk, must be carried out. Next, there is a need to identify the key risks. Each individual and population may differ, allowing for specific methods and interventions to be implemented. There must be effective communication with stakeholders to present the appropriate steps and recommended procedures to provide beneficial actions. While doing so, resources are researched for positive outcomes, including those that may be considered barriers. Finally, an evaluation of measures that support and enhance successful behavior change is noted (RHIhub, 2023c).

Pender's Health Promotion Model

Nola Pender developed the HPM to assist with understanding health promotion and healthy behaviors. Looking at the needs of individuals to successfully perform methods to promote health and actively participate in positive health behaviors can be stressful. However, by doing so, their quality of life can be supported. Assisting in self-care is essential and can help an individual throughout their lifespan. The HPM

BOX 4.6 ACTIVE REFLECTION ACTIVITY ON PENDER'S HPM

Watch the video on Pender's HPM, which includes an explanation of health promotion, https://study.com/academy/lesson/what-is-the-health-promotion-model-definition-theory.html

1. How do you see the HPM compared with the goals of HP 2030?
2. Present a scenario in which you could apply this model.
3. Name three ways to use this model in your future nursing practice.

AACN *Essentials* (2021): Domains: #1; #3; #5; #7; #9

- Competencies: 1.1; 1.3; 3.1; 5.1; 7.3; 9.3
- Subcompetencies: 1.1a; 1.1b; 1.3a; 1.3b; 3.1b; 3.1c; 3.1d; 3.1e; 3.1h; 5.1a; 5.1b; 7.3b; 9.3a

Spheres of Care: Wellness/Disease prevention

Concepts: Evidence-based practice; Clinical judgment

Source: Study.com, 2023.

can be applied to many health conditions and health promotion concerns, such as hypertension, myocardial infarction, safety, aging, hemodialysis, and adherence (Nursing-Theory.org, 2023a; Box 4.6).

Khodaveisi et al. (2017) used Pender's HPM to look at the behaviors of overweight and obese women. The ability to use health-promoting behaviors was implemented to assist women in self-help, enable health monitoring to lose weight, and promote healthy behaviors. An additional study by Ibrahim and Qalawa (2022) studied the stress with which student nurses with chronic illnesses were affected during the COVID-19 pandemic. This model allowed the identification of unhealthy behaviors to be changed and overall support and control of healthy behaviors to be implemented.

Orem's Self-Care Deficit Nursing Theory

The SCDNT was developed by Dorothea Orem and viewed as a broad theory that could be used in various nursing settings. This theory focuses on individuals who provide self-care concepts to perform activities to assist with recovery from those that have caused dependency. Orem identified the need for independence into three categories. The first category is universal self-care, which includes the areas of air, water, food, activity, rest, and hazard prevention. Secondary are the developmental self-care requisites of maturational and situational. Maturational looks at the advancement of growth to a higher level, while situational focuses on the development and the possibility of harmful effects that can develop (Nursing-Theory.org, 2023b).

Another area related to health deviations may become apparent with an individual's condition. Self-care deficits can occur when an individual cannot meet their self-care requisites, leading to such support being compensated, partially compensated, or needing education and help. Overall, Orem's theory has been successful in helping individuals and their caregivers make a more effective transition from the hospital setting to their home or long-term care facility (Nursing-Theory.org, 2023b; Figure 4.5).

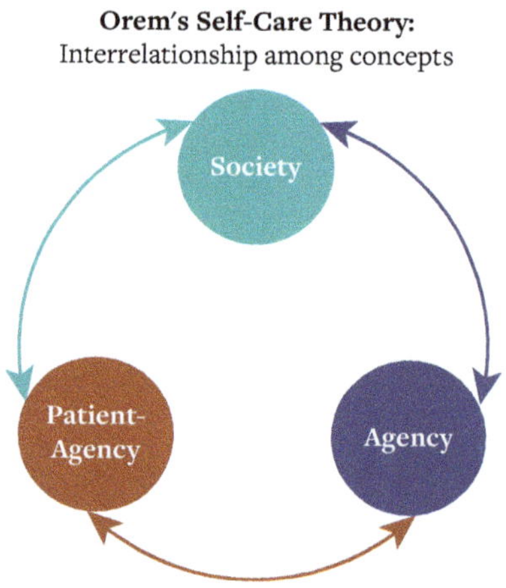

Orem's Self-Care Theory:
Interrelationship among concepts

FIGURE 4.5 Orem's Self-Care Model (Visual)

Health Literacy

Health literacy and communication between health professionals and clients are vital to improving health and healthcare quality. The ODPHP (2021a) creates, promotes, and curates evidence-based health literacy and communication tools, practices, and research for health professionals. The use of resources to find effective strategies for sharing health information in ways people can understand and use are necessary interventions (ODPHP, 2021a).

Health Literacy/Health Disparities/SDOH/HP 2030

Health disparities are situations through which individuals can be exposed to inequitable political, economic, social, environmental, educational, and behavioral resources. *Health literacy* focuses on communicating content to improve the quality and currency of health and reduce health disparities regarding health information (ODPHP, 2021a).

An individual's language and literacy skills are essential to avoid problems with the SDOH. Individuals need to find, understand, and effectively use knowledge to make positive decisions for themselves, their families, and their communities. With the development of HP 2030 activities, the changes and updates focused on several areas. Areas include the following: emphasizing the utilization of the information; making decisions that are decided by being sufficiently informed and not just what would be correct decisions; and needing to view health through the eyes of the public (ODPHP, n.d.b.).

Arguably, the National Academy of Medicine, formally called the Institute of Medicine (IOM) presents one of the most influential models of health literacy.

The IOM model contains four underlying constructs: knowledge of culture and concepts, health literacy (printed using writing and reading skills), verbal/oral (using the ability to listen and speak), and numerical presentations (Liu et al., 2020). The diverse needs of individuals, individual relationships with the public, those providing healthcare, and the existing healthcare systems are invested in the total picture.

When incorporating the SDOH, the need to view the determinants such as education, income, and access to healthcare play a key role in facilitating disease prevention and methods to make the most confident decisions for care. Simmons et al. (2017) looked into training for health literacy with an emphasis on easy-to-understand wording so that the everyday individual could focus on simple client education techniques. The use of written materials in various languages, along with the use of the teach-back method, has been identified as a successful method. In the teach-back process, the client/caregiver is assessed for their acquired knowledge in a manner that they could understand the information (Farris, 2015). The inclusion of visual prompts and web-based content emphasizing the presentation of cultural needs is stressed.

HP 2030 signifies one specific goal, noting the importance of health literacy. Health literacy is an essential overlying principle in the new version of HP 2030 (Santana et al., 2021). That goal is to focus on eliminating health disparities, achieving health equity, and attaining health literacy to improve the health and well-being of all (HP 2030, n.d.b.; Box 4.7).

BOX 4.7 ACTIVE LEARNING REFLECTION ON HEALTH LITERACY

Watch the following video on health literacy: https://odphp.health.gov/healthypeople/priority-areas/health-literacy-healthy-people-2030

1. Name the five things to know about health literacy. Use evidence-based practices to support your answer.
2. Name two vulnerable populations who might have trouble with adequate health literacy. Reflect on two interventions to assist with health literacy based on evidence-based practice.

AACN *Essentials* (2021): Domains: #2; #3; #4; #6; #7; #8

- Competencies: 2.2; 2.8; 3.1; 3.2; 4.2; 6.1; 7.2; 8.1; 8.3
- Subcompetencies: 2.2c; 2.2e; 2.8b; 3.1c; 3.1f; 3.1g; 3.2c; 4.2c; 6.1b; 6.1d; 7.2b; 8.1a; 8.3c

Spheres of Care: Wellness/Disease prevention

Concepts: Communication; DEI; SDOH; Evidence-based practice

Source: ODPHP, n.d.b.

TABLE 4.3 HP 2030 Objectives Related to Health Literacy

- Increase the proportion of adults whose healthcare provider checked their understanding—HC/HIT-01
- Decrease the proportion of adults who report poor communication with their healthcare provider—HC/HIT-02
- Increase the proportion of adults whose healthcare providers involved them in decisions as much as they wanted—HC/HIT-03
- Increase the proportion of people who say their online medical record is easy to understand—HC/HIT-D10
- Increase the proportion of adults with limited English proficiency who say their providers explain things clearly—HC/HIT-D11
- Increase the health literacy of the population—HC/HIT-R01

Source: ODPHP, n.d.b.

DHSS has separated two health literacy categories and defined them as personal and organizational. *Personal health literacy* refers to when individuals can find and understand health information, whereas *organizational health literacy* is when equitable access is available for those individuals (ODPHP, n.d.b.). There are six specific HP 2030 objectives related to health literacy (Table 4.3).

Health Literate Care Model

The Health Literate Care Model (HLCM) assists with health improvements related to prevention, making positive decisions, and overall self-care management. It provides the needed understanding of health through effective and clear communication and directions and ensures that each individual understands what is being discussed. If the HLCM is used to present knowledge, there becomes an organizational approach to assess, plan, implement, and evaluate the process to ensure learning. The model calls for all healthcare providers to approach all clients who risk not understanding valuable health information, provide a range of clear communication strategies, and confirm that the client understands what is being said and taught (ODPHP, 2021b; Figure 4.6).

SMART Objectives/Goals

Goals are developed to evaluate teaching. However, assessing effective teaching requires goals to be measurable and obtainable. There are five components to a compelling goal—*s*pecific, *m*easurable, *a*ttainable, *r*elevant, and *t*imely (CDC, 2022a)—and they comprise the acronym often used: *SMART* (Figure 4.7).

Nurses must assist clients with setting short- and long-term goals related to their health and well-being. By doing so, clients can achieve positive health outcomes (White, 2022). By using SMART goal components, clients will improve their ability to provide direction, develop a clear focus, clarify decision-making, offer a sense of purpose, gain control over their health, and encourage motivation (White, 2022).

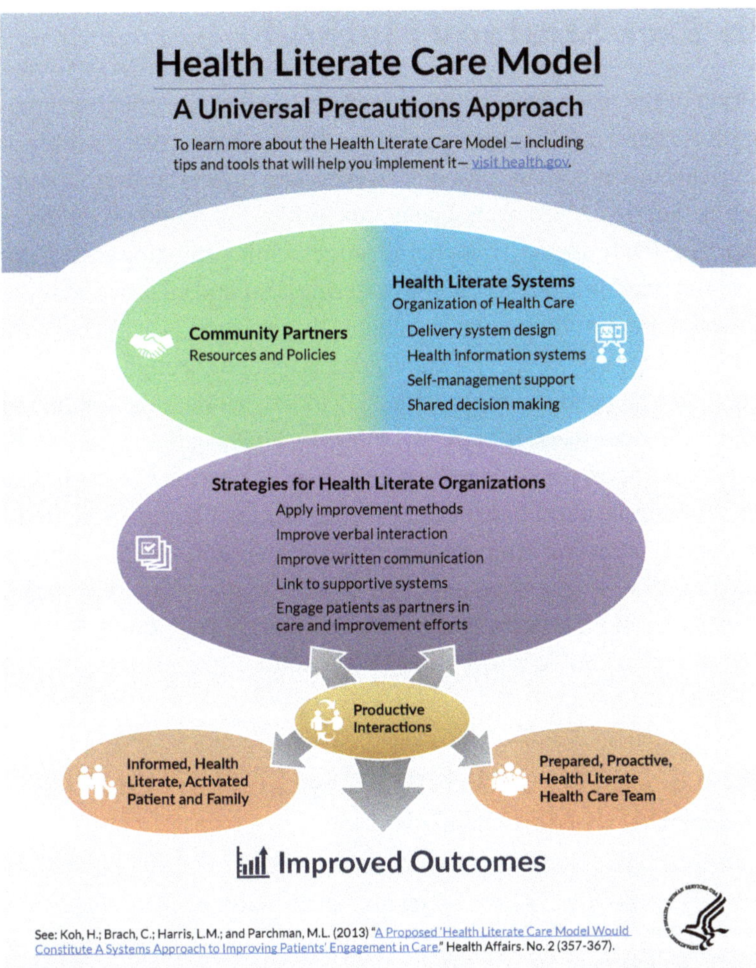

FIGURE 4.6 Health Literate Care Model

S	**Specific** Clearly State your Goal
M	**Measurable** Ensure you can Measure Success
A	**Attainable** Set Goals you know you can Achieve
R	**Relevant** Set Goals Relevant to your Career or Education
T	**Time-Based** Set a Deadline for Completion

FIGURE 4.7 SMART Objectives/Goals

Teach-Back Strategy Method

The addition of the teach-back strategy method has been an effective intervention to engage clients and families better to understand follow-up with healthcare activities. Using this technique can give one an adequate understanding of step-by-step instructions. Farris (2015) stated that this method is based on evidence-based knowledge to actively engage those being taught while providing safety, promoting adherence, and providing quality care. By offering clear and effective communication and ensuring understanding from the client, this method is available without the need for technology and cost. The knowledge is gained through an explanation of the process, skill, or need in simple words. HCPs can validate the understanding by having the individual teach it back. By doing so, HCPs can ensure that there is a clear understanding of the information and client education has been understood correctly. An example may be that of a heart failure client being instructed to weigh themselves every morning after voiding, wearing the same clothing and recording it in a journal. The weight then needs to be compared with the trending of the previous weights, and if shortness of breath or a gain of 2–3 pounds is noted in one week, the individual should notify their HCP (AHRQ, 2021; Farris, 2015; Box 4.8).

BOX 4.8 ACTIVE LEARNING REFLECTION ON THE TEACH-BACK METHOD

Use your knowledge about the concept of the teach-back method and the following link for the following two scenarios: https://www.ahrq.gov/sites/default/files/wysiwyg/professionals/quality-patient-safety/patient-family-engagement/pfeprimarycare/teach-back_quickstart_full.pdf.

1. Your client is being placed on warfarin for atrial fibrillation, and you are using the teach-back method strategy to educate the client about the drug and implications that should be stressed. Name three specific details that you want them to repeat back to you.
2. A client is scheduled for a computed tomography (scan of the abdomen and upper gastrointestinal series). Use the teach-back method strategy to educate the client about preparation for each test. Name two specific details you want them to repeat back to you.

AACN *Essentials* (2021): Domains: #1; #2; #3; #4; #6; #8

- Competencies: 1.1; 2.2; 2.4; 2.8; 3.3; 4.2; 6.1; 8.1; 8.3
- Subcompetencies: 1.1b; 2.2e; 2.4d; 2.8a; 2.8b; 2.8c; 3.3b; 4.2c; 6.1b; 8.1b; 8.1d; 8.3c

Spheres of Care: Wellness/Disease prevention; Chronic disease management

Concepts: Communication; Evidence-based practice; SDOH

Sources: AHRQ, n.d.; 2021; Farris, 2015.

Chapter Highlights

- Discussion about the definitions of *health promotion* and *disease prevention*
- Discussion about health literacy, domains of learning, learning styles, stages of change, health promotion and disease prevention models, SMART goals, and the teach-back method
- Active learning reflections for health promotion, VARK learning styles, domains of learning, teach-back method, and health promotion models
- Active learning exercise related to Intervention Wheel and writing SMART goals
- Case studies on health promotion/disease prevention, health literacy, and primary prevention

Active Learning Exercises

Application to Intervention Wheel/SMART Goals

The nurse presents at a senior center about vaccinations for adults older than age 60.

1. Develop a PowerPoint presentation applicable to the target population, limiting the presentation to a maximum of 10 slides. Include a title page, two SMART goals/objectives, and a reference slide.
2. Apply two population-based interventions to this presentation using the community-focused approach discussed in Chapter 1. Use the resource for the intervention wheel to assist.

https://www.health.state.mn.us/communities/practice/ research/phncouncil/docs/PHInterventions.pdf

AACN *Essentials* (2021): Domains: #1; #2; #3; #6; #8

- Competencies: 1.1; 1.2; 2.2; 2.5; 2.8; 2.9; 3.1; 3.3; 3.4; 6.1; 6.1; 6.4; 8.3
- Subcompetencies: 1.1a; 1.1b; 1.2c; 2.2b; 2.2c; 2.5d; 2.5g; 2.8a; 2.9b; 3.1a; 3.1b; 3.1c; 3.1e; 3.3b; 3.4c; 6.1e; 6.2e; 6.4d; 8.3a; 8.3e

Spheres of Care: Wellness/Disease prevention

Concepts: Communication; Evidence-based practice; Health policy; SDOH

Sources: CDC, 2022a; Minnesota Department of Health, 2019; White, 2022.

Case Studies

Case Study #1: Application to Health Promotion/ Disease Prevention

Watch the following video to understand a clinician's role in disease prevention and health promotion: https://www.youtube.com/watch?v=DtWE2Ft7ACk.

1. After watching the video, document three ways in which you could discuss health and promotion for each of the following scenarios:
   a. A 10-year-old obese child (https://esmed.org/MRA/mra/article/view/2152/193545601)
   b. A 37-year-old man who just purchased a gun for family protection (https://injepijournal.biomedcentral.com/articles/10.1186/s40621-021-00319-9)
   c. A 65-year-old woman with a history of hypertension and osteoarthritis (https://journals.humankinetics.com/view/journals/japa/29/2/article-p207.xml)

AACN *Essentials* (2021): Domains: #1; #2; #3 ;#4; #6; #7; #8; #9

- Competencies: 1.1; 1.2; 1.3; 2.2; 2.4; 2.5; 2.6; 2.8; 2.9; 3.1; 3.3; 4.2; 6.1; 7.1; 8.3; 9.2
- Subcompetencies: 1.1b; 1.2c; 1.3b; 2.2c; 2.2e; 2.4b; 2.5a; 2.5e; 2.6b; 2.8a; 2.8b; 2.8c; 2.8d; 2.8e; 2.9a; 2.9c; 3.1c; 3.1f; 3.1g; 3.3b; 4.2c; 6.1b; 7.1c; 8.3c; 9.2b; 9.2g

Spheres of Care: Wellness/Disease prevention; Chronic disease management; Regenerative/restorative care

Concepts: Clinical judgment; Communication; Compassionate care; Ethics; SDOH

Sources: Ketabchi et al., 2021; Perry, 2022; Schlenk et al., 2020; USPSTF Info, 2018.

Case Study #2: Application to Health Literacy

Many individuals are highly educated but have health literacy issues. Watch the following video: https://www.youtube.com/watch?v=BgTuD7l7LG8. How would you answer the following questions?

1. How could you effectively prepare clients to understand their disease process and the prescribed medications? What education would be needed to read and understand medication bottle labels? Give three specific examples that can be provided to clients.

2. Many clients you may encounter need help to read and/or understand written words. How could you best assess clients to determine their ability to understand health issues? How can you intervene to assist these clients and ensure their complete understanding? Name three ways.

AACN *Essentials* (2021): Domains: #1; #2; #3 ;#4; #6; #8; #9

- Competencies: 1.1; 1.2; 1.3; 2.2; 2.4; 2.5; 2.6; 2.8; 2.9; 3.1; 3.3; 4.2; 6.1; 8.3; 9.2
- Subcompetencies: 1.1b; 1.2c; 1.3a; 1.3b; 2.2c; 2.2e; 2.4b; 2.5a; 2.5e; 2.6b; 2.8a; 2.8b; 2.8c; 2.8d; 2.8e; 2.9a; 2.9c; 3.1c; 3.1f; 3.1g; 3.3b; 4.2c; 6.1b; 8.3c; 9.2b; 9.2g

Spheres of Care: Wellness/Disease prevention; Chronic disease management

Concepts: Clinical judgment; Communication; Compassionate care; SDOH; Evidence-based practice

Source: WisLit, 2010.

Case Study #3: Primary Prevention Exercise

Review the following blog on primary prevention for CVD: https://www.nursingcenter.com/blogs-plus/blogs/blogs-post#/post/Case-Study-Primary-Prevention-of-Cardiovascular-Di

1. A 25-year-old man with a family history of heart disease was present with both parents' lineage. Develop a handout to guide him in giving the client three primary prevention interventions.
2. Four-year-old children are learning about dental care prevention/oral health issues. As a classroom assignment, plan an active learning exercise to present this information to them. In addition, a one-page handout can be developed for parents to reinforce the presentation.

AACN *Essentials* (2021): Domains: #1; #2; #3; #4; #7; #8

- Competencies: 1.1; 1.2; 1.3; 2.2; 2.4; 2.5; 2.6; 2.8; 2.9; 3.1; 3.3; 4.2; 7.1; 7.2; 8.2; 8.3
- Subcompetencies: 1.1b; 1.2c; 1.3b; 2.2c; 2.2e; 2.4b; 2.5a; 2.5e; 2.6b; 2.8a; 2.8b; 2.8c; 2.8d; 2.8e; 2.9a; 2.9c; 3.1a; 3.1c; 3.1f; 3.1g; 3.3b; 4.2c; 7.1c; 7.2b; 8.2b; 8.3c; 8.3e

Spheres of Care: Wellness/Disease prevention

Concepts: Clinical judgment; Communication; Compassionate care; SDOH; Evidence-based practice

Source: Waronker, 2020.

NCLEX Questions

1. A client enters the local health clinic and states, "I've noticed how many people are out walking in my neighborhood. Is walking good for you?" What is the best response to help the client through the stages of change for exercise?
   a. "Walking is OK; running is better."
   b. "Yes, walking is great exercise. Could you go for a five-minute walk next week?"
   c. "Yes, I want you to begin walking. Walk 30 minutes daily and eat more fruits and vegetables."
   d. "They probably aren't walking fast or far enough. You may need to spend at least 45 minutes if you want to do any good."
2. Upon their initial visit to a healthcare provider, your client comments regarding the need to fill out numerous forms, including health history information. Which of the following would be the most appropriate reply?
   a. The insurance company will need this information to bill you.
   b. The healthcare provider will see you only if the forms are complete.
   c. The healthcare provider must know your health background information to care for you effectively.
   d. It is just a routine to do paperwork when you go to a new healthcare provider.

References

Agency for Healthcare Research and Quality. (n.d.). *Implementation quick start guide: Teach-back*. https://www.ahrq.gov/sites/default/files/wysiwyg/professionals/quality-patient-safety/patient-family-engagement/pfeprimarycare/teach-back_quickstart_full.pdf

Agency for Healthcare Research and Quality. (2021). *Teach-back interventions*. https://www.ahrq.gov/patientsafety/reports/engage/interventions/teachback.html

American Association of Colleges of Nursing. (2021). *The essentials: Core competencies for professional nursing education*. https://www.aacnnursing.org/Essentials

Baixinho, C., Dixe, M., Madeira, C., Alves, S., & Henriques, M. (2019). Falls in institutionalized elderly with and without cognitive decline: A study of some factors. *Dementia & Neuropsychologia, 13*(1), 116–121. https://doi.org/10.1590/1980-57642018dn13-010014

Boston University School of Public Health. (2022a). *The Health Belief Model*. https://sphweb.bumc.bu.edu/otlt/MPHModules/SB/BehavioralChangeTheories/BehavioralChangeTheories2.html

Boston University School of Public Health. (2022b). *The Transtheoretical Model (Stages of Change)*. https://sphweb.bumc.bu.edu/otlt/MPH-Modules/SB/BehavioralChangeTheories/BehavioralChangeTheories6.html

Cardoso, T., Martins, M., & Monteiro, M. (2017). Community care unit and elderly health promotion: An intervention program. *Revista de Enfermagem Referência, IV*, 103–114. https://doi.org/10.12707/RIV16071

Centers for Disease Control and Prevention. (n.d.). *Domains of learning.* https://www.cdc.gov/healthyschools/professional_development/videos/pd201/04-domains_of_learning.pdf

Centers for Disease Control and Prevention. (2018). *Adult learning theories.* https://www.cdc.gov/healthyschools/professional_development/e-learning/pd201/section_02.html

Centers for Disease Control and Prevention. (2022a). *Develop SMART objectives.* https://www.cdc.gov/publichealthgateway/phcommunities/resourcekit/evaluate/develop-smart-objectives.html

Centers for Disease Control and Prevention. (2022b). *What is health literacy?* https://www.cdc.gov/healthliteracy/learn/

Centers for Disease Control and Prevention. (2023b). *Advisory Committee on Immunization Practices (ACIP).* https://www.cdc.gov/vaccines/acip/index.html

Centers for Disease Control and Prevention. (2023a). *National Center for Chronic Disease Prevention and Health Promotion (NCCDPHP).* https://www.cdc.gov/chronicdisease/index.htm

Chung, S., Romanelli, R. J., Stults, C. D., & Luft, H. S. (2018). Preventive visit among older adults with Medicare's introduction of Annual Wellness Visit: Closing gaps in underutilization. *Preventive Medicine, 115*, 110–118. https://doi.org/10.1016/j.ypmed.2018.08.018

Department of Health and Human Services. (2022). *Preventive care.* March 17, 2022. https://www.hhs.gov/healthcare/about-the-aca/preventive-care/index.html

Drew, C. (2022). *SMART goals in education.* HelpfulProfessor.com. https://helpfulprofessor.com/smart-goals-in-education/

Drew, C. (2023). *Bloom's taxonomy.* HelpfulProfessor.com. https://helpfulprofessor.com/blooms-taxonomy-examples/

EducationPlanner.org. (n.d.). *What's your learning style?* http://www.educationplanner.org/students/self-assessments/learning-styles-styles.shtml

Farris, C. (2015). The teach back method. *Home Healthcare Now, 33*(6), 344–345. https://doi.org/10.1097/nhh.0000000000000244

Ferreira, R., Baixinho, C., Ferreira, Ó., Nunes, A., Mestre, T., & Sousa, L. (2022). Health promotion and disease prevention in the elderly: The perspective of nursing students. *Journal of Personalized Medicine, 12*(2), 1–14. https://doi.org/10.3390/jpm12020306

Gallaway, M. S., Aseret-Manygoats, T., & Tormala, W. (2022). Disparities of access, use, and barriers to seeking health care service in Arizona. *Medical Care, 60*(2), 113–118. https://doi.org/10.1097/mlr.0000000000001665

Gonzalo, A. (2024). *Dorthea Orem: Self-care deficit theory.* Nurseslabs, April 30, 2024. https://nurseslabs.com/dorothea-orems-self-care-theory/

Hoque, E. (2016). Three domains of learning: Cognitive, affective and psychomotor. *Journal of EFL Education and Research, 2*(2), 45–52

Huot, S., Hob, H., Kob, A., Lamb, S., Tactayb, P., MacLachlan, J., & Raanaas, R. (2019). Identifying barriers to healthcare delivery and access in the Circumpolar North: Important insights for health professional. *International Journal of Circumpolar Health, 78*(1), 1–8. https://doi.org/10.1080/22423982.2019.1571385

Ibrahim, N., & Qalawa, S. A. A. (2022). Perceived stress using Pender's Health Promotion Model among student nurses with chronic diseases during COVID-19 outbreak. *Journal of Positive School Psychology, 6*(6). https://journalppw.com/index.php/jpsp/article/view/9251

Ketabchi, B., Gittelman, M.A., Southworth, H., Arnold, M., Denny, S., & Pomeranz, W. (2021). Attitudes and perceived barriers to firearm safety anticipatory guidance by pediatricians:

A statewide perspective. *Injury Epidemiology*, 8(Suppl 1; 21), 1–7. https://doi.org/10.1186/s40621-021-00319-9

Khodaveisi, M., Omidi, A., Farokhi, S., & Soltanian, A. (2017). The effect of Pender's Health Promotion Model in improving the nutritional behavior of overweight and obese women. *International Journal of Community Based Nursing & Midwifery*, 5(2), 165–174. https://pubmed.ncbi.nlm.nih.gov/28409170/

Liu, C., Wang, D., Liu, C., Jiang, J., Wang, X., Chen, H., Ju, X., & Zhang, X. (2020). What is the meaning of health literacy? A systematic review and qualitative synthesis. *Family Medicine and Community Health*, 8(2), e000351. https://doi.org/10.1136/fmch-2020-000351

Mallillin, L. (2020). Different domains in learning and the academic performance of the students. *Journal of Educational System*, 4(1), 2020, 1–11. http://dx.doi.org/10.13140/RG.2.2.13320.16640

McEnroe-Petitte, D. (2020). Caring for patients who are homeless. *Nursing 2020*, 50(3), 24–30. https://doi.org/10.1097/01.nurse.0000654600.98061.61

McLean, S., Francis, M., Lacy, N., & Alvarado, A. (2019). Point-of-encounter assessment: Using Health Belief Model constructs to change grading behaviors. *Journal of Medical Education and Curricular Development*, 6, 2382120519840358. https://doi.org/10.1177/2382120519840358

Minnesota Department of Health. (2019). *Public health interventions: Application for nursing practice* (2nd ed.). https://www.health.state.mn.us/communities/practice/research/phncouncil/docs/PHInterventions.pdf

Nouri, S., Barnes, D., Volow, A., McMahan, R., Kushel, M., Jin, C., Boscardin, J., & Sudore, R. (2019). Health literacy matters more than an experience for advance care planning knowledge among older adults. *Journal of American Geriatric Society*, 67(10), 2151–2156. https://doi.org/10.1111/jgs.16129

Nursing-Theory.org. (2023b). *Dorothea E. Orem—nursing theorist.* https://nursing-theory.org/nursing-theorists/Dorothea-E-Orem.php

Nursing-Theory.org. (2023a). *Pender's Health Promotion Model.* https://nursing-theory.org/theories-and-models/pender-health-promotion-model.php

Nutbeam, D., McGill, B., & Premkumar, P. (2018). Improving health literacy in community populations: A review of progress. *Health Promotion International*, 33(5), 901–911. https://doi.org/10.1093/heapro/dax015

Office of Disease Prevention and Health Promotion. (n.d.a.). *Access to health services.* Healthy People 2030. https://health.gov/healthypeople/priority-areas/social-determinants-health/literature-summaries/access-health-services#cit11

Office of Disease Prevention and Health Promotion. (n.d.b.). *Health literacy in Healthy People 2030.* Healthy People 2030. https://health.gov/healthypeople/priority-areas/health-literacy-healthy-people-2030

Office of Disease Prevention and Health Promotion. (2021a). *Health literacy.* https://health.gov/our-work/national-health-initiatives/health-literacy

Office of Disease Prevention and Health Promotion. (2021b). *Health Literate Care Model.* https://health.gov/our-work/national-health-initiatives/health-literacy/health-literate-care-model

Office of Disease Prevention and Health Promotion. (2023). *What is MyHealthfinder?* https://health.gov/myhealthfinder

Perry, A. (2022). Primary prevention of obesity: Active interventions in school age populations. *Medical Research Archives*, 8(6), 1–9. https://esmed.org/MRA/mra/article/view/2152/193545601

Pronk, N., Kleinman, D., Goekler, S., Ochiai, E., Blakey, C., & Brewer, K. (2021). Promoting health and well-being in Healthy People 2030. *Journal of Public Health Management and Practice*, 27(6), S242–S248. https://doi.org/10.1097/phh.0000000000001254

Ross, A., Bevans, M., Brooks, A., Gibbons, S., & Wallen, G. (2017). Nurses and health-promoting behaviors: Knowledge may not translate into self-care. *AORN Journal, 105*(3), 267–275. https://doi.org/10.1016/j.aorn.2016.12.018

Rural Health Information Hub. (2023a). *Health promotion and disease prevention models.* https://www.ruralhealthinfo.org/toolkits/health-promotion/2/theories-and-models

Rural Health Information Hub. (2023b). *Stages of Change Model (Transtheoretical Model).* https://www.ruralhealthinfo.org/toolkits/health-promotion/2/theories-and-models/stages-of-change

Rural Health Information Hub. (2023c). *The Health Belief Model.* https://www.ruralhealthinfo.org/toolkits/health-promotion/2/theories-and-models/health-belief

Santana, S., Brach, C., Harris, L., Ochiai, E., Blakey, C., Bevington, F., Kleinman, D., & Pronk, N. (2021). Updating health literacy for Healthy People 2030: Defining its importance for a new decade of public health. *Journal of Public Health Management and Practice, 27*(Suppl 6), S258–S264. https://doi.org/10.1097/phh.0000000000001324

Schlenk, E., Fitzgerald, G. K., Rogers, J., Kwoh, C. K., & Sereika, S. (2021). Promoting physical activity in older adults with knee osteoarthritis and hypertension: A randomized controlled trial. *Journal of Aging and Physical Activity, 29*(2), 207–218. https://doi.org/10.1123/japa.2019-0498

Simmons, R. A., Cosgrove, S. C., Romney, M. C., Plumb, J. D., Brawer, R. O., Gonzalez, E. T., Fleisher, L. G., & Moore, B. S. (2017). Health literacy: Cancer prevention strategies for early adults. *American Journal of Preventive Medicine, 53*(3S1), S73–S77. https://doi.org/10.1016/j.amepre.2017.03.016

Study.com. (2023). *Pender's Health Promotion Model: Overview, theory & examples.* https://study.com/academy/lesson/what-is-the-health-promotion-model-definition-theory.html

United States Preventive Services Task Force. (n.d.a.). *Aspirin use to prevent cardiovascular disease: Preventive medication.* https://www.uspreventiveservicestaskforce.org/uspstf/recommendation/aspirin-to-prevent-cardiovascular-disease-preventive-medication

United States Preventive Services Task Force. (n.d.b.). *Home.* https://www.uspreventiveservicestaskforce.org/uspstf/

United States Preventive Services Task Force. (n.d.c.). *Reports to Congress.* https://www.uspreventiveservicestaskforce.org/uspstf/about-uspstf/reports-congress

USPSTF Info. (2018). *Overview of the U.S. Preventive Services Task Force.* YouTube, February 15, 2018. https://www.youtube.com/watch?v=DtWE2Ft7ACk

USPSTF Info. (2024). *Screening for breast cancer: USPSTF Final recommendation.* YouTube, April 30, 2024. https://www.youtube.com/watch?v=r6olpv75gnM

Vector Solutions. (2023a). *Teaching attitudes: The affective domain of learning and learning objectives.* https://www.vectorsolutions.com/resources/blogs/teaching-attitudes-the-affective-domain-of-learning-and-learning-objectives/

Vector Solutions. (2023b). *Teaching skills: The psychomotor domain of learning and learning objectives.* https://www.vectorsolutions.com/resources/blogs/teaching-skills-the-psychomotor-domain-of-learning-and-learning-objectives/

Visual, Aural, Reading, Kinesthetic. (2023a). *VARK modalities: What do visual, aural, read/write & kinesthetic really mean?* https://vark-learn.com/introduction-to-vark/the-vark-modalities/

Visual, Aural, Reading, Kinesthetic. (2023b). *The VARK questionnaire—How do you learn best?* https://vark-learn.com/the-vark-questionnaire/

Waronker, L. (2020). *Case study: Primary prevention of cardiovascular disease. Lippincott nursing center blog.* https://www.nursingcenter.com/ncblog/february-2020/case-study-primary-prevention-of-cardiovascular-di

White, A. (2022). *The use of SMART goals in nursing.* https://nursingcecentral.com/the-use-of-smart-goals-in-nursing/#:~:text=The%20acronym%20SMART%20refers%20to,%E2%80%93%20Relevant%3B%20T%20%E2%80%93%20Timely

WisLit. (2010). *AMA health literacy video—Short version.* YouTube, December 22, 2010. https://www.youtube.com/watch?v=BgTuD7l7LG8

Women's Preventive Services Initiative. (2022). *Home.* https://www.womenspreventivehealth.org

World Health Organization. (2023). *About us.* http://www.emro.who.int/about-who/public-health-functions/health-promotion-disease-prevention.html

Zajacova, A., & Lawrence, E. M. (2018). The relationship between education and health: Reducing disparities through a contextual approach. *Annual Review of Public Health, 39,* 273–289. https://doi.org/10.1146/annurev-publhealth-031816-044628

Credits

Fig. 4.1: Copyright © by Vanderbilt University Center for Teaching (CC BY 2.0) at https://commons.wikimedia.org/wiki/File:Bloom%27s_Revised_Taxonomy.jpg.

Fig. 4.2: Adapted from Vector Solutions, https://www.vectorsolutions.com/resources/blogs/teaching-attitudes-the-affective-domain-of-learning-and-learning-objectives/. Copyright © 2023 by Vector Solutions.

Fig. 4.3: Adapted from Vector Solutions, https://www.vectorsolutions.com/resources/blogs/teaching-skills-the-psychomotor-domain-of-learning-and-learning-objectives/. Copyright © 2023 by Vector Solutions.

Fig. 4.4: Boston University of Public Health, https://sphweb.bumc.bu.edu/otlt/MPH-Modules/SB/BehavioralChangeTheories/BehavioralChangeTheories6.html. Copyright © 2022 by Boston University School of Public Health.

Fig. 4.5: Nurselabs, https://nurseslabs.com/dorothea-orems-self-care-theory/. Copyright © 2023 by Nurseslabs.

Fig. 4.6: Office of Disease Prevention and Health Promotion, "Health Literature Care Model," https://health.gov/our-work/national-health-initiatives/health-literacy/health-literate-care-model, 2021.

Fig. 4.7: Adapted from Chris Drew, https://helpfulprofessor.com/smart-goals-in-education/. Copyright © 2022 by Helpful Professor.

CHAPTER 5

Healthcare Delivery

"Access to basic quality health care is one of the most important domestic issues facing our nation."

—Ed Pastor

Learning Outcomes

After reading this chapter, students should be able to:

1. Compare and contrast the U.S. healthcare delivery system with other global healthcare systems
2. Compare and contrast Medicare, Medicaid, Indian Health Service (IHS), and TRICARE
3. Distinguish between a health maintenance organization (HMO), a preferred provider organization (PPO), and third-party payers (TTPs)
4. Understand the details of the Patient Protection and Affordable Care Act (ACA)
5. Understand the gross domestic product (GDP) and its effect on healthcare delivery

Keywords and Concepts

Patient Protection and Affordable Care Act (ACA), gross domestic product (GDP), healthcare delivery (global and United States), health maintenance organization (HMO), Indian Health Service (IHS), Medicare, Medicaid, preferred provider organization (PPO), TRICARE

Definitions of the Keywords

ACA: An insurance program providing affordable health insurance for individuals with household incomes between 100% and 400% of the federal poverty level (HealthCare.gov, n.d.a.)

GDP: Value of goods and services produced through the national economy minus the overall value of goods and services used (U.S. Department of Commerce, n.d.)

Healthcare delivery (global and United States): Forms the most visible function of the health system, both to clients and the general public (European Observatory on Health Services and Policies, n.d.)

HMO: Type of insurance coverage emphasizing integrated care and prevention/wellness (HealthCare.gov, n.d.b.)

IHS: An agency within the Department of Health and Human Services (DHHS) responsible for providing healthcare services to American Indians and Alaska Natives (IHS, n.d.)

Medicare: Federal health insurance program for those older than age 65, certain young people with disabilities, and individuals with end-stage renal disease (ESRD; Medicare.gov, n.d.a.)

Medicaid: Public insurance program that provides health coverage to low-income families and individuals, funded jointly by federal and state monies (Center on Budget and Policy Priorities, 2020)

PPO: An insurance plan that covers individuals in a network of selected healthcare providers (Centers for Disease Control and Prevention [CDC], 2023)

TRICARE: An insurance healthcare program for military service members and family members (TRICARE, 2023)

Introduction

Everyone deserves effective healthcare services and resources for optimal health. High-quality healthcare that provides primary care services and a robust public health service are warranted. The need for global universal healthcare coverage that covers the entire continuum of essential health services at all three levels of prevention should be a staple for all (World Health Organization [WHO], n.d.).

Healthcare delivery issues affecting population health include barriers such as lack of access, improper management of chronic disease conditions, inadequate preventative services, and health disparities and inequality (Schwartz et al., 2022).

With the various forms of groups, networks, and independent practices, whether in the public or private sectors or for-profit or not-for-profit, healthcare delivery systems assist with communication and collaboration to provide the best for their participants (Office of Disease Prevention and Health Promotion [ODPHP], n.d.b.). Healthcare providers should look at patient-centered continuity of care while coordinating and communicating, meeting all cultural and ethical care resources and services for the population (ODPHP, n.d.a.). This chapter will address issues related to healthcare delivery through the presentation of various insurance and financial means to provide healthcare services and meet payment requirements. Additional discussion about the types of healthcare delivery and their relationship to the social determinants of health (SDOH), poverty, and access to care will be discussed.

Background of the Concepts

Approximately one in 10 individuals in the United States does not have health insurance (ODPHP, n.d.b.). With health insurance, populations could have higher primary care visits, assistance with preventive care and screenings, and decreased care for chronic illness conditions (Berchick et al., 2018). Optimal health could be in jeopardy without the ability to provide proper preventive methods.

Schwarz et al. (2022) researched barriers to adequate healthcare. Individuals with chronic conditions noted a lack of care coordination and ineffective patient-healthcare provider communications. Other barriers included being in a rural rather than urban setting, lack of holistic care, and obstacles with the healthcare delivery process. Clients' perceptions of inadequate healthcare included their socioeconomic status, low health literacy, and inability to pay for services as factors. Enhancing better care coordination by increasing access to care, availability, and capacity for health insurance could relieve these issues.

Healthcare Delivery

Healthcare delivery is the visible foundation of the health system. How a client flows through the health care process, services dealing with the diagnosis and treatment of disease, or the promotion, maintenance, and restoration of health are important aspects to consider. The primary healthcare delivery service areas include all factors, such as public health, acute care, specialties, primary care, urgent care, pharmaceutical care, dental care, and long-term care (European Observatory on Health Systems and Policies, n.d.).

Healthcare Delivery Global

Healthcare delivery worldwide is provided through many different avenues. The efficacy and efficiency of the delivery methods must also be more consistent.

Long-term investments in human resources, infrastructure, and primary care, such as in Israel, provide a more holistic approach (Thomas, 2023). Comparing healthcare characteristics and pros and cons will help illustrate the vast differences in global healthcare delivery (Table 5.1).

TABLE 5.1 Healthcare Delivery Around the Globe

Country/Nation/Region	Characteristics	Pros and Cons
United Kingdom	• National Health System (79% publicly financed from taxes and operated by the Department of Health) • About 20% is paid for by national insurance, and private clients and copayments make up the rest	• Pros: Universal healthcare/ free for all • Cons: Ethnic minorities and the poor face inequality in the healthcare system; social care measures are not implemented
European Union	• Include all citizens irrespective of paying capacity. • Funded mainly by taxes paid by the employer and by the public • Healthcare is free, except for some elective and specialist services	• Pros: Controls costs better; high approval from clients • Cons: Inequalities in health status and healthcare finance and delivery
Singapore	Three M's system: a public statutory insurance system, MediShield Life for large hospital bills, and some high-end outpatient treatments, but not primary or specialist care at the outpatient level	• Pros: A compulsory national health savings account called MediSave; MediFund is a social welfare program for poor citizens who cannot pay for out-of-pocket expenses even with MediSave • Cons: 30% out-of-pocket expenses
China	Almost universal publicly funded medical insurance, with urban employees enrolled in employment-based programs	• Pros: Ceiling on reimbursement • Cons: Wide inequalities in public health services
India	• Universal free outpatient and inpatient care at government clinics and hospitals • Newer system called the *National Health Protection Scheme* (Ayushman Bharat-Pradhan Mantri Jan Arogya Yojana) to help with staffing	• Pros: Grassroots health and wellness centers provide cashless hospital care for the 40% of people (approximately 100 million) who live below the poverty line • Cons: Government facilities are understaffed and ill-equipped, so most pay out of pocket for private healthcare

(*Continued*)

TABLE 5.1 *(Continued)*

Country/Nation/Region	Characteristics	Pros and Cons
Australia	• Tax-funded universal free public health insurance program called Medicare • All citizens receive free care, physician services, and drugs at public hospitals	• Pros: Jointly run by federal, state, and territorial governments • Cons: Research not well-aligned with national priorities
South America (Chili, Brazil, Colombia, Costa Rica, Argentina)	• Universal and publicly funded in countries such as Chile and Columbia • Progressed since only employees in the formal labor market received public health insurance, to which employers, employees, and the government contributed	• Pros: Overall, cheaper medical services • Cons: Capacity of the systems is low, and drug shortages are common
Africa	• Some countries (Ghana, Kenya, and Rwanda have some type of national health insurance • Most Africans are either low- or middle-income and turn to the public health system or traditional healers	• Pros: Universal healthcare is a right • Cons: Lack of money in several countries for healthcare spending; poor have no healthcare in most countries
Canada	Has 13 provincial and territorial healthcare insurance plans (no single plan); called *Medicare*	• Pros: The federal government provides healthcare funding to the provinces and territories • Cons: The provincial and territorial healthcare insurance plans consult with respective physician colleges or groups; together, they decide which services are medically necessary for healthcare insurance

Sources: Adapted from Government of Canada, 2023; Thomas, 2023.

Investments in information technology, research, and development are vital to making healthcare systems more accessible and improving health outcomes. Attention to the care of older adults, seen effectively in Japan, and mental well-being are prominent components in Australia and other areas that need to be addressed globally (Thomas, 2023).

With the many changes in healthcare systems and delivery, especially since the COVID-19 pandemic, several efforts have been incorporated to meet the barriers encountered. The worldwide focus is on the use of technology, both virtual and distance modalities. The use of technology in several countries has been met with positive responses, effective results, and approval from the population. The pandemic also allowed access to those who may not have been able to obtain healthcare before this time (Kelly et al., 2020).

Kelly et al. (2020) support using the Internet of Things (IoT), a wireless, interrelated, and connected digital device system that can collect, send, and store data without requiring human-to-human or human-to-computer interaction. The IoT assists in providing improved access and incorporating primary, secondary, and tertiary care. By doing so, healthcare can be seen as being more proactive, a continuous process, and more effectively coordinated. The IoT is an implementation that can be followed by many and will enable flexible healthcare delivery, providing care to many and relieving gaps within the current care provisions. The continued need for more innovative and effective healthcare delivery models will enhance the global community.

Healthcare Delivery United States

The U.S. healthcare delivery system is complex and chaotic. Unlike most other developed countries, the United States does not have universal health coverage. The U.S. healthcare system combines privately and publicly funded programs (Thomas, 2023). Most hospitals and clinics are privately owned, with about 60% nonprofit and another fifth for-profit. Coverage by federal and state programs is partial, and most insured Americans have employment-based private insurance (Thomas, 2023). About one-third of the United States is covered by three publicly funded programs: Medicare, Medicaid, and the Children's Health Insurance Programs (CHIP; Thomas, 2023).

There are many issues with the U.S. healthcare system. Extensive use of procedures such as hip replacements and specialized tests such as computed tomography and magnetic resonance imaging has increased costs (Thomas, 2023). Equity in healthcare delivery is an issue in terms of access and efficiency. Preventing diseases is not a focus; chronic diseases have increased due to the lack of extensive primary care services (Thomas, 2023).

The American College of Physicians (ACP) has remained a voice for high-quality healthcare in the United States and advocates for universal health coverage. The ACP recommends more patient-centered, equitable, technology-driven, and affordable healthcare delivery methods (Erickson et al., 2020). The ACP wants improved client outcomes and additional areas addressing healthcare inequalities, especially those associated with the SDOH.

> The American College of Physicians envisions a health care system where payment and delivery systems put the interests of patients first, by supporting physicians and their care teams in delivering high-value and patient centered care.
>
> The American College of Physicians envisions a health care system where primary care is supported with a greater investment of resources; where payment levels between complex cognitive care and procedural care are equitable; and where payment systems

support the value that internal medicine specialists offer to patients in the diagnosis, treatment, and management of team-based care, from preventive health to complex illness.

The American College of Physicians envisions a health care system where financial incentives are aligned to achieve better patient outcomes, lower costs, and reduce inequities in health care.

The American College of Physicians envisions a health care system where patients and physicians are freed of inefficient administrative and billing tasks, documentation requirements are simplified, payments and charges are more transparent and predictable, and delivery systems are redesigned to make it easier for patients to navigate and receive needed care conveniently and effectively.

The American College of Physicians envisions a health care system where value-based payment programs incentivize collaboration among clinical care team-based members and use only appropriately attributed, evidence-based, and patient-centered measures.

The American College of Physicians envisions a health care system where health information technologies enhance the patient-physician relationships, facilitate communication across the care continuum, and support improvements in patient care.

Source: Shari M. Erickson et al., Selection from "Envisioning a Better U.S. Health Care System for All: Health Care Delivery and Payment System Reforms," *Annals of Internal Medicine*, vol. 172, no. 2 Supplement.

Anderlini (2018) notes the negative perceptions of U.S. healthcare. The high healthcare costs imply negative impacts on the total population. Many issues need to be approached by placing influential multidisciplinary leaders in roles related to medical education, research, funding development, planning, and publications to disseminate valuable information (Boxes 5.1 and 5.2).

BOX 5.1 ACTIVE LEARNING REFLECTION ACTIVITY

What Is Health Insurance?

Watch the following video and reflect on the questions asked: https://www.youtube.com/watch?v=dF3Dcol5XLgo.asp.

1. What two items that you learned from the video are still valid today?
2. Why did universal healthcare, proposed by President Harry Truman, not become the norm?
3. What is the difference between the concept of in-network and out-of-network?
4. What is the concept of a deductible, and why is this done?
5. What is the concept of a copay, and what does that mean to you?

American Association of Colleges of Nursing (AACN) *Essentials* (2021): Domains: #1; #2; #3; #7; #9

- Competencies: 1.2; 2.1; 2.3; 2.4; 2.8; 2.9; 3.2; 3.3; 7.1; 7.2; 9.1; 9.3
- Subcompetencies: 1.2c; 2.1c; 2.3f; 2.4b; 2.8e; 2.9a; 2.9b; 3.2a; 3.3a; 7.1c; 7.2a; 7.2b; 7.2c; 7.2d; 7.2e; 9.1a; 9.1g; 9.3g

Spheres of Care: Wellness/Disease prevention; Chronic disease management

Concepts: Diversity, Equity, and Inclusion (DEI); Health policy; SDOH; Clinical judgment

Source: Healthcare Triage, 2013.

BOX 5.2 ACTIVE LEARNING REFLECTION ACTIVITY

How Good Is the U.S. Healthcare System?

Watch the following video about the state of the U.S. healthcare system: https://www.healthsystemtracker.org/health-of-the-healthcare-system/.

There are four areas addressed in this video. Reflect by answering the following questions:

1. Name one area noted in the health portion of the video.
2. Name one area noted in the quality portion of the video.
3. Name one area noted in the cost portion of the video.
4. Name one area noted in the access portion of the video.
5. Reflect on two conclusions from the video that are priorities for the U.S. healthcare system.

AACN *Essentials* (2021): Domains: #1; #2; #3; #7; #8

- Competencies: 1.2; 2.1; 2.3; 2.4; 2.8; 2.9; 3.2; 3.3; 7.1; 7.2; 8.1
- Subcompetencies: 1.2c; 2.1c; 2.3f; 2.4b; 2,8e; 2.9a; 2.9b; 3.2a; 3.3a; 3.3b; 7.1c; 7.2a; 7.2b; 7.2c; 7.2d; 7.2e; 8.1b

Spheres of Care: Wellness/Disease prevention; Chronic disease management

Concepts: DEI; Health policy; SDOH

Source: Cox et al., 2015.

Comparison of the U.S. Healthcare System and Global

Comparing the U.S. healthcare system with those of other countries brings even a more chaotic viewpoint and the need to solve certain issues. Matthews-Trigg et al. (2019) identified five areas: communication and client interactions with those in low-income countries, refugees, and immigrants; reducing healthcare expenses; understanding the SDOH; comprehending the U.S. healthcare system and its interaction with other countries; and identifying the motivation of healthcare workers toward global healthcare. They summarized that engaging international healthcare providers with those from the United States will be most valuable for all populations, especially the United States. Positive and improved patient care can be provided using these five concepts. Providers can reformulate successful programs and policies by examining the SDOH and other challenges healthcare policies present. The researchers were able to signify that the obtained global health work will help understand the strengths and weaknesses of the U.S. healthcare system. Therefore, by evaluating the international healthcare experiences practiced in the United States, healthcare providers will be better positioned to reevaluate their current practices (Matthews-Trigg et al., 2019).

One of the best ways to identify the healthcare status of a country is by comparing infant mortality rates. The Organisation for Economic Co-operation and Development (OECD) consists of 38 democracies around the world involved in market-based economies. Examples of other countries that belong to the OECD are Canada, the United Kingdom, Australia, and Germany (United Health Foundation [UHF], 2022). The United States ranks 33 out of 38 OECD countries, with a slight improvement over the past 50 years, but still falls short of other countries (UHF, 2022).

Another prominent issue is life expectancy at birth. The United States ranks 31 out of 47, with the average rate at 77 years. However, the average life expectancy for the OECD is 80.5 years (UHF, 2022). During the COVID-19 pandemic, life expectancy dropped for all OECD countries, with many delaying care and increasing mental health issues (UHF, 2022).

Healthcare spending also differs between the United States and other OECD countries. The average total expenditure on health in OECD countries was $6,414 U.S. dollars (USD) per capita in 2022. The United States spent nearly three times that amount, totaling $12,555 USD per capita (OECD, 2022; Peter G. Peterson Foundation [PGPF], 2023b; Figure 5.1).

Even with more spending, U.S. healthcare outcomes are far worse than other developed countries. The problems with life expectancy and infant mortality rates were already discussed, but other issues, such as unmanaged diabetes, safety during childbirth, heart attack mortality, and unmanaged asthma, rank lower than other OECD countries (OECD, 2022; PGPF, 2024).

U.S. healthcare spending per capita is almost twice the average of other wealthy countries
Healthcare Costs per Capita ($)
United State
$12,742
Switzerland
$9,044
Germany
$8,541
Netherlands
$7,277
Sweden
$7,009
Belgium
$6,994
France
$6,924
Average
$6,850
Canada
$6,845
Australia
$6,807
Ireland
$6,730
United Kingdom
$5,867
Japan
$5,424
Italy
$4,736

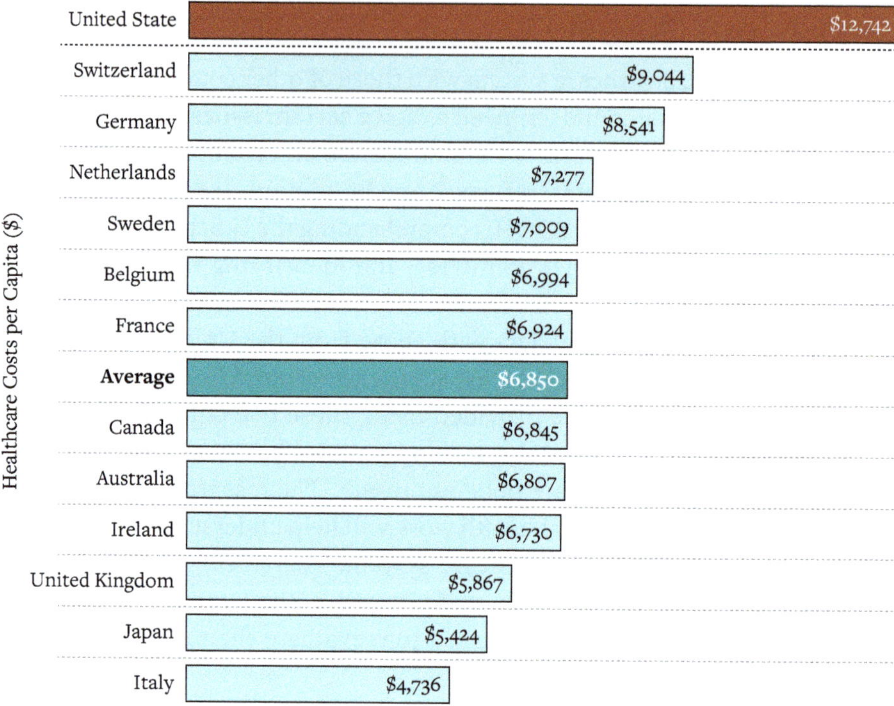

FIGURE 5.1 U.S. Healthcare Spending Versus Other Countries

Types of Care in the United States

The United States has both public and private healthcare options. In 1965, President Lyndon Johnson signed legislation that introduced Medicare and Medicaid. The change included health insurance for the older population, physicians' insurance for older adults (Medicare), and federal expansion assistance to states to assist people experiencing poverty (Medicaid; U.S. Senate, n.d.). Private health insurance entails mostly employer-sponsored plans, covering nearly half of the United States (Healthinsurance.org, n.d.).

Medicare

Medicare consists of two choices: traditional and advantage. Traditional Medicare consists of Part A, hospital insurance, and Part B, medical insurance. Medicare Advantage Plans (MAPs) are Part C, an alternative to original Medicare but Medicare-approved plans from a private company (Medicare.gov, n.d.c.). Individuals are eligible for Medicare based on specific criteria (Table 5.2).

TABLE 5.2 Medicare Criteria

- People ages 65 and older
- People younger than age 65 with specific disabilities (e.g., amyotrophic lateral sclerosis)
- People of all ages with ESRD (permanent kidney failure requiring dialysis or a kidney transplant)

Source: Medicare.gov, n.d.f.

Medicare Part A helps cover hospital inpatient care, including critical access to hospitals and skilled nursing facilities (not custodial or long-term care). It also helps cover hospice care and some home healthcare. Beneficiaries must meet certain conditions to receive these benefits. Most people don't pay a premium for Part A because they or a spouse already paid it through their payroll taxes while working (Medicare.gov, n.d.f.).

Medicare Part B helps cover doctors' services and outpatient care. It also covers other medical services that Part A doesn't, such as physical and occupational therapy services and home healthcare. Part B helps pay for these covered services and supplies when they are medically necessary (Medicare.gov, n.d.f.). Most people pay a monthly premium for Part B. The premium cost for 2025 was about $185 per month (Medicare.gov, n.d.a.).

If you have Parts A and B, you can join an MAP or Medicare Part C. This type of Medicare health plan is offered by Medicare-approved private companies that must follow the rules set by Medicare. Most MAPs include drug coverage (Part D; Medicare.gov, n.d.d.).

Medicare Part D consists of prescription drug coverage and is available to everyone with Medicare. To get Medicare prescription drug coverage, people must join a plan approved by Medicare that offers Medicare drug coverage. Most people pay a monthly premium for Part D. The premium cost is based on your income and tax filing status (Medicare.gov, n.d.b.; Figure 5.2).

Medicaid

Medicaid is a federal and state healthcare program mainly associated with impoverished individuals and families. Currently, this program covers about 87 million U.S. citizens, primarily disabled persons, pregnant women, low-income elderly adults, low-income households with children, and those in nursing homes who qualify based on low income, making it the primary payer for long-term care. Unfortunately, Medicaid represents the fastest-growing component of the states' budgets (Medicaid.gov, n.d.b.).

Each state has different criteria and rules for Medicaid coverage, unlike the federal Medicare program, which is the same in every state. One example is Florida's Medicaid criteria (Benefits.gov, n.d.; Table 5.3).

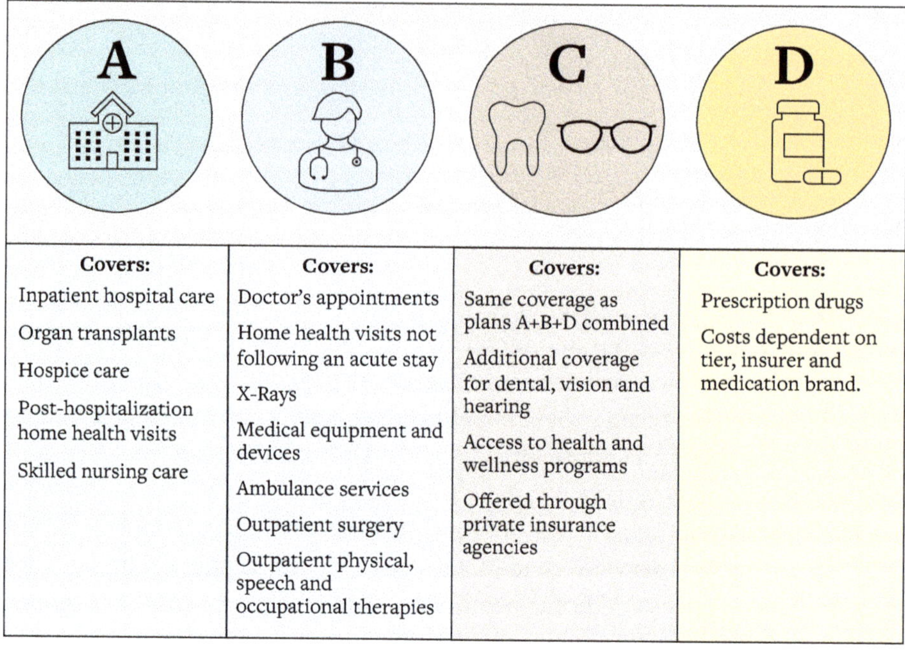

FIGURE 5.2 Parts of Medicare

TABLE 5.3 Example of Florida Medicaid Criteria

- Resident of the state of Florida
- U.S. national, citizen, permanent resident, or legal alien needing healthcare/insurance assistance, whose financial situation is low or exceptionally low
- Must also be one of the following:
  - Pregnant
  - Be responsible for a child age 18 or younger
  - Blind
  - Have a disability or a family member in your household with a disability
  - Be age 65 or older
- Also, income is a factor; for example, a family of four must have a combined income of less than $39,900

Source: Benefits.gov, n.d.

Children's Health Insurance Program (CHIP)

CHIP is another state and federal program that provides healthcare to eligible children. CHIP was signed into law in 1997 and provides federal matching funds to states to provide health coverage to children in families with incomes too high to qualify for Medicaid but who can't afford private coverage. All states have expanded children's coverage significantly through their CHIPs (Medicaid.gov, n.d.b.; Figure 5.3).

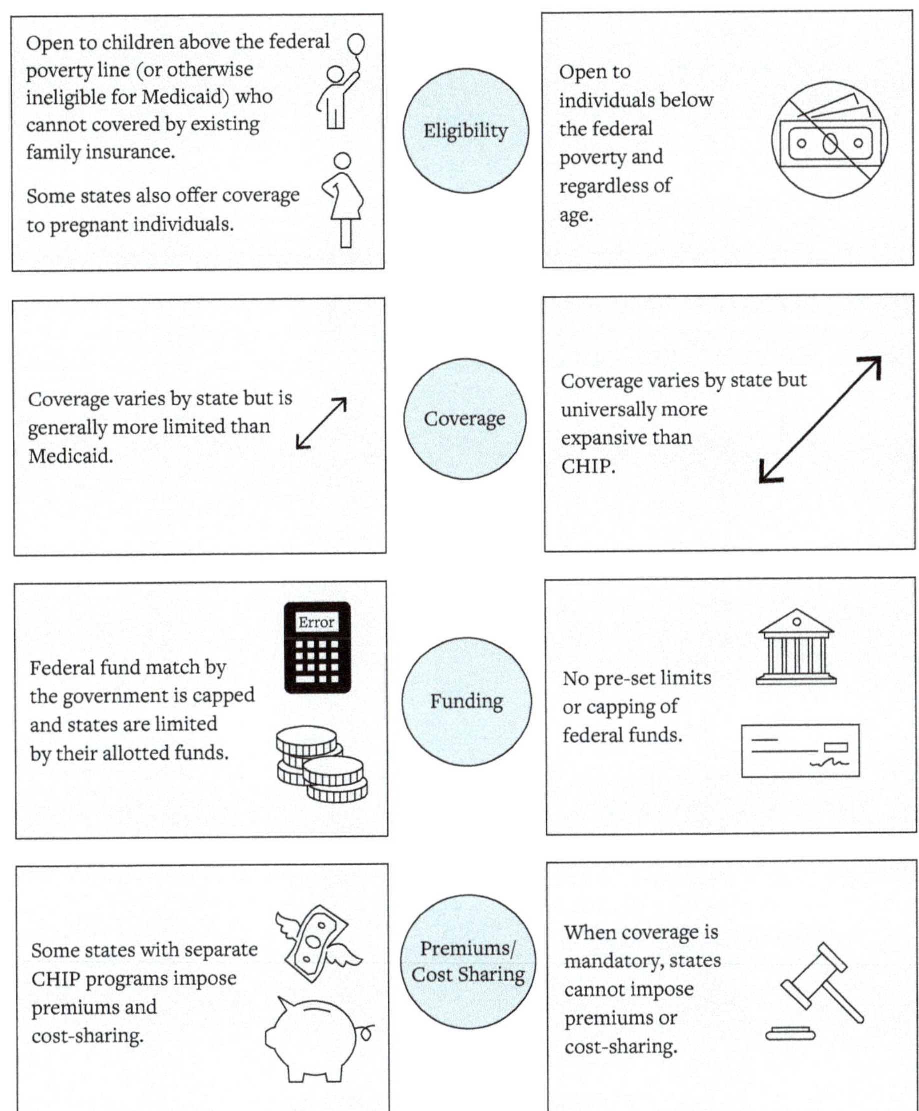

FIGURE 5.3 CHIP Versus Medicaid

TRICARE

TRICARE is a healthcare program for uniformed service members, retirees, and their families worldwide. TRICARE provides comprehensive coverage to all beneficiaries, including health plans, prescriptions, and dental plans. The Defense Health Agency manages it under the leadership of the assistant secretary of defense (Health Affairs; TRICARE, 2023; Figure 5.4).

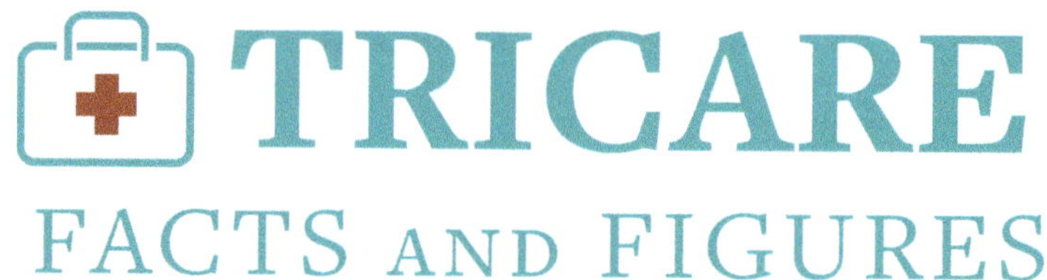

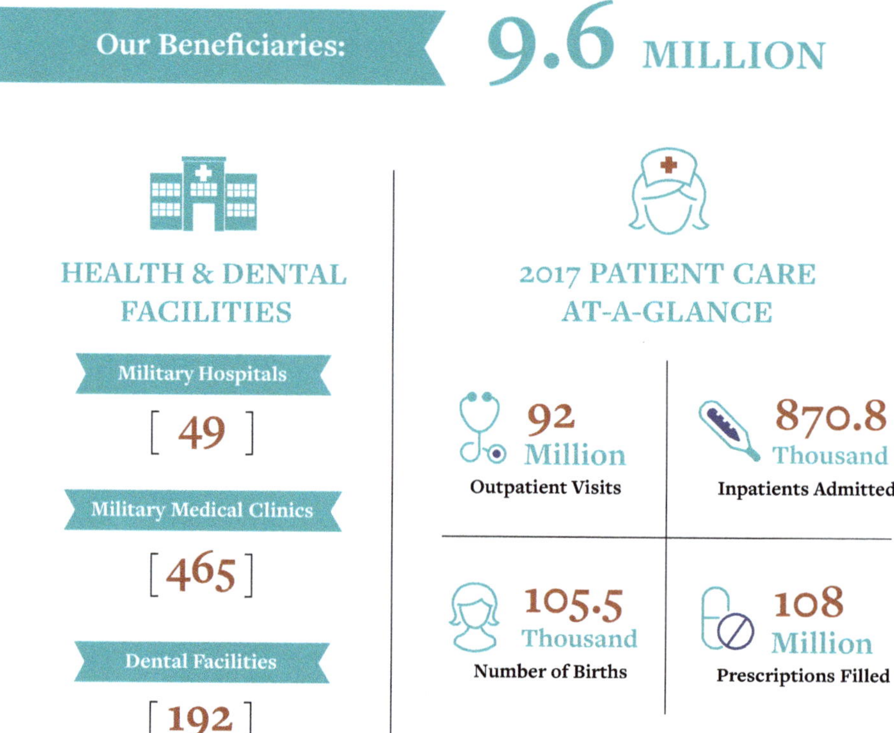

FIGURE 5.4 Facts and Numbers Related to TRICARE

Indian Health Service

The IHS, an agency within DHHS, provides federal health services to American Indians and Alaska Natives. Established in 1787 and based on articles in the Constitution, IHS provides a comprehensive health service delivery system for approximately 2.6 million American Indians and Alaska Natives who belong to 574 federally recognized tribes in 37 states (IHS, n.d.).

Factors That Affect the U.S. Healthcare Delivery System

The United States spends much more money per person on healthcare costs than other countries. Challenges such as limited appointment abilities, decreased primary care options, restricted hours of operation, transportation barriers, lack of education about the different care sites, and SDOH factors affect access and health outcomes (Heath, 2022).

Gross Domestic Product

With a substantially expensive healthcare system comes the need to spend more to pay for the expenses. The GDP is the annual value of a nation's final goods and services (Fernando, 2023). In the United States, a large percentage of the GDP is used for healthcare expenditures (Figure 5.5). With the increased GDP spending toward healthcare, fewer people could likely be covered.

SDOH and Healthcare Delivery

Healthcare delivery and its relationship to SDOH primarily focus on the met and unmet needs of others. Gurewich et al. (2020) worked on the conceptual framework for developing the Outcomes from Addressing SDOH in Systems (OASIS) to work on presenting positive outcomes for populations. Through this system, those involved in the political arena, healthcare administration, clinicians, and researchers can work together to identify concerns and appropriate interventions to achieve the best methods to assist populations in various ways by looking at ways to provide health equity to meet the unmet interventions that affect health and its outcomes. Gurewich et al. (2020) incorporated Maslow's hierarchy of needs as specific concepts to base the framework on and specifically included the areas

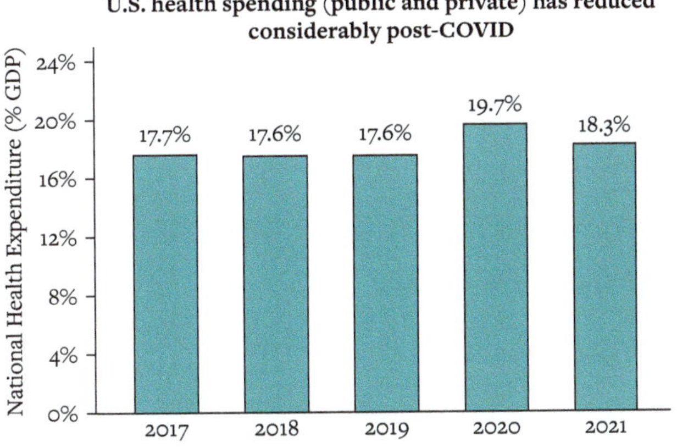

FIGURE 5.5 U.S. Health Spending (GDP Percentage)

of basic physiological needs. By using OASIS, a systematic approach is followed to identify relationships with unmet needs and develop a more unified method to meet the unmet social needs of individuals. This method of evidence-based research can simplify the processes of providing adequate healthcare (Gurewich et al., 2020).

Poverty and Healthcare Delivery

DHHS publishes updated federal poverty guidelines annually. These guidelines are used to determine:

- Eligibility for Medicaid and CHIP
- Eligibility for ACA premium tax credits and cost-sharing reductions (subsidies)
- Eligibility for Medicare Savings Programs and the Low-Income Subsidy for Medicare Part D (Healthinsurance.org, 2022; Box 5.3)

BOX 5.3 ACTIVE LEARNING REFLECTION ACTIVITY

CDC Policies: Food Assistance Programs for Older Adults

Go to the following website: https://www.usa.gov/food-help.

Scroll down and open the "Food Assistance Programs for Older Adults" section. Open the section titled "Federal Poverty Income Guidelines." Review the information related to the poverty guidelines specific to the state in which you live.

(https://aspe.hhs.gov/topics/poverty-economic-mobility/poverty-guidelines).

1. An elderly individual whom you care for needs financial and food security. How can you assist them in learning about governmental processes for applying for assistance? Name two ways you can help them.
2. Name two local resources to assist with food insecurity. Detail how they could gain access and what requirements are needed.

AACN *Essentials* (2021): Domains: #2; #3; #6; #7; #8; #9

- Competencies: 2.1; 2.2; 2.4; 2.8; 2.9; 3.1; 3.2; 3.3; 3.5; 6.3; 6.4; 7.2; 8.4; 9.1; 9.2; 9.3; 9.6
- Subcompetencies: 2.1a; 2.1b; 2.2d; 2.4d; 2.8c; 2.8e; 2.9a; 3.1c; 3.1e; 3.2b; 3.3b; 3.5c; 3.5d; 6.3c; 6.4d; 7.2a; 7.2b; 7.2c; 7,2e; 8.4b; 9.1c; 9.2b; 9.2g; 9.3g; 9.6a

Spheres of Care: Wellness/Disease prevention; Chronic disease management

Concepts: Compassionate care; SDOH; DEI

Source: Assistant Secretary for Planning and Evaluation, 2023; USA.gov, n.d.

Primary prevention is less costly than delivering secondary or tertiary interventions. Unfortunately, the current fee-for-service healthcare delivery model has led to the mitigation of poor health outcomes due to poverty (Jones, 2022). How can individuals and communities afford the healthcare needed to prevent chronic diseases?

Poverty is the fourth leading cause of death in the United States (Managed Healthcare Executive [MHE], 2023). In 2019, roughly 183,000 deaths were associated with poverty in the United States among people ages 15 and older (MHE, 2023). People with an income less than 50% of the U.S. median income have roughly the same survival rates until after age 40. The death rate is significantly higher than that of individuals with more adequate incomes and resources (MHE, 2023).

Access to Care and Healthcare Delivery

Medicaid and CHIP provide critical health coverage for millions of people. Through these programs, the Centers for Medicare & Medicaid Services (CMS) supports access to care in many ways. Most importantly, people gain access to healthcare services that may not be affordable without Medicaid or CHIP. Additionally, some programs and benefits include special protections—such as provider networks and payment methods—that help ensure accessible services (Medicaid.gov, n.d.a.).

Preventive care and other services help people stay healthy and avoid more costly care. CMS offers materials, toolkits, and other resources for states to administer Medicaid and CHIP beneficiaries to learn about these services and how to access them. CMS also supports many efforts to measure access, share the results, and promote progress (Medicaid.gov, n.d.a.).

The WHO believes in universal healthcare. This means that people can access the full range of quality health services they need, when and where they need them, without financial hardship (WHO, 2023). Health inequalities and disparities will continue unless all individuals and communities have fair and equitable healthcare and resources.

Different Aspects of the Healthcare System

The U.S. healthcare system is complex and chaotic. Many lay individuals need help navigating the different avenues of getting and receiving affordable and effective healthcare access and delivery. Following are some aspects and terms noted within the U.S. healthcare system.

Patient Protection and Affordable Care Act

The ACA was developed in 2010 to include comprehensive healthcare insurance available to individuals, families, businesses, other insurers, tax-exempt organizations, and governmental entities. Specifically, tax provisions indicate how individuals and families will file their taxes. DHHS had three primary goals for ACA provisions, as noted in Table 5.4 (2022).

The ACA provided several changes to reduce racial and ethnic health disparity issues. It allowed lower-income individuals to afford healthcare and improved access to care. However, further expansion of Medicaid is needed to positively affect health disparities (Buchmueller et al., 2016; Table 5.5; Box 5.4).

TABLE 5.4 Primary Goals of the ACA

- Make affordable health insurance available to more people.; the law provides consumers with subsidies (premium tax credits) that lower costs for households with incomes between 100% and 400% of the federal poverty level (FPL)
- Expand the Medicaid Program to cover all adults with income below 138% of the FPL; not all states have expanded their Medicaid programs
- Support innovative medical care delivery methods designed to lower healthcare costs generally.

Source: DHHS, 2022.

BOX 5.4 ACTIVE LEARNING REFLECTION ACTIVITY

What Is So Special About the ACA?

Watch the following YouTube video and review the following website:

DHHS: 5 things about the Affordable Care Act (ACA): https://www.youtube.com/watch?v=j9tRVESzJ1M&t=39s

DHHS: Preventive care: https://www.hhs.gov/healthcare/about-the-aca/preventive-care/index.html

1. In what three ways have the ACA made the most impact and why? Provide a rationale for your answer.
2. How would you briefly explain three ways the ACA has affected those with chronic diseases?
3. How would you briefly explain two ways the ACA has affected cancer care?
4. Research the amount by which the ACA has reduced the number of uninsured individuals in the United States since 2010.

AACN *Essentials* (2021): Domains: #2; #3; #7

- Competencies: 2.1; 2.9; 3.3; 7.2
- Subcompetencies: 2.1a; 2.1b; 2.9a; 3.3a; 3.3b; 7.2a; 7,2b; 7.2c; 7.2e

Spheres of Care: Wellness/Disease prevention; Chronic disease care; Regenerative/restorative care; Hospice/palliative/supportive care

Concepts: Communication; Compassionate care; DEI; Evidence-based practice; Health policy; SDOH

Sources: DHHS, n.d.; 2021.

TABLE 5.5 What Changed With the ACA

- Insurers cannot all charge, limit, or deny coverage in the area of a preexisting condition.
- Young adult coverage occurs under a parental plan until age 26. After age 26, an individual can enroll through an open enrollment plan.
- There are no limits for yearly or lifetime coverage.
- Preventative care is commonly obtained at no cost to the individual and includes checking blood pressure, diabetes, and cholesterol tests; cancer screenings, including mammograms and colonoscopies; counseling on various topics; well-baby and well-child visits and immunizations.
- Insurance companies can no longer cancel your coverage just because you or your employer made a mistake on your insurance application.
- Medicaid was expanded.
- Limitations were placed on out-of-pocket expenses.
- Women can no longer be charged more for insurance and are guaranteed coverage for services essential to women's health.

Source: DHHS, 2022.

Third-Party Payers

TPPs developed with the introduction of the ACA. To save money, TPPs are paid for by the enrolled insurees. As these are either public or private groups, the client pays a premium, and then the organization pays the medical costs on the client's behalf. Gosalia (2019) researched the use of hearing aids and the increased demand for coverage. Various insurance companies covered full or partial costs, but the large number of individuals filing for claims became costly. TPPs became the popular choice for clients at this time as the price was lower, along with coverage for the expenses of follow-up care (Gosalia, 2019).

The U.S. Department of Veterans Affairs (VA) uses TPPs to pay for healthcare. TPPs must pay the VA bills charged, and federal regulations regulate them. The VA has set guidelines for reasonable charges that individual VA medical facilities adjust based on geographical area adjustment factors. These changes relate to inpatient, outpatient, skilled nursing facilities, physicians, and nonphysician providers. Prescription drug plans are also available (VA, 2023).

Preferred Provider Organization

PPOs are plans in which healthcare providers in a network offer care to members. These plans are popular and permit in-network or out-of-network providers, specialists, and hospital facilities to be used. There is no need for referrals or a set primary care provider (PCP). The cost for a PPO plan includes higher out-of-pocket costs, copays, and an annual deductible to be met. PPO plans may hinder individuals using medical care as PPOs, which do not require a client to have a PCP, in considering whether care is necessary, leading to reduced costs. PPO plans include flexibility as specialists can be chosen per client whether the provider is not in the network (Humana, 2022; Medical Mutual, 2023).

Health Maintenance Organization

An HMO is a health insurance plan with limited coverage provided to healthcare professionals with contracts with the HMO. In-network providers are covered, while out-of-network providers, only cover an emergency, out-of-area urgent care, or a temporary out-of-area dialysis facility. Some HMOs may have point-of-service plans, covering some out-of-network services at a higher premium (HealthCare.gov, n.d.c.; MetLife, 2023).

Prevention and wellness are the focus and may require the individual to live in a specific location for their coverage. For HMOs, the individual will need a PCP who is in the network. This will allow for coordinating medical plans, treatments, and other services and specifying referrals as needed and can help lower costs (MetLife, 2023).

No Surprises Act

Effective January 1, 2022, the No Surprises Act, which Congress passed as part of the Consolidated Appropriations Act of 2021, was designed to protect clients from surprise bills for emergency services at out-of-network facilities or for out-of-network providers at in-network facilities, holding them liable only for in-network cost-sharing amounts. The No Surprises Act also enables uninsured clients to receive a reasonable-faith estimate of the cost of care (CMS, 2023).

Chapter Highlights

- Understanding the differences between Medicare, Medicaid, TRICARE, IHS, PPOs, HMOs, and TPPs
- Comparing healthcare delivery around the globe
- Active learning reflection activity on ACA
- Active learning reflection activity on healthcare delivery
- Active learning reflection activity on health insurance
- Active learning reflection activity related to the Intervention Wheel
- Case studies related to homelessness and healthcare delivery, understanding Medicare, and comparing the Canadian and U.S. healthcare delivery systems

Active Learning Exercises

Intervention Wheel Active Learning Strategy (Addressing Application of the Intervention Wheel)

Use the Minnesota Department of Health's *Public health interventions: Applications for public health nursing practice* (2nd ed.; "The Wheel Manual") to complete the following application. Please use the Outreach intervention to assist with the assignment.

How could you use the Intervention Wheel to provide a U.S. target population of lower-income and lower health literacy improvement in healthcare access and quality at the community, systems, and individual levels?

AACN *Essentials* (2021): Domains: #1; #2; #3; #5; #6; #7; #8; #9

- Competencies: 1.2; 2.1; 2.2; 2.3; 2.8; 2.9; 3.1; 3.2; 3.3; 5.1; 6.4; 7.1; 7.2; 8.2; 9.2; 9.3; 9.4; 9.5; 9.6
- Subcompetencies: 1.2c; 1.2e; 2.1a; 2.1b; 2.1c; 2.2b; 2.2d; 2.2e; 2.3c; 2.8a; 2.8b; 2.8c; 2.8d; 2.8e; 2.9a; 3.1a; 3.1b; 3.1c; 3.1e; 3.1i; 3.2a; 3.3b; 5.1c; 6.4d; 7.1c; 7.2a; 7.2b; 7.2c; 7.2e; 8.2d; 9.2d; 9.3g; 9.4a; 9.5c; 9.6a

Spheres of Care: Wellness/Disease prevention; Chronic disease management

Concepts: DEI; Ethics; Evidence-based practice; Health policy; SDOH

Source: Minnesota Department of Health, 2019.

Case Studies

Case Study #1: Homelessness and Healthcare Delivery

Go to https://www.ihi.org/resources/Pages/CaseStudies/default.aspx. Review the case study titled *A Downward Spiral: A Case Study in Homelessness*. Answer the discussion questions at the end of the scenario.

AACN *Essentials* (2021): Domains: #1; #2; #3; #6; #7; #8; #9

- Competencies: 1.2; 2.1; 2.2; 2.3; 2.8; 2.9; 3.1; 3.2; 3.3; 6.4; 7.1; 7.2; 8.2; 9.2; 9.3; 9.4; 9.5; 9.6
- Subcompetencies: 1.2c; 1.2e; 2.1a; 2.1b; 2.1c; 2.2b; 2.2d; 2.2e; 2.3c; 2.8a; 2.8b; 2.8c; 2.8d; 2.8e; 2.9a; 3.1a; 3.1b; 3.1c; 3.1e; 3.1i; 3.2a; 3.3b; 6.4d; 7.1c; 7.2a; 7.2b; 7.2c; 7.2e; 8.2d; 9.2d; 9.3g; 9.4a; 9.5c; 9.6a

Spheres of Care: Wellness/Disease prevention; Chronic disease management

Concepts: Compassionate care; DEI; Ethics; Evidence-based practice; Health policy; SDOH

Source: Institute for Healthcare Improvement, 2023.

Case Study #2: Understanding Medicare

A retired client receives Medicare benefits Parts A and B. Use the following website to help you answer the following questions: https://www.medicare.org/what-is-medicare-parts-a-and-b/.

1. Develop a PowerPoint presentation identifying these benefits.
2. Determine whether these benefits meet your client's needs.
3. Present to the client about additional MAPs and Medicare Part D benefits.
4. Estimate the potential costs for at least two MAPs, indicating which one you would advise the client to enroll in.

AACN *Essentials* (2021): Domains: #2; #3; #7; #9

- Competencies: 2.1; 2.3; 2.8; 2.9; 3.1; 3.3; 3.5; 7.1; 7.2; 9.3; 9.4
- Subcompetencies: 2.1c; 2.3a; 2.3f; 2.8a; 2.8c; 2.8d; 2.8e; 2.9a; 2.9b; 3.1a; 3.1c; 3.1d; 3.1e; 3.3a; 3.3b; 3.5d; 7.1c; 7.1d; 7.2a; 7.2b; 7.2c; 7.2d; 9.3a; 9.3g; 9.4a

Spheres of Care: Wellness/Disease prevention; Chronic disease care; Regenerative/restorative care

Concepts: Compassionate care; DEI; Evidence-based practice; Health policy; SDOH

Source: Medicare.org, 2023.

Case Study #3: Compare U.S. and Canadian Healthcare Systems

Use the following website to help you answer the following questions: https://www.pbs.org/newshour/health/how-canada-got-universal-health-care-and-what-the-u-s-could-learn.

The United States and Canada share a border but have different healthcare systems. Compare the following items between the United States and Canada and answer the questions proposed:

1. How does healthcare funding differ in the two countries?
2. What are two advantages and two disadvantages of these other approaches to funding healthcare delivery?
3. What effects do they have on the populations' health status?
4. What effects, if any, would they have on the role of the population health nurse?

AACN *Essentials* (2021): Domains: #2; #3; #7; #9

- Competencies: 2.1; 2.3; 2.8; 2.9; 3.1; 3.3; 3.4; 3.5; 7.1; 7.2; 9.3; 9.4
- Subcompetencies: 2.1c; 2.3a; 2.3f; 2.8a; 2.8c; 2.8d; 2.8e; 2.9a; 2.9b; 3.1a; 3.1c; 3.1d; 3.1e; 3.3a; 3.3b; 3.4e; 3.5d; 7.1c; 7.1d; 7.2a; 7.2b; 7.2c; 7.2d; 9.3a; 9.3g; 9.4a

Spheres of Care: Wellness/Disease prevention; Chronic disease care; Regenerative/restorative care

Concepts: Compassionate care; DEI; Evidence-based practice; Health policy; SDOH

Source: Public Broadcasting System, 2020.

NCLEX Questions

1. Medicare Parts A and B include which of the following benefits? **Select all that apply.**
   a. Inpatient hospital costs
   b. Vision costs
   c. Dental costs
   d. Medication costs
   e. Skilled nursing home costs
   f. Hospice care
   g. Home healthcare
2. Who may apply for benefits of the ACA? **Select all that apply.**
   a. Women
   b. Children
   c. Older adults
   d. Those receiving Medicare
   e. Individuals who are not U.S. citizens
   f. Incarcerated individuals

References

American Association of Colleges of Nursing. (2021). *The essentials: Core competencies for professional nursing education*. https://www.aacnnursing.org/Essentials

Anderlini, D. (2018). The United States health care system is sick: From Adam Smith to over-specialization. *Cureus, 10*(5), e2720. https://doi.org/10.7759/cureus.2720

Assistant Secretary for Planning and Evaluation. (2023). *Poverty guidelines*. https://aspe.hhs.gov/topics/poverty-economic-mobility/poverty-guidelines

Benefits.gov. (n.d.). *Florida Medicaid*. https://www.benefits.gov/benefit/1625.

Berchick, E. R., Hood, E., & Barnett, J. C. (2018). *Health insurance coverage in the United States: 2017.* https://www.census.gov/content/dam/Census/library/publications/2018/demo/p60-264.pdf

Buchmueller, T. C., Levinson, Z. M., Levy, H. G., & Wolfe, B. L. (2016). Effect of the Affordable Care Act on racial and ethnic disparities in health insurance coverage. *American Journal of Public Health, 106*(8), 1416–1421. https://ajph.aphapublications.org/doi/10.2105/AJPH.2016.303155

Centers for Disease Control and Prevention. (2023). *Preferred provider organization (PPO)*. https://www.cdc.gov/nchs/hus/sources-definitions/ppo.htm

Center on Budget and Policy Priorities. (2020). *Policy basics: Introduction to Medicaid*. https://www.cbpp.org/research/health/introduction-to-medicaid

Centers for Medicare and Medicaid Services. (2023). *No Surprises Act*. https://www.cms.gov/NoSurprises

Cox, C., Gonzalez, S., & Kamal, R. (2015). *Health of the healthcare system: An overview*. https://www.healthsystemtracker.org/health-of-the-healthcare-system/

Department of Health and Human Services. (n.d.). *Preventive care*. https://www.hhs.gov/healthcare/about-the-aca/preventive-care/index.html

Department of Health and Human Services. (2021). *5 things about the Affordable Care Act (ACA)*. YouTube, March 23, 2021. https://www.youtube.com/watch?v=j9tRVESzJ1M&t=39s

Department of Health and Human Services. (2022). *About the ACA*. https://www.hhs.gov/healthcare/about-the-aca/index.html

Erickson, S., Outland, B., Joy, S., Rockwern, B., Serchen, J., Mire, R., & Goldman, J. (2020). Envisioning a better U.S. health care system for all: Health care delivery and payment system reforms. *Annuals of Internal Medicine, 2*, S1–S67. https://doi.org/10.7326/M19-2407

European Observatory on Health Systems and Policies. (n.d.). *Health care delivery*. https://eurohealthobservatory.who.int/themes/health-system-functions/health-care-deliverY

Fernando, J. (2023). *Gross domestic product*. https://www.investopedia.com/terms/g/gdp.asp

Gosalia, A. (2019). Third-party payers. ... The silver bullet? *Seminars in Hearing, 40*(3), 207–213. https://doi.org/10.1055/s-0039-1693490

Government of Canada. (2023). *Canada's healthcare system*. https://www.canada.ca/en/health-canada/services/canada-health-care-system.html

Gurewich, D., Garg, A., & Kressin, N. R. (2020). Addressing social determinants of health within healthcare delivery systems: A framework to ground and inform health outcomes. *Journal of General Internal Medicine*, 35, 1571–1575. https://doi.org/10.1007/s11606-020-05720-6

HealthCare.gov. (n.d.a.). *Affordable Care Act*. https://www.healthcare.gov/glossary/affordable-care-act/

HealthCare.gov. (n.d.b.). *Health maintenance organization (HMO)*. https://www.healthcare.gov/glossary/health-maintenance-organization-hmo/

HealthCare.gov. (n.d.c.). *How to pick a health insurance plan*. https://www.healthcare.gov/choose-a-plan/plan-types/

Healthinsurance.org. (n.d.). *What is private health insurance?* https://www.healthinsurance.org/glossary/private-health-insurance/

Healthinsurance.org. (2022). *What is the federal poverty level?* https://www.healthinsurance.org/glossary/federal-poverty-level/

Healthcare Triage. (2013). *What is health insurance, and why do you need it? Health Care Triage #2*. YouTube, November 3, 2013. https://www.youtube.com/watch?v=dF3Dcol5XLgo.asp

Heath, S. (2022). *Top challenges impacting patient access to healthcare*. TechTarget, February 22, 2022. https://patientengagementhit.com/news/top-challenges-impacting-patient-access-to-healthcare

Humana. (2022). *What is a PPO?* https://www.humana.com/medicare/medicare-resources/what-is-ppo?kc=0300041012

Indian Health Service. (n.d.). *About IHS*. https://www.ihs.gov/aboutihs/

Institute for Healthcare Improvement. (2023). *A downward spiral: A case study in homelessness.* https://www.ihi.org/education/IHIOpenSchool/resources/Pages/CaseStudies/HomelessnessS-toppingADownwardSpiral.aspx

Investopedia. (n.d.). *Medicaid vs. CHIP.* https://www.investopedia.com/articles/health-insurance/091016/medicaid-vs-chip-understanding-differences.asp

Jones, D. D. (2022). Medicalization of poverty: A call to action for America's healthcare workforce. *Family Medicine and Community Health, 10*(3), e001732. https://doi.org/10.1136/fmch-2022-001732

Kelly, J. T., Campbell, K. L., Gong, E., & Scuffham, P. (2020). The Internet of Things: Impact and implications for health care delivery. *Journal of Medical Internet Research, 22*(11), e20135. https://doi.org/10.2196/20135

Managed Healthcare Executive. (2023). *Poverty is the fourth leading cause of death in the United States, study finds.* https://www.managedhealthcareexecutive.com/view/poverty-is-the-fourth-leading-cause-of-death-in-the-united-states-study-finds

Matthews-Trigg, N., Citrin, D., Halliday, S., Acharya, B., Maru, S., Bezruchka, S., & Maru, D. (2019). Understanding perceptions of global healthcare experiences on provider values and practices in the USA: A qualitative study among international health physicians and program directors. *British Medical Journal Open*, 9, e026020. https://bmjopen.bmj.com/content/9/4/e026020

Medicaid.gov. (n.d.a.). *Access to care.* https://www.medicaid.gov/medicaid/access-care/index.html

Medicaid.gov. (n.d.b.). *Medicaid.* https://www.medicaid.gov/medicaid/index.html

Medicaid.gov. (n.d.c.). *Program history.* https://www.medicaid.gov/about-us/program-history/index.html

Medical Mutual. (2023). *What is a PPO? Understanding PPO health plans.* https://www.medmutual.com/Individuals-and-Families/Understanding-PPO-Health-Plans

Medicare.gov. (n.d.a.). *2023 Medicare costs.* https://www.medicare.gov/Pubs/pdf/11579-medicare-costs.pdf

Medicare.gov. (n.d.b.). *Monthly premium for drug plans.* https://www.medicare.gov/drug-coverage-part-d/costs-for-medicare-drug-coverage/monthly-premium-for-drug-plans

Medicare.gov. (n.d.c.). *Parts of Medicare.* https://www.medicare.gov/basics/get-started-with-medicare/medicare-basics/parts-of-medicare

Medicare.gov. (n.d.d.). *Your coverage options.* https://www.medicare.gov/health-drug-plans/health-plans/your-coverage-options

Medicare.gov. (n.d.e.). *Your guide to understanding Medicare Parts A-D.* https://www.medicare.org/articles/your-guide-to-understanding-medicare-parts-a-d/

Medicare.gov. (n.d.f.). *What's Medicare?* https://www.medicare.gov/what-medicare-covers/your-medicare-coverage-choices/whats-Medicare

Medicare.org. (2023). *What is Medicare Parts A & B?* https://www.medicare.org/what-is-medicare-parts-a-and-b/

MetLife. (2023). *What is an HMO insurance plan*? https://www.metlife.com/stories/benefits/hmo-insurance/

Minnesota Department of Health. (2019). *Public health interventions: Applications for public health nursing practice* (2nd ed.). https://www.health.state.mn.us/communities/practice/research/phncouncil/docs/PHInterventions.pdf

Office of Disease Prevention and Health Promotion. (n.d.a.). *Healthcare.* Healthy People 2030. https://health.gov/healthypeople/objectives-and-data/browse-objectives/health-care

Office of Disease Prevention and Health Promotion. (n.d.b.). *Health care access and quality.* Healthy People 2030. https://health.gov/healthypeople/objectives-and-data/browse-objectives/health-care-access-and-quality

Organisation for Economic Co-operation and Development. (2022). *Health statistics.* https://www.oecd.org/health/health-data.htm

Peter G. Peterson Foundation. (2023a). *Healthcare spending in the United States remains high.* April 5, 2023. https://www.pgpf.org/blog/2023/04/healthcare-spending-in-the-united-states-remains-high#

Peter G. Peterson Foundation. (2024). *How does the U.S. healthcare system compare to other countries?* July 12, 2023. https://www.pgpf.org/article/how-does-the-us-healthcare-system-compare-to-other-countries/

Public Broadcasting System. (2020). *How Canada got universal health care and what the U.S. could learn.* https://www.pbs.org/newshour/health/how-canada-got-universal-health-care-and-what-the-u-s-could-learn

Schwarz, T., Schmidt, A., Bobek, J., & Ladurner, J. (2022). Barriers to accessing health care for people with chronic conditions: A qualitative interview study. *BMC Health Service Research, 22,* 1–15. https://doi.org/10.1186/s12913-022-08426-z

Thomas, L. (2023). *Healthcare systems around the world.* https://www.news-medical.net/health/Healthcare-Systems-Around-the-World.aspx

TRICARE. (2021). *Facts and figures.* https://www.tricare.mil/About/Facts

TRICARE. (2023). *TRICARE 101.* https://www.tricare.mil/Plans/New

United Health Foundation. (2022). *Annual report 2022: Special edition.* American Health Rankings. https://assets.americashealthrankings.org/app/uploads/ahr_2022annualreport.pdf

USA.gov. (n.d.). *Food assistance.* https://www.usa.gov/food-help

USA.gov. (2024). *How to apply for Medicaid and CHIP.* November 27, 2024. https://www.usa.gov/medicaid-chip-insurance?utm_source=usa_benefits-gov&utm_medium=redirect&utm_campaign=redirect_benefits-gov

U.S. Department of Commerce. (n.d.). *Gross domestic product.* https://www.commerce.gov/tags/gross-domestic-product-gdp

U.S. Department of Veterans Affairs. (2023). *Community care: Third party billing.* https://www.va.gov/COMMUNITYCARE/revenue-ops/payer-info.asp

U.S. Senate. (n.d.). *Medicare signed into law.* https://visaguide.world/international-health-insurance/us/

World Health Organization. (n.d.). *Universal healthcare coverage.* https://www.who.int/health-topics/universal-health-coverage#tab=tab_1

Credits

Fig. 5.1: Peter G. Peterson Foundation, https://www.pgpf.org/blog/2023/07/how-does-the-us-health-care-system-compare-to-other-countries. Copyright © 2023 by Peter G. Peterson Foundation.

Fig. 5.2: Adapted from Medicare.org, https://www.medicare.org/articles/your-guide-to-understanding-medicare-parts-a-d/. Copyright © by Medicare.org.

Fig. 5.2a: Copyright © by Microsoft.

Fig. 5.3: Adapted from Investopedia, https://www.investopedia.com/articles/health-insurance/091016/medicaid-vs-chip-understanding-differences.asp. Copyright © 2022 by Investopedia, LLC.

Fig. 5.3a: Copyright © by Microsoft.

Fig. 5.4: Defense Health Agency, https://www.tricare.mil/About/Facts, 2021.

Fig. 5.5: Peter G. Peterson Foundation, https://www.pgpf.org/blog/2023/04/healthcare-spending-in-the-united-states-remains-high#. Copyright © 2023 by Peter G. Peterson Foundation.

CHAPTER 6

Epidemiological Principles

"As our world continues to generate unimaginable amounts of data, more data lead to more correlations, and more correlations can lead to more discoveries."

—Hans Rosling

Learning Outcomes

After reading this chapter, students should be able to:

1. Discuss the meaning and use of epidemiology
2. Identify the steps of the epidemiologic process
3. Understand the statistical principles of epidemiology in healthcare
4. Apply disease incidence and prevalence
5. Distinguish between the meanings of morbidity and mortality
6. Apply the concept of surveillance
7. Apply the terms *epidemic*, *endemic*, and *pandemic*

Keywords and Concepts

Endemic; epidemic; epidemiology; incidence; morbidity; mortality; pandemic; prevalence; surveillance

Definitions of the Keywords

Epidemic: Affecting a large number of individuals within a population simultaneously (Merriam-Webster Dictionary, n.d.a.)

Epidemiology: Medical science branch involving the distribution and control of disease in a specific population (Merriam-Webster Dictionary, n.d.b.)

Endemic: Something belonging to or in a particular people or community (Intermountain Health, 2020)

Incidence: Identifying new cases that could affect a condition's characteristics, behaviors, or circumstances (Merriam-Webster Dictionary, n.d.c.)

Morbidity: The frequency of a disease that occurs within a population of individuals (Merriam-Webster. (n.d.d.)

Mortality: The number of individuals who die from a particular disease process (Merriam-Webster Dictionary, n.d.e.)

Pandemic: Occurring over a wide geographic area, affecting a significant proportion of the population (Merriam-Webster Dictionary, n.d.f.)

Prevalence: Relationship to the frequency that a population becomes affected by a specific disease or condition (Merriam-Webster Dictionary, n.d.g.)

Statistical principles: Statistics using mathematics for data collection, analysis, and interpretation of the findings (Zorić, 2021)

Surveillance: The systematic process of investigating diseases or conditions (Merriam-Webster Dictionary, n.d.h.)

Introduction

Healthcare has evolved in many ways through the study of epidemiology processes. By doing so, the need to investigate the causes, provide dissemination of information, and perform disease control in national and international populations is vital. The statistical process began with Florence Nightingale, who started by documenting the conditions of soldiers during the Crimean War (Science Museum, 2019). Nightingale found that many of the soldiers perished from preventable illnesses that were not due to the actual injuries of war. By placing the conditions that affected the soldiers' health outcomes, Nightingale could share interventions to change many healthcare practices (Science Museum, 2019).

Nursing students need to learn about the distribution and determinants of health and illness across populations. The 2019 Campaign for Action report noted the importance of a basic understanding of the distribution and determinants of health and disease across people, including recognizing changes across a population. Knowing their significance and outcome implications is even more critical as outbreaks and disease distribution changes occur. This chapter will address the concept of epidemiology and its principles, the importance of surveillance, and the application of these principles.

Background of the Concepts

Epidemiologists are those individuals who focus on the study of epidemiology. This form of research is used to disseminate the means of conditions and how to prevent the spread of diseases. The epidemiologist's role is multifaceted and includes the collection of data and the relationship to the diseases. This includes information about the environment, cultures, ethnicities, ages, sexes, and lifestyles. Looking at the trends of infections and the transmission of organisms plays an important role, as is the need for the development of vaccinations, laboratory testing, and other functions for prevention (Science Museum, 2019).

Epidemiologists use evidence-based practice to identify and study health and what contributes to their prominence in the population. Using statistics assists in understanding the knowledge gained, allowing for the development of new interventions for meeting the needs of individuals and communities. Real-life data collections have found successful solutions to disease and how to focus on and evaluate genetic, social, environmental, and other conditions to eradicate diseases. An example of such efforts includes the need for hand hygiene by Ignac Semmelweis in 1847 and his collection of data on women who died from childbed fever. The autopsy findings looked at the illnesses they developed, leading to the intervention of a handwashing policy for physicians and medical students (Tyagi & Barwal, 2020).

Scientists must include genetics, social, environmental, and biological factors by studying causes, distributions, and controlling disease conditions that affect populations (Rouz, 2022). Multifaceted approaches include using avenues such as social drivers of health, understanding the health impacts of systemic racism and policy complications, and big data to achieve more positive health outcomes (Roux, 2022).

Epidemiological Principles

There are many aspects to understanding the world of epidemiology. Epidemiologic principles and their respective processes can be used to investigate and study any health-related issue. Although this is an informative process, the ability to prevent or at least minimize the effects of diseases that contribute to any population's health problems is addressed. It is often thought that epidemiologic means are only utilized for epidemics or pandemics. This view is inaccurate as epidemiologists look at current situations that are prominent in the world but also at lifestyle and even occupational conditions that lead to the development of chronic diseases such as diabetes and lung cancer (Science Museum, 2019).

Epidemiology Definition

Epidemiology is the study of factors that assist in determining the contribution of conditions or disease processes specifically researched by epidemiologists

(National Institute on Deafness and Other Communication Disorders, 2011). The method uses specific data and a systematic approach to probe diseases and issues affecting populations. The epidemiological process steps have been designed to be performed orderly. As a means to study public health developments, many factors become entwined to allow for significant findings and inclusions of data to examine such areas to uncover the necessary knowledge to facilitate positive outcomes.

Epidemiology is a discipline that has evolved with the changes in society and the emergence of new diseases and fields related to epidemiology (Frerot et al., 2018). Maynard (1978) conceived the first definition of *epidemiology* as "a method of reasoning about disease that deals with biological inference derived from observations of disease phenomena in population groups" (p. 87). Today, the definition has evolved to include many other disciples, avenues, and aspects. Understanding all factors encompassing epidemiology is essential for population health (Frerot et al., 2018; Box 6.1).

BOX 6.1 ACTIVE LEARNING REFLECTION ACTIVITY

What Is Epidemiology?

Watch the following video regarding epidemiology: https://www.youtube.com/watch?v=q-17icRTMyY.

1. Reflect on three items that you learned from watching this video.
2. Name three ways you could apply this to today's world and issues.

American Association of Colleges of Nursing (AACN) *Essentials* (2021): Domains: #1; #3; #6; #8

- Competencies: 1.1; 1.2; 3.1; 3.2; 3.3; 3.5; 3.6; 6.3; 6.4; 8.4
- Subcompetencies: 1.1a; 1.2a; 3.1a; 3.1b; 3.1c; 3.1d; 3.1e; 3.1h; 3.2a; 3.3b; 3.5c; 3.6c; 3.6e; 6.3a; 6.4d; 8.4c

Spheres of Care: Wellness/Disease prevention; Chronic disease management

Concepts: Communication; Evidence-based practice; Clinical judgment

Source: LiveScience, 2020.

Epidemiological Triad

Balasubramanian (2022) noted the traditional way of explaining how infectious diseases cause and spread through the epidemiological triad. The three components of this triad are host, environment, and agent. An example of a host is an individual. The agent could be the flu, while the environment could be a crowded elementary school where several students have the disease (Figure 6.1).

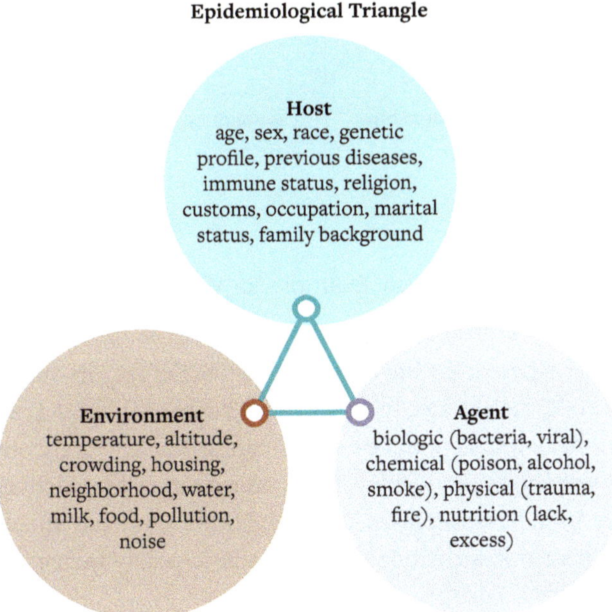

FIGURE 6.1 Epidemiological Triad

Other concepts that address the spread include direct and indirect transmission. *Direct transmission* is where the agent directly infects the host and causes the disease. An example is the bacteria that causes tuberculosis. *Indirect transmission* occurs through avenues such as mosquitoes carrying malaria. These are known as *vectors*, as they carry diseases from one host to another but do not cause them (Balasubramanian, 2022). Transmission will be discussed more in Chapter 7.

Ecological Model

In defining an ecological model, the key is the importance of the interconnection between factors across all health issue levels and people's relationship with their physical and sociocultural surroundings (Rural Health Information Hub [RHIhub], 2018). Levels of influence on health behaviors include community, public policy, institutional and organizational, intrapersonal, and interpersonal factors (RHIhub, 2018).

The Centers for Disease Control and Prevention (CDC, 2022b) provides an example of an ecological model that uses a social aspect. The social-ecological model framework is a prime prevention framework mentioned in violence prevention. This framework aims to identify all elements that could influence violence and provide intervention strategies to reduce its risk (Figure 6.2).

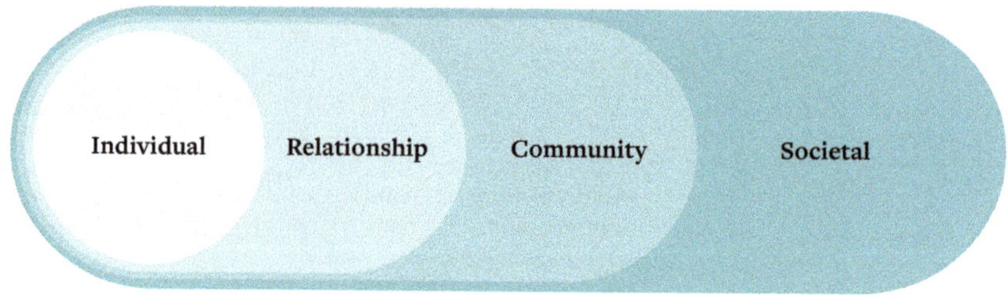

FIGURE 6.2 Social-Ecological Example for Violence Prevention

An individual aspect identifies personal and belief factors that could increase the risk for violence, such as age, income, and substance abuse. A relationship notes close associations, such as peers or significant others, which could perpetuate the expanded probability of violence. The community acknowledges the settings, such as schools, homes, workplaces, and neighborhoods, that affect the situation. The societal aspect notes the health or economic policy factors that increase a violent climate (CDC, 2022b).

Web of Causation

Often many factors play into the actual cause of a disease or an illness. The *web of causation* explores multiple causative factors, giving each equal prominence in identifying determinants and relevant interventions and disputing that it is not a linear event (Ventriglio et al., 2016). The web of causation offers a helpful way to understand the etiology and link the social determinants of health (SDOH), social factors, and biomedical etiological factors (Ventriglio et al., 2016; Figure 6.3).

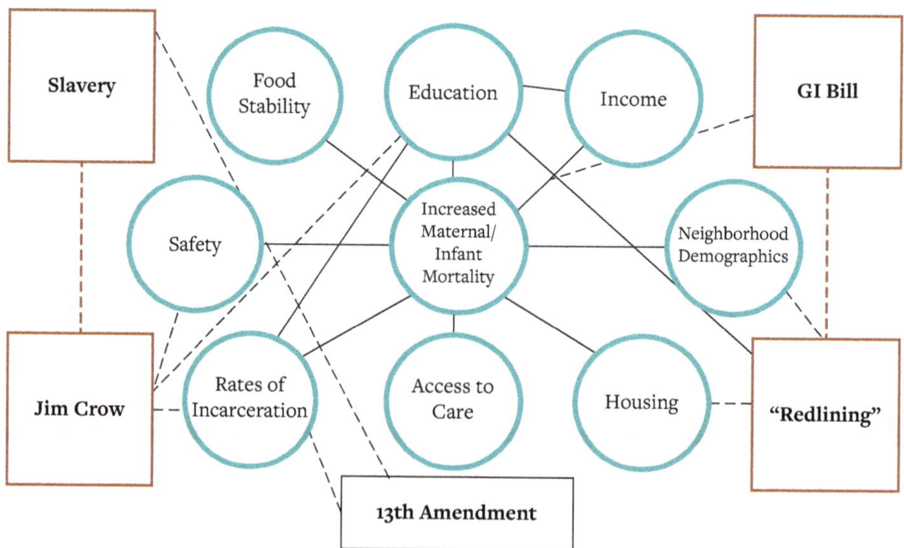

FIGURE 6.3 Example of Web of Causation (Maternal/Infant Mortality and SDOH)

Epidemiology Types/Studies

Epidemiologists who study epidemiology use many data sources for epidemiological studies of diseases or illnesses. Primary data is collected from initial data, such as interviewing individuals who became sick at a restaurant. Secondary data has been obtained for other purposes, such as birth and death records, public health cases, and population census records (Britannica, n.d.).

The epidemiology process includes distribution and determinants, focusing on the frequency of the events about a number from that affected population. Another aspect is that of the patterns. By doing so, epidemiologists can look specifically at the times diseases or injuries occur, such as seasonal, weekly, daily, hourly, and on weekends, illustrating descriptive epidemiology (Fox et al., 2022). Other aspects may include health inequalities, disparities, and racial and ethnic groups that affect disease distribution, noting the components of a social epidemiology study (Roux, 2022).

Other epidemiological studies report a comparison to analyze the possible causes and effects. Analytical epidemiological studies evaluate hypotheses to learn whether statistical associations exist between suspected causal factors and disease occurrence (Brittanica, n.d.). Another type of study, *experimental*, contains data manipulation through control and another group (Biradar & Divya, 2018; Table 6.1).

TABLE 6.1 Types of Epidemiological Studies

Types	Meaning	Example
Descriptive	Various methods are used to collect disease occurrence from all relevant sources; the data are then collated by time, place, and person	Seasonal trends of flu
Social	Focuses on understanding how social organization shapes the distribution of health and disease	How race and poverty (e.g., African American) could affect the United States maternal mortality rates
Analytic	Analysis of disease determinants for possible causal relations	Whether access to healthcare affects Hispanic diabetes rates
Experimental	A hypothesis is developed, and a model is constructed in which one or more selected factors are manipulated; the effect of the manipulation will either confirm or disprove the hypothesis	Some people with diabetes are given a new drug, whereas others receive a placebo

Sources: Biradar & Divya, 2018; Brittanica, n.d.; Fox et al., 2022; Roux, 2022.

Lau et al. (2020) looked specifically at the future of epidemiology. Their presentation shows that the field has changed and needs to be planned differently for public health needs. Reviewing current practices and incorporating new topics and challenges, specifically with unique needs for public health research, is a focus. Nationally and internationally, the broad and diverse situations that may occur and the means to collect significant data will be vital. Areas to be included surround the application of epidemiology, biological/genetic aspects, the SDOH, communications, collaboration with others, advanced statistical techniques, and research study designs. In the past, public health issues have had a different approach. In the future, problems will evolve, and there will need to be monitoring of such situations as climate change, gun violence, the opioid epidemic, and social health disparities (Box 6.2).

BOX 6.2 ACTIVE LEARNING REFLECTION

Further Understanding Epidemiology

Go to the following website: https://www.environmentalscience.org/epidemiology.

Scroll down to the section titled "What are the present and future challenges for epidemiology?" and read the content.

1. Focus on one of the six heading topics.
2. Name two ways that the nursing profession can prepare and implement assistance in understanding future epidemiologic challenges.

AACN *Essentials* (2021): Domains: #1; #3; #6; #8

- Competencies: 1.1; 1.2; 3.1; 3.2; 3.3; 3.5; 3.6; 6.3; 6.4; 8.4
- Subcompetencies: 1.1a; 1.2a; 3.1a; 3.1b; 3.1c; 3.1d; 3.1e; 3.1h; 3.2a; 3.3b; 3.5c; 3.6c; 3.6e; 6.3a; 6.4d; 8.4c

Spheres of Care: Wellness/Disease prevention; Chronic disease management

Concepts: Communication; Evidence-based practice, SDOH

Source: Mason, 2023.

Statistical Principles

The ability to study epidemiological practices includes statistical analysis. This process focuses on data collection, interpretation, and presentation of the findings. The orderly process is followed to study simple to complex issues and be significant in identifying identifiable results and researching the data that may be insignificant or irrelevant to the study. The collected data is analyzed by locating specific patterns or trends resulting from the events (Monaghan et al., 2021).

Evidence-based practice is a leading measure to study various situations or issues. Using this form of research, epidemiologists can investigate many different areas, looking at multiple variables to apply the findings from clinicians and other scientific/medical researchers. This multidisciplinary approach can interpret, synthesize, and apply knowledge from different disciplines. This will inhibit the presentation of errors or inappropriate conclusions, along with consistent use of terms and communication in presenting the overall information (Barlett & Gagnon, 2016).

Multidisciplinary approaches to statistical principles promise to yield more extraordinary scientific advances by understanding and improving human performance. All departments and professionals are integrated in treating a specific condition or situation. This guarantees full and continued support and is positive for individuals and communities. The continuous use of multidisciplinary teams has been implemented in many countries and is now considered standard for research (Taberna et al., 2020; Zajac et al., 2021).

Incidence and Prevalence

Understanding disease, illness, or issue rates is critical. One such significant rate is incidence. The definition of *incidence* notes the number of new cases or situations that occur over a specific time (Tenny & Boktar, 2022). Incidence often needs to be more adequately identified as the populations at risk. If the population changes, the incidence will also change. Ensuring that the correct population is used is essential when reporting the numbers (Tenny & Boktor, 2022; Box 6.3).

Following is the proper way to calculate an incidence rate:

$$\text{Incidence} = \frac{\text{Number of } \textit{new} \text{ people in the sample with the characteristic}}{\text{Total number of people in the sample}}$$

BOX 6.3 ACTIVE LEARNING ACTIVITY

Incidence Rate Calculation

In one year, there are 795,000 new strokes in the United States. The population of the United States is 324 million people. Please calculate the rate per 100,000.

AACN *Essentials* (2021): Domains: #2; #3; #5

- Competencies: 2.5; 3.1; 5.1
- Subcompetencies: 2.5e; 3.1a; 3.1b; 5.1d

Spheres of Care: Chronic disease management

Concepts: Clinical judgment; Evidence-based practice

Source: Tenny & Boktor, 2022.

Prevalence is the total number of people affected by a specific condition at a particular time, regardless of when they developed the characteristic (Monaghan et al., 2021; Westreich, 2019). There are several ways to measure and report prevalence depending on the time frame of the estimate. *Point prevalence* is the proportion of a population with the characteristic at a specific point in time. *Period prevalence* is the proportion of a population that has the aspect at any point during a given period of interest with a typical period in the past 12 months. *Lifetime prevalence* is the proportion of a population who has had the characteristic at some point in life (National Institute of Mental Health, n.d.).

Following is the proper way to calculate a prevalence rate:

$$\text{Prevalence} = \frac{\textit{Total}\text{ number of people in the sample with the characteristic (new plus existing)}}{\text{Total number of people in the sample}}$$

A common factor must be present to express rates and compare populations regarding incidence and prevalence. Rates are typically expressed per 1,000, 10,000, or 100,000 population to make it easier to understand and compare. The conversion is simple: multiply the raw rate by the population unit. The following example converts the rate from the previous model to a rate per 100,000: 0.001042 x 100,000 = 104.2 cases per 100,000 population (CDC, n.d.; Box 6.4).

Understanding the relationship between incidence and prevalence is critical. An easy way to understand incidence and prevalence is by understanding how water enters and leaves a bathtub through the following video (Public Health Agency, 2022; Figure 6.4; Box 6.5).

BOX 6.4 ACTIVE LEARNING REFLECTION ACTIVITY

Understanding Incidence and Prevalence

Review the video at the following link: https://www.youtube.com/watch?v=1jzZe3ORdd8.

1. How can increased prevalence rates be a good situation? Name one specific way and give an example.

AACN *Essentials* (2021): Domains: #2; #3; #4; #5

- Competencies: 2.5; 3.1; 4.2; 5.1
- Subcompetencies: 2.5e; 3.1a; 3.1h; 4.2a; 5.1d

Spheres of Care: Chronic disease management

Concepts: Clinical judgment; Evidence-based practice

Source: Rahul Patwari [Rahul's EM], 2013.

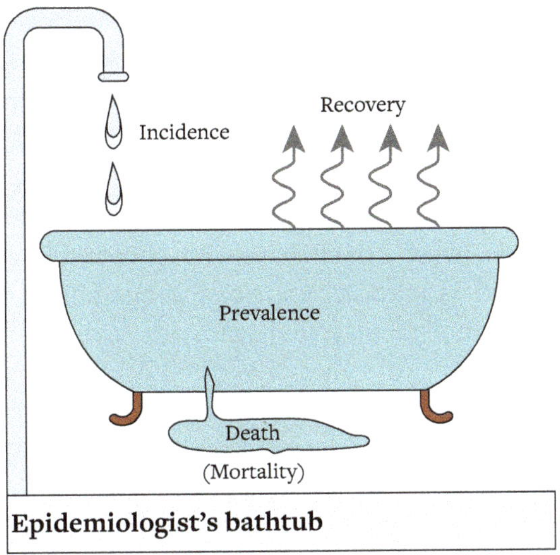

FIGURE 6.4 The Epidemiologist's Bathtub

BOX 6.5 ACTIVE LEARNING REFLECTION EXERCISE

Further Incidence and Prevalence Calculations

Calculate the following problems for incidence and prevalence:

1. There are 44,232 new cases of acquired immunodeficiency syndrome (AIDS) reported in the United States. The estimated midyear population of the United States was approximately 290,809,777. Calculate the incidence rate of AIDS: ____________________ per 100,000.
2. In a survey of 1,150 women who gave birth in Maine, 468 reported taking a multivitamin at least four times a week during the month before becoming pregnant. Calculate the prevalence of frequent multivitamin use in this group: ____________________ x 100 = ______________ %.

AACN *Essentials* (2021): Domains: #2; #3; #4; #5

- Competencies: 2.5; 3.1; 4.2; 5.1
- Subcompetencies: 2.5e; 3.1a; 4.2a; 5.1d

Spheres of Care: Chronic disease management

Concepts: Clinical judgment; Evidence-based practice

Source: Developed by authors.

Morbidity and Mortality

In the study of epidemiology, there is the need to measure two specific statistical concepts for occurrence rates: morbidity and mortality. Both of these share essential relationships in the field of public health. *Morbidity* is the ratio of the number of cases of a specific disease or condition to the number of people in a particular population. *Mortality* is the ratio of deaths from a specific disease or illness to the number of people in a particular population (Hernandez & Kim, 2022).

Morbidity rates tend to be estimated and use the prevalence or incidence of the cases. An example includes individuals with diabetes of a certain age or ethnic background. Mortality is stated as a rate or absolute number and is often called the *death rate*. One example is maternal death rates over a set period. Accurately determining these numerical values allows epidemiologists to actively study and prioritize which health events may be most important to focus resources towards and effectively manage the condition (Hernandez & Kim, 2022).

It is essential to ensure consistent statistical analysis of morbidity and mortality. Concerns about the possibility of information needing to be included or completed can skew the findings. Some other barriers include language, methods of collecting and analyzing data, use of census for samples, and the incorporation of bias (Hernandez & Kim, 2022).

Zylke and Bauchner (2020) studied the effects of the COVID-19 pandemic related to morbidity and mortality. They identified that only using mortality as a pandemic factor overlooks the direct and indirect impacts of morbidity. Several conditions, such as cardiac conditions, respiratory ailments, and multisystem inflammatory syndromes, have surfaced but are still being evaluated. Following the guidelines and restrictions for COVID-19 spread, pandemic interventions may have decreased the virus's communication but provided the development of other conditions that lead to morbidity. Such examples include mental health conditions, social isolation, and nutritional deficiencies (Boserup et al., 2020; McGinty et al., 2020; Box 6.6).

BOX 6.6 ACTIVE LEARNING REFLECTION ACTIVITY

Application of Morbidity and Mortality Using Maternal Mortality and Morbidity

Watch the following video: https://www.youtube.com/watch?v=9MJh-oREOU8. Reflect on the following questions:

1. Which race/ethnicity has the highest maternal morbidity rates?
2. Which SDOHs (name two) could affect the rates?
3. In the video, what percentage of deaths could be preventable?
4. What percentage of maternal morbidity after delivery could be preventable?
5. What two primary prevention interventions need to be implemented to address this issue?

AACN *Essentials* (2021): Domains: #1; #2; #3; #4; #5; #7; #8; #9

- Competencies: 1.1; 1.3; 2.8; 2.9; 3.1; 3.3; 3.4; 4.2; 5.1; 7.2; 8.3; 9.3
- Subcompetencies: 1.1a; 1.3b; 2.8c; 2.8e; 2.9d; 3.1a; 3.1b; 3.1d; 3.1e; 3.1g; 3.1h; 3.1i; 3.3a; 3.3b; 3.4b; 4.2c; 5.1c; 7.2a; 7.2b; 7.2c; 8.3e; 9.3g

Spheres of Care: Wellness/Disease prevention; Chronic disease prevention

Concepts: Evidence-based practice; Clinical judgment; SDOH, Diversity, equity and inclusion (DEI)

Source: DPCPSI, 2020.

Epidemic, Endemic, and Pandemic

Diseases have usual incidence, prevalence, morbidity, and mortality rates. But what if these rates change or become an issue in a particular area? A disease increase is noted, but a sudden rise in a specific population could become a problem. A sudden disease spread or uptake to a group or population is called an *epidemic* (American Lung Association [ALA], 2023). An example of an epidemic is the rise in childhood obesity.

A *pandemic* is an epidemic that has spread or increased in several areas and countries (ALA, 2023; Roberts & Landowski, 2022). Pandemics cause disruptions to economies and social factors. The most recent example was COVID-19 in 2020.

There is a belief that COVID-19 will continue to be present but will be noted in certain areas. The term *endemic* is used when a disease or an issue is constant in a particular population. Although an endemic is a continuous presence in a community, it differs from a pandemic or epidemic because it is somewhat contained, does not spread or increase out of control, and does not stress the healthcare infrastructure (ALA, 2023). Another example of an endemic issue is Lyme disease, which is prevalent in some regions of the United States (Figure 6.5; Box 6.7).

What's the difference between an endemic, epidemic and pandemic disease?

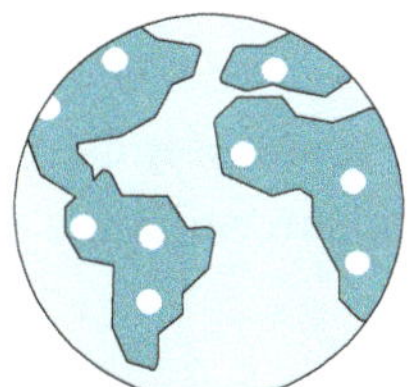

Endemic disease
is constantly present in a certain population or region, with relatively low spread (or there may be periods when it doesn't affect people at all, if it is only present in the environment).

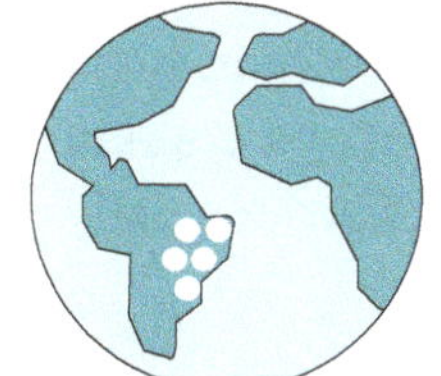

Epidemic disease
is when there is a sudden increase in cases spreading through a large population like a country (an outbreak is similar, but usually covers a smaller geographic area).

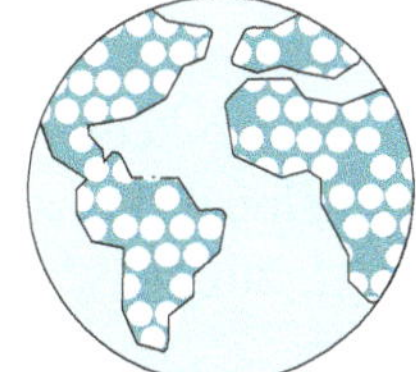

Pandemic disease
is when there is a sudden increase in cases spreading through several countries, continents, or the whole world.

FIGURE 6.5 Differences Between an Epidemic, an Endemic, and a Pandemic

BOX 6.7 ACTIVE LEARNING REFLECTION ACTIVITY

Epidemics, Pandemics, and Endemics

Watch the following video and answer the following questions: https://www.youtube.com/watch?v=nclAnJXdgqs.

1. Name two examples used in the video regarding endemic issues.
2. Name two examples used in the video regarding epidemic issues.
3. Apply two positive interventions to decrease epidemics and pandemics.

AACN *Essentials* (2021): Domains: #2; #3; #4; #5; #6

- Competencies: 2.5; 3.1; 3.2; 3.3; 3.4; 3.6; 4.2; 5.1; 5.2; 6.3; 6.4
- Subcompetencies: 2.5e; 3.1a; 3.1c; 3.1e; 3.1h; 3.2a; 3.3b; 3.4b; 3.6c; 3.6e; 4.2a; 5.1d; 5.2a; 6.3a; 6.3c; 6.4d

Spheres of Care: Wellness/Disease prevention; Chronic disease management

Concepts: Evidence-based practice; Health policy; SDOH; Clinical judgment

Source: 2 Minute Classroom, 2020.

Surveillance

Surveillance of diseases and issues is critical to public health. Monitoring the incidence and prevalence of specific health issues is vital to protecting the public. Certain conditions are required by law to be reported to local, state, and territory authorities to contain outbreaks (CDC, 2023; Table 6.2).

The CDC constantly monitors the National Notifiable Diseases Surveillance System (NNDSS). Health departments gather and use data to protect their local communities and report/notify them of any issues. The CDC uses the NNDSS to keep individuals and communities healthy and defends America from global threats through strategically placed regional surveillance centers (CDC, 2023).

Data Sources/Types of Surveillance Systems

Evidence-based and reliable data must be obtained and secured to monitor certain diseases and issues. *Passive surveillance* is routine data collection from fixed sites (World Health Organization, 2023). *Active surveillance* is the collection of reported cases by health authorities. *Sentinel surveillance* is a network of purpose-built reporting sites where more detailed information and samples are collected from people who fit the surveillance criteria. Sentinel surveillance can supplement existing passive systems with more detailed information without overburdening existing national disease surveillance systems (Murray & Cohen, 2017; Table 6.3; Box 6.8).

TABLE 6.2 Reportable Versus Notifiable: What Is the Difference?

Reportable Diseases and Conditions	Notifiable Diseases and Conditions
Each state or territory sets local laws and rules for reporting diseases and conditions.	The Council of State and Territorial Epidemiologists and the CDC identify the list of notifiable diseases and conditions.
Healthcare professionals, laboratories, hospitals, and other providers must tell public health departments when a person is diagnosed.	States voluntarily inform the CDC when a person meets specific criteria to become a case.
Public health departments collect information about the person and how they became ill.	Case records do not contain personally identifiable information.
This information is used to locate the source of an outbreak and prevent its spread.	The CDC uses data to monitor, measure, and alert individual communities or nations to outbreaks and other public health threats.
The list of diseases and conditions can change every year.	The list of about 120 diseases and conditions is updated every year.

Source: CDC, 2023.

TABLE 6.3 Types of Surveillance Systems/Meaning/Examples

Type	Meaning	Examples
Passive	Routine data collection from fixed sites	Hospitals Outpatient facilities
Active	Group of reported cases reported to health authorities	Measle cases Flu cases
Sentinel	Network of purpose-built reporting sites where more detailed information and samples are collected from people who fit the surveillance criteria	NNDSS

Source: Adapted from Murray & Cohen, 2017.

BOX 6.8 ACTIVE LEARNING REFLECTION ACTIVITY

Application of Epidemiology Surveillance

Class Active Learning Strategy

Please use a reliable source to find answers/statistics regarding the following issues on your assigned topic. Use the most recent year located unless stated.

1. Compare the national suicide rates for older adults versus adolescents.
2. Compare infant mortality rate in ZIP codes 46806 versus 33914.
3. Compare the rate of pregnant women in the United States who drink alcohol versus those in Ireland.
4. Compare the sudden infant death syndrome rates in the United States in 1998 versus 2023 (or the last year available).

AACN *Essentials* (2021): Domains: #1; #2; #3; #4; #5; #7; #8; #9

- Competencies: 1.1; 1.3; 2.4; 2.7; 2.8; 2.9; 3.1; 3.3; 3.4; 4.2; 5.1; 7.2; 8.3; 9.3
- Subcompetencies: 1.1a; 1.3b; 2.4d; 2.7d; 2.8c; 2.8e; 2.9d; 3.1a; 3.1b; 3.1d; 3.1e; 3.1g; 3.1h; 3.1i; 3.3a; 3.3b; 3.4b; 4.2c; 5.1c; 7.2a; 7.2b; 7.2c; 8.3e; 9.3g

Spheres of Care: Wellness/Disease prevention; Chronic disease management; Regenerative/Restorative care

Concepts: Evidence-based practice; SDOH; Clinical judgment

Source: Developed by author.

Chapter Highlights

- Discussion on epidemiology in public health
- Application of incidence and prevalence
- Discussion of morbidity and mortality
- Active learning exercises related to epidemiology
- Active learning exercises related to prevalence
- Active learning exercises related to morbidity and mortality
- Active learning exercises related to surveillance
- Case studies related to the intervention wheel, incidence and prevalence, mortality, and current laws and policies

Active Learning Exercises

Intervention Wheel Active Learning Strategy (Addressing Application of the Intervention Wheel)

Local law enforcement agencies have identified a significant increase in deaths from opioid and xylazine usage in the community. A community group has been formed to investigate the situation and develop collaborative measures to decrease this issue.

Use the following link to complete the following application: https://www.health.state.mn.us/communities/practice/research/phncouncil/docs/PHInterventions.pdf.

The orange section of the intervention wheel contains three intervention levels (collaboration, coalition-building, and community organizing).

Complete the following items using one of the intervention levels:

1. Note the particular intervention used and why.
2. List two objectives at the community level.
3. List at least four needed community leaders.
4. Note two ways to collect data.
5. Name two ways in which the dissemination of the issue will occur.
6. How will you assess/evaluate the process?

AACN *Essentials* (2021): Domains: #2; #3; #4; #5; #6; #8; #9

- Competencies: 2.6; 2.7; 3.1; 3.3; 3.5; 4.1; 4.2; 5.1; 6.1; 8.1; 8.2; 8.3; 8.4; 9.3
- Subcompetencies: 2.6a; 2.6b; 2.7a; 3.1b; 3.1c; 3.1d; 3.1e; 3.1h; 3.3a; 3.3b; 3.5c; 3.5d; 4.1g; 4.2d; 5.1g; 6.1b; 8.1a; 8.1d; 8.1e; 8.2c; 8.2d; 8.3a; 8.4a; 8.4b; 9.3a

Spheres of Care: Wellness/Disease prevention; Chronic disease management; Regenerative/Restorative care

Concepts: Communication; Evidence-based practice; Clinical judgment

Source: Minnesota Department of Health, 2019.

Case Studies

Case Study #1: Application of Surveillance

As a public health nurse practitioner in your community, you frequently participate in routine health physicals. Throughout the summer months, you have begun noticing that several children from grades six through 12 have weights exceeding 20 pounds.

1. What measures can you take to identify the incidence and prevalence of this issue?
2. Plan a 30-minute presentation for low-income parents that can be given at a parental meeting. Offer interventions that can be implemented along with surveillance data collection for each child. Use the following website to assist with this active learning exercise: https://www.cdc.gov/scienceambassador/educational/active-activities.html#chronic-disease.

AACN *Essentials* (2021): Domains: #1; #2; #3; #4; #5; #6; #7; #8

- Competencies: 1.3; 2.3; 2.4; 2.8; 3.1; 3.2; 3.3; 4.2; 5.1; 6.4; 7.2; 8.2
- Subcompetencies: 1.3a; 1.3b; 1.3c; 2.3a; 2.3b; 2.3f; 2.3g; 2.4b; 2.8a; 2.8c; 2.8d; 2.8e; 3.1a; 3.1e; 3.2a; 3.2b; 3.3b; 4.2c; 5.1b; 6.4b; 7.2a; 7.2b; 7.2e; 8.2b

Spheres of Care: Wellness/Disease prevention; Chronic disease management

Concepts: Evidence-based practice; SDOH; Clinical judgment

Source: CDC, 2022a.

Case Study #2: Application of Statistical Principles

Florida Health Charts allow for the application of specific surveillance data.

Go to the following website: https://www.flhealthcharts.gov/ChartsDashboards/rdPage.aspx?rdReport=LeadingCausesofDeath.Report.

Click on the tab "Chronic Diseases" under "Health Indicators." Then click on "Leading Causes of Death Profile." Choose the latest year. Open the "COVID-19" tab and answer the following questions:

1. Which gender has the highest rate of age-adjusted death rate per 100,000? What does the term *age-adjusted* mean?
2. Which race has the highest age-adjusted death rate per 100,000? Apply two rationales for these data.

AACN *Essentials* (2021): Domains: #3; #7; #8

- Competencies: 3.1; 7.3; 8.1; 8.2; 8.3
- Subcompetencies: 3.1a; 3.1b; 3.1c; 3.1d; 7.3b; 8.1a; 8.1c; 8.2c; 8.3c

Spheres of Care: Chronic disease management

Concepts: Evidence-based practice; Clinical judgment

Source: Florida Department of Health, 2021.

Case Study #3: Applying Web of Causation

A client comes to an outpatient health clinic reporting shortness of breath, dizziness, and fatigue that have worsened over the past week. The client has an albuterol inhaler from a past respiratory issue and has been using it more.

1. What five questions might you want to ask the client?
2. How would asking the client where they live, work, and play help you?
3. What other specific questions could you ask regarding work and occupation that could help you during the assessment?
4. What do you want to know about past medical history and prior/current medications?

AACN *Essentials* (2021): Domains: #1; #2; #3; #5; #6; #7

- Competencies: 1.1; 1.3; 2.2; 2.3; 2.4; 2.5; 2.6; 2.7; 2.8; 2.9; 3.1; 3.3; 5.1; 6.3; 7.2
- Subcompetencies: 1.1b; 1.3c; 2.2e; 2.3c; 2.3d; 2.3e; 2.3g; 2.4a; 2.4b; 2.4d; 2.5b; 2.6d; 2.7a; 2.7c; 2.8a; 2.8b; 2.8c; 2.9a; 2.9d; 2.9e; 3.1e; 3.1h; 3.3a; 3.3b; 5.1c; 5.1f; 6.3a; 7.2a

Spheres of Care: Wellness/Disease prevention; Chronic disease management

Concepts: Clinical judgment; Evidence-based practice

Sources: Swift, 2022; adapted from Wolters Kluwer.

NCLEX Questions

1. In Jonesboro, there is a population of 1,000 individuals. Fifteen residents have already been diagnosed with breast cancer; nine residents were diagnosed with breast cancer during a recent screening event. Which answer is the correct prevalence number?

    a. Twenty-four residents
    b. Nine residents
    c. Fifteen residents
    d. Six residents

2. Which data would be considered passive surveillance? **Select all that apply.**

    a. The local number of flu cases
    b. Infection rates from an outpatient clinic
    c. COVID-19 deaths at a local hospital
    d. Data from the NNDSS

References

American Association of Colleges of Nursing. (2021). *The essentials: Core competencies for professional nursing education.* https://www.aacnnursing.org/Essentials

American Lung Association. (2023). *Epidemic, pandemic and endemic: What's the difference?* https://www.lung.org/blog/epidemic-pandemic-endemic-covid

Balasubramanian, C. (2022). *Epidemiological triad.* https://www.gideononline.com/blogs/epidemiological-triad/

Bartlett, G., & Gagnon, J. (2016). Physicians and knowledge translation of statistics: Mind the gap. *Canadian Medical Association Journal, 188*(1), 11–12. https://www.ncbi.nlm.nih.gov/pmc/articles/PMC4695343/pdf/1880011.pdf

Biradar, S., & Divya, S. (2018). Experimental epidemiology—A review. *Asian Journal of Pharmaceutical Technology & Innovation, 6*(27), 10–35. https://www.asianpharmtech.com/articles/experimental-epidemiology--a-review.pdf

Boserup, B., McKenney, M., & Elkbuli, A. (2020). Alarming trends in US domestic violence during the COVID-19 pandemic. *American Journal of Emergency Medicine, 38*(12), 2753–2755. https://doi.org/10.1016/j.ajem.2020.04.077

Brittanica. (n.d.). *Sources of epidemiological data.* https://www.britannica.com/science/epidemiology

Campaign for Action. (2019). *Nursing education and the path to population health improvement.* https://campaignforaction.org/wpcontent/uploads/2019/03/NursingEducationPathtoHealth-Improvement.pdf

Centers for Disease Control and Prevention. (n.d.). *Expression of rates.* https://www.cdc.gov/STD/Sassi/Module2/expression_of_rates.html

Centers for Disease Control and Prevention. (2022a). *Science Ambassador Program: Index of educational activities organized by topic.* https://www.cdc.gov/scienceambassador/educational/active-activities.html#chronic-disease

Centers for Disease Control and Prevention. (2022b). *The social-ecological model: A framework for prevention.* https://www.cdc.gov/violenceprevention/about/social-ecologicalmodel.html

Centers for Disease Control and Prevention. (2023). *What is case surveillance*? https://www.cdc.gov/nndss/about/index.html

DPCPSI. (2020). *Maternal morbidity and mortality: What do we know? How are we addressing it?* National Institutes of Health. YouTube, November 13, 2020. https://www.youtube.com/watch?v=9MJh-oREOU8

Florida Department of Health. (2021). *COVID-19: Leading causes of death.* Florida Health Charts. https://www.flhealthcharts.gov/ChartsDashboards/rdPage.aspx?rdReport=LeadingCausesofDeath.Report

Fox, M., Murray, E., Lesko, C., & Sealey-Jefferson, S. (2022). On the need to revitalize descriptive epidemiology. *American Journal of Epidemiology, 191*(7), 1174–1179. https://doi.org/10.1093/aje/kwac056

Frerot, M., Lefebvre, A., Aho, S., Callier, P, Astruc, K., & Aho Glele, L. (2018). What is epidemiology? Changing definitions of epidemiology 1978-2017. *PLoS ONE, 13*(12), e0208442. https://doi.org/10.1371/journal.pone.0208442

Hernandez, J. B. R., & Kim, P. Y. (2022). *Epidemiology morbidity and mortality.* StatPearls. https://www.ncbi.nlm.nih.gov/books/NBK547668/

Intermountain Health. (2020). *What's the difference between a pandemic, an epidemic, endemic, and an outbreak?* https://intermountainhealthcare.org/blogs/whats-the-difference-between-a-pandemic-an-epidemic-endemic-and-an-outbreak

Lau, B., Duggal, P., Ehrhardt, S., Armenian, H., Branas, C. C., Colditz, G. A., Fox, M. P., Hawes, S. E., He, J., Hofman, A., Keyes, K., Ko, A. I., Lash, T. L., Levy, D., Lu, M., Morabia, A., Ness, R., Nieto, F. J., Schisterman, E. F., ... & Celentano, D. D. (2020). Perspectives on the future of epidemiology: A framework for training. *American Journal of Epidemiology, 189*(7), 634–639. https://doi.org/10.1093/aje/kwaa013

LiveScience. (2020). *What is epidemiology?* YouTube, April 15, 2020. https://www.youtube.com/watch?v=q-17icRTMyY

Mason, M. (2023). *Epidemiology 101.* EnvironmentalScience.org. https://www.environmentalscience.org/epidemiology

Maynard, J. E. (1978). Passive immunization against Hepatitis B: A review of recent studies and comment on current aspects of control. *American Journal of Epidemiology, 107*(2), 87–90. https://doi.org/10.1093/oxfordjournals.aje.a112520

McGinty, E., Presskreischer, R., Han, H., & Barry, C. L. (2020). Psychological distress and loneliness reported by US adults in 2018 and April 2020. *Journal of the American Medical Association, 324*(1), 93–94. https://jamanetwork.com/journals/jama/fullarticle/2766941

Merriam-Webster Dictionary. (n.d.a.). *Epidemic definition.* https://www.merriam-webster.com/dictionary/epidemic

Merriam-Webster Dictionary. (n.d.b.). *Epidemiology definition.* https://www.merriam-webster.com/dictionary/epidemiology

Merriam-Webster Dictionary. (n.d.c.). *Incidence definition.* https://www.merriam-webster.com/dictionary/incidence

Merriam-Webster Dictionary. (n.d.d.). *Morbidity.* https://www.merriam-webster.com/dictionary/morbidity

Merriam-Webster Dictionary. (n.d.e.). *Mortality.* https://www.merriam-webster.com/dictionary/mortality

Merriam-Webster Dictionary. (n.d.f.). *Pandemic definition.* https://www.merriam-webster.com/dictionary/pandemic

Merriam-Webster Dictionary. (n.d.g.). *Prevalence definition.* https://www.merriam-webster.com/dictionary/prevalence

Merriam-Webster Dictionary. (n.d.h.). *Surveillance definition.* https://www.merriam-webster.com/dictionary/surveillance

Minnesota Department of Health. (2019). *Public health interventions: Application for nursing practice* (2nd ed.). https://www.health.state.mn.us/communities/practice/research/phncouncil/docs/PHInterventions.pdf

Monaghan, T., Rahman, S., Agudelo, C., Wein, A., Lazar, J., Everaert, K., & Dmochowski, R. (2021). Foundational statistical principles in medical research: A tutorial on odds ratios, relative risk, absolute risk, and number needed to treat. *International Journal of Environmental Research and Public Health, 18*(11), 1–11. https://doi.org/10.3390/ijerph18115669

Murray, J., & Cohen, A. (2017). Infectious disease surveillance. *International Encyclopedia of Public Health, 4*, 222–229. http://dx.doi.org/10.1016/B978-0-12-803678-5.00517-8

National Institute on Deafness and Other Communication Disorders. (2011). *What is epidemiology?* https://www.nidcd.nih.gov/health/statistics/what-epidemiology

National Institute of Mental Health. (n.d.). *What is prevalence?* https://www.nimh.nih.gov/health/statistics/what-is-prevalence

Northern Inter-Tribal Health Authority. (n.d.). *Epidemiology.* https://www.nitha.com/epidemiology/

Public Health Agency. (2022). *Incidence vs. prevalence and the epidemiologist's bathtub.* https://www.publichealth.hscni.net/node/5277

Rahul Patwari (Rahul's EM). (2013). *The relationship between incidence and prevalence.* YouTube, July 26, 2013. https://www.youtube.com/watch?v=1jzZe3ORdd8

Roach, J. (2016). *ROOTT's theoretical framework of the web of causation between structural and social determinants of health and wellness—2016.* https://www.roottrj.org/web-causation

Roberts, W., & Landowski, J. (2022). *Endemics, pandemics and epidemics explained.* https://www.baptistjax.com/juice/stories/covid-19/epidemiology-101

Roux, A. (2022). Social epidemiology: Past, present, and future. *Annual Review of Public Health, 43*, 79–98. https://doi.org/10.1146/annurev-publhealth-060220-042648

Rural Health Information Hub. (2018). *Ecologic models.* https://www.ruralhealthinfo.org/toolkits/health-promotion/2/theories-and-models/ecological

Science Museum. (2019). *Epidemiology: The public health science.* https://www.sciencemuseum.org.uk/objects-and-stories/medicine/epidemiology-public-health-science

Swift, H. (2022). *Web of causation: What is it and how to incorporate it?* Wolters Kluwer. https://www.wolterskluwer.com/en/expert-insights/web-of-causation-what-is-it-and-how-to-incorporate-it

Taberna, M., Gil Moncayo, F., Jané-Salas, E., Antonio, M., Arribas, L., Vilajosana, E., Peralvez Torres, E. P., & Mesía, R. (2020). The multidisciplinary team (MDT) approach and quality of care. *Frontiers in Oncology, 10*(85), 1–16. https://doi.org/10.3389/fonc.2020.00085

Tenny, S., & Boktor, S. (2022). *Incidence.* https://www.ncbi.nlm.nih.gov/books/NBK430746/

Tyagi, U., & Barwal, K. C. (2020). Ignac Semmelweis—Father of hand hygiene. *Indian Journal of Surgery, 82*(3), 276–277. https://doi.org/10.1007/s12262-020-02386-6

Ventriglio, A., Bellomo, A., & Bhugra, D. (2016). Web of causation and its implications for epidemiological research. *International Journal of Social Psychiatry, 62*(1), 3–4. https://doi.org/10.1177/0020764015587629

Westreich, D. (2019). *Epidemiology by design: A Monaghan in causal approach to the health sciences.* Oxford University Press.

World Health Organization. (2023). *Influenza surveillance.* https://www.emro.who.int/health-topics/influenza/influenza-surveillance.html

Zajac, S., Woods, A., Tannenbaum, S., Salas, E., & Holladay, C. (2021). Overcoming challenges to teamwork in healthcare: A team effectiveness framework and evidence-based guidance. *Frontiers in Communication, 6,* 1–20. https://doi.org/10.3389/fcomm.2021.606445

Zorić, A. B. (2021). Applied statistics: Basic principles and application. *International Journal of Innovation and Economic Development, 7*(3), 27–33. https://ideas.repec.org/a/mgs/ijoied/v7y2021i3p27-33.html

Zylke, J. W., & Bauchner, H. (2020). Mortality and morbidity: The measure of a pandemic. *Journal of the American Medical Association, 324*(5), 458–459. https://jamanetwork.com/journals/jama/fullarticle/2768085

2 Minute Classroom. (2020). *Endemic vs epidemic vs pandemic. How epidemiologists classify disease prevalence.* YouTube, March 22, 2020. https://www.youtube.com/watch?v=nclAnJXdgqs

Credits

Fig. 6.1: Adapted from Northern Inter-Tribal Health Authority (NITHA), https://www.nitha.com/epidemiology/. Copyright © by Northern Inter-Tribal Health Authority (NITHA).

Fig. 6.2: Centers for Disease Control and Prevention, https://www.cdc.gov/violence-prevention/about/?CDC_AAref_Val=https://www.cdc.gov/violenceprevention/about/social-ecologicalmodel.html, 2022.

Fig. 6.3: ROOTT, https://www.roottrj.org/web-causation. Copyright © 2016 by Restoring Our Own Through Transformation.

Fig. 6.4: Adapted from Public Health Agency, "Epidemiologist's Bathtub," https://www.publichealth.hscni.net/node/5277. Copyright © 2022 by Public Health Agency.

Fig. 6.5: Copyright © by Wellcome (CC BY 4.0) at https://wellcome.org/news/how-can-world-adapt-covid-19-long-term-endemic#gid=ab18&pid=0.

CHAPTER 7

Infectious and Communicable Diseases

The world is slowly transforming into the vaccine haves and the vaccine have-nots. ... This inequity is not just a moral failure but a scientific failure.

—Professor Madhukar Pai, Canada research chair in epidemiology and global health

Learning Outcomes

After reading this chapter, students should be able to:

1. Understand communicable and infectious diseases
2. Apply the six stages of the chain of infection
3. Differentiate between the modes of transmission
4. Apply active, passive, and herd immunity
5. Distinguish between isolation and quarantine
6. Understand the concept of an R-naught value and its importance
7. Distinguish between a nosocomial and a community-acquired infection

Keywords and Concepts

Communicable diseases, community-acquired infection, immunity, infectious diseases, isolation, nosocomial infection, quarantine, R-naught (Ro) values, susceptibility, transmission

Definitions of the Keywords

Communicable diseases: Conditions that cause illnesses and spread from one person to another from individuals or animals (Centers for Disease Control and Prevention [CDC], 2023b)

Community-acquired infection: Infection that occurs without recent inpatient healthcare (CDC, n.d.a.)

Immunity: The ability to resist disease and its related microorganisms (Merriam-Webster, n.d.a.)

Infectious diseases: Diseases that are caused by such microorganisms as bacteria, viruses, parasites, or fungi (World Health Organization [WHO], 2023)

Isolation: the act of separating beings to prevent a crossing of transmission of organisms (Merriam-Webster, n.d.b.)

Nosocomial infection: Subset of infectious diseases acquired in a healthcare facility (Cheung, 2024)

Quarantine: Activities to limit or restrict individuals or products to prevent the spread of disease, especially when a contagious disease is involved (Merriam-Webster, n.d.c.)

R-naught (Ro) value: Values to represent the average number of individuals who can infect, transmit, or spread a communicable disease to a single person (Gunderson & Woskie, 2023)

Susceptibility: Without the ability to resist a pathogen or condition (Merriam-Webster, n.d.d.)

Transmission: The act of transmitting, passing, or sharing a disease process from one to another (Merriam-Webster, n.d.e.)

Introduction

It is essential to understand that "while all communicable diseases are infectious, not all infectious diseases are communicable" (Correll, 2023, para 4). An example of this is tetanus, which can occur when an individual comes in contact with dirt or dust and enters the body through cuts or punctures, spreading the bacteria *Clostridium tetani*. The production of the toxin develops into painful symptoms in the neck and jaw muscles. This leads to an infection but is not a communicable disease (CDC, 2022c). This chapter will discuss aspects of infectious and communicable diseases while looking into how populations can become susceptible to acquiring conditions through transmission. Stages of infection, modes of transmission, and emerging trends will also be discussed.

Background of the Concepts

Vaccinating individuals is essential as new viruses continue to affect the world. The WHO states that as of May 2022, COVID-19 had affected almost 1 billion people in lower-income countries compared with countries with high incomes. Overall, this identified the need to continue providing education and vaccinations to all individuals, emphasizing those older than age 60, healthcare workers, and those with underlying chronic conditions (WHO, 2024b).

The recent increase in monkeypox incidence has become an additional concern worldwide. Its initial presentation was in 1958 through a shipment of rodents from Ghana, Africa; overall, the prevalence recently declined. Luckily, with the availability and administration of vaccines providing protective benefits, a wide outbreak could be prevented (CDC, 2023a; 2023f).

Global communicable diseases have recently increased. International measles cases soared by 79% in the first two months of 2022 compared with 2021. In 2020, 23 million children missed essential childhood vaccines through routine healthcare services, the highest number since 2009 (WHO, 2022b). For example, 13 African countries reported new yellow fever outbreaks in 2021, compared with nine in 2020 and three in 2019 (Johns Hopkins Bloomberg School of Public Health, 2022; WHO, 2022a; WHO, 2022b).

WHO reports an overall issue with infectious disease prevention. The risk for large outbreaks worldwide has increased as communities relaxed social distancing practices and implemented other preventive measures for COVID-19 during the height of the pandemic. In addition, millions of people are being displaced from their homes due to emergency disasters and conflicts. These factors disrupt the routine vaccination schedules of children and adults, and overcrowding in some areas will raise the risk of vaccine-preventable disease outbreaks (WHO, 2022b).

Historical Perspectives

Throughout history, communicable diseases have affected humanity. As the world becomes more populated and connected, so will the risk of more virulent infections, much like the impact of the COVID-19 pandemic (Moore, 2021).

The first recorded pandemic occurred during the Peloponnesian War in Athens, Greece, in 430 B.C., killing almost two-thirds of the population (Moore, 2021). From there, the Antonine Plague emerged in 163 A.D. and is now considered to be an early version of smallpox (Moore, 2021).

Recent history of pandemics included the infamous Black Death of the 14th century. This second and largest outbreak of the bubonic plague claimed the lives of 30%–60% of the European population (Moore, 2021). The Great Plague of London in 1665 caused the deaths of 20% of London's population (Moore, 2021).

Further outbreaks of cholera and human immunodeficiency virus (HIV) have shaped the world's issue with pandemics. There were 50 million deaths resulting from the Spanish flu pandemic in 1918 (Moore, 2021).

The most recent history of a pandemic is COVID-19. The first indication of a new infection was in late 2019 from Wuhan, China. An atypical new pneumonialike illness that wasn't responding to standard treatments was noted. Cases began to spread across the globe, and on March 11, 2020, the WHO declared COVID-19 a pandemic. Since COVID-19 is a virus, it has mutated many times and continues to be a global problem (CDC, 2023c).

Infectious Diseases

Infectious diseases can be grouped into three categories: illnesses that cause high levels of mortality, diseases that place on populations heavy burdens of disability, and diseases that, owing to the rapid and unexpected spread, can have serious global repercussions (WHO, 2023). Many of the critical determinants of health and causes of infectious diseases lie outside the direct control of the health sector. Other sectors involved are sanitation and water supply, environmental and climate change, education, agriculture, trade, tourism, transport, industrial development, and housing (WHO, 2023).

The *natural history of disease* refers to how a disease develops and progresses over time without intervention. Understanding disease progression is essential for implementing prevention measures and understanding how the disease develops. This will allow for identifying the best approaches for screening and diagnosing the disease. Disease progression occurs in four stages (Frontier Nursing University, 2022; Table 7.1).

TABLE 7.1 Stages of a Disease, an Infection, or a Health Condition

Stages	Definitions/Context
Susceptibility	Does not have the disease but is susceptible to it
Preclinical disease, pre-symptomatic, subclinical, or latent	Disease has not started yet, and there are no symptoms. May be detected by screening tests
Clinical disease	Experiences, signs, and symptoms of the disease are clinically apparent; most diseases are diagnosed during this stage
Recovery, disability, or death	Person recovers or dies from the disease; if the person recovers, they may not experience the disease's short- and long-term sequelae

Source: Frontier Nursing University, 2022.

Nosocomial/Community-Acquired Infections

Where infections are acquired can be differentiated between nosocomial and community. *Nosocomial infections* are obtained in a healthcare setting and are referred to as *healthcare-associated infections* (HAI; Monegro et al., 2023). *Community-acquired infections* occur outside of a healthcare facility (SingHealth, 2021). A thorough assessment of the client upon admission or during an initial encounter is critical to understanding where the infection originated.

R-Naught Values

R-naught (Ro) values provide needed insight into the potential spread of a disease that local, state, and national governments and public health authorities can use to factor into their decision-making to control the disease best. Also, since it can be calculated for various diseases, it allows us to contextualize an outbreak with ones we have seen previously, such as severe acute respiratory syndrome (SARS), Middle Eastern respiratory syndrome (MERS), Ebola, acquired immunodeficiency syndrome (AIDS), seasonal flu, and the 2009 H1N1 flu pandemic (Gunderson & Woskie, 2023).

There are three main factors used to calculate Ro. Factors include the infectious period of the disease, mode of transmission, and contact rate. The *infectious period* is when an infected person can transmit that infection to another human, meaning the length of time for which a person with the disease is contagious. Longer infectious periods mean higher Ro values. The *mode of transmission* is how the disease spreads. Airborne infections, such as the flu, will spread more quickly than those requiring physical contact to be transmitted, such as HIV and Ebola. Therefore, airborne infections have higher Ro values (Gunderson & Woskie, 2023).

The *contact rate* refers to how many people a person with the disease can be expected to come into contact with it. This variable is not specific to a disease like the first two. Instead, it is affected by numerous factors, including location and public health measures in place, such as quarantines and travel bans. This factor is modifiable (Gunderson & Woskie, 2023; Box 7.1).

BOX 7.1 ACTIVE LEARNING REFLECTION ACTIVITY

Investigating the Ro Values of Common Infectious Diseases

Investigate the Ro values of the following infectious diseases. Use the following websites to complete the activity:

- https://transportgeography.org/contents/applications transportation-pandemics/basic-reproduction-number- r0-of-major-infectious-diseases/
- https://doi.org/10.1186/s40001-023-01047-0

Disease	**Number/Range**
Measles:	______________
Pertussis:	______________
Ebola:	______________
Chickenpox:	______________
Rubella:	______________
COVID-19 (first version):	______________
COVID-19 (later version):	______________

Follow-up: Based on your findings, create a social marketing flyer emphasizing the importance of averting an epidemic for the disease with the highest Ro number. Use two evidence-based sites/articles to support your position.

American Association of Colleges of Nursing (AACN) *Essentials* (2021): Domains: #1; #3; #4

- Competencies: 1.1; 1.2; 1.3; 3.1; 3.3; 3.6; 4.2
- Subcompetencies: 1.1b; 1.2a; 1.3a; 1.3b; 3.1b; 3.1c; 3.1f; 3.3b; 3.6a; 3.6c; 3.6d; 3.6e; 4.2c

Spheres of Care: Wellness/Disease prevention

Concepts: Communication; Clinical judgment; Evidence-based practice

Sources: Karimizadeh et al., 2023; Geography of Transport Systems, 2023.

Immunity

Immunity to a disease is achieved through antibodies in a person's system. *Antibodies* are proteins the body produces to neutralize or destroy toxins or disease-carrying organisms. Antibodies are disease specific. For example, measles antibodies will protect a person exposed to measles but have no effect if exposed to mumps (CDC, 2021b).

Active Immunity (Natural Versus Acquired)

Active immunity occurs when exposure to a disease organism triggers the immune system to produce antibodies to that disease. Active immunity can be acquired through natural or vaccine-induced immunity (CDC, 2021b).

- Natural active immunity is acquired from exposure to the disease organism through infection with the actual disease.
- Vaccine-induced natural immunity is acquired through vaccination by introducing a killed or weakened form of the disease organism (CDC, 2021b).

Either way, if an immune person comes into contact with that disease in the future, their immune system will recognize it and immediately produce the antibodies needed to fight it. Active immunity is long-lasting and sometimes lifelong (CDC, 2021b).

Passive Immunity (Natural Versus Acquired)

Passive immunity is provided when a person is given antibodies to a disease rather than producing them through their immune system (CDC, 2021b).

- A newborn baby acquires passive natural immunity from its mother through the placenta.
- People can also receive passive acquired immunity through antibody-containing blood products such as immune globulin, which may be given when immediate protection from a specific disease is needed (CDC, 2021b).

The significant advantage of passive immunity is that protection is immediate, whereas active immunity takes time (usually several weeks) to develop. However, passive immunity lasts only for a few weeks or months. Only active immunity is long-lasting (CDC, 2021b; Box 7.2).

BOX 7.2 ACTIVE LEARNING REFLECTION ACTIVITY

Different Types of Immunity

Use the following two links to complete the activity:

- https://www.youtube.com/watch?v=yvKENnMUxLA
- https://www.cdc.gov/vaccines/vac-gen/immunity-types.htm

Active natural: ______________________________

Active acquired: ______________________________

Passive natural: ______________________________

Passive acquired: ______________________________

Follow-up: Create a detailed teaching plan for future mothers on the importance of passive natural immunity. Use two evidence-based resources to support your teaching plan and the importance of passive natural immunity.

AACN *Essentials* (2021): Domains: #1; #2; #3; #4; #5

- Competencies: 1.3; 2.2; 2.5; 3.1; 4.2; 5.1
- Subcompetencies: 1.3a; 1.3b; 1.3c; 2.2e; 2.5c; 2.5d; 3.1a; 3.1c; 3.1f; 4.2c; 5.1c; 5.1f

Spheres of Care: Wellness/Disease prevention

Concepts: Evidence-based practice; Clinical judgment

Sources: CDC, 2021b; Dr Matt & Dr Mike, 2019.

Herd Immunity

Herd immunity is the indirect protection from an infectious disease that happens when a population is immune through vaccination or an immunity developed through previous infection. The WHO supports achieving herd immunity through vaccination rather than allowing disease to spread through any population segment, as the latter would result in unnecessary cases and deaths. Achieving herd immunity with safe and effective vaccines makes diseases rarer and saves lives (WHO, 2023).

Achieving herd immunity for a particular disease differs for each one, depending on the Ro value. For example, herd immunity against measles requires about 95% of the population to be vaccinated. The remaining 5% will be protected because measles will not spread among vaccinated people. For polio, the threshold is about 80%. The proportion of the population who must be immunized against COVID-19 to begin inducing herd immunity is unknown (WHO, 2020a).

Communicable Diseases

Communicable diseases spread from one person or animal to another or from a surface to a person. They are the result of pathogens, such as viruses and bacteria. Communicable diseases include colds and the flu. They can be transmitted through bodily fluids, insect bites, contaminated surfaces, water, food, or the air (Medical News Today, 2023).

Spreading of Communicable Diseases

Three things are required for an infection to occur. First, a source (e.g., the infectious agent) must exist. Examples of infectious agents are viruses or bacteria. Next, there needs to be a way for the agent to cause the infection (e.g., a susceptible person). Lastly, there must be a means for the agent to be moved from the susceptible person (e.g., contact, spraying, or inhalation; CDC, 2016).

The chain of infection is a set of six intertwined links that describe how communicable diseases spread. Each step of the chain is required to transmit infectious illness effectively. Breaking any of the six links inhibits the spread of an infectious disease (Texas Health and Human Services [THHS], 2021a; Figure 7.1).

Pathogens

Four main types of *pathogens* cause infection. These are viruses, bacteria, fungi, and protozoa. These pathogens are different in many ways, but they have one main similarity: Once they are inside you, they can damage cells or interfere with the body's everyday activities (Koo, 2023; Figure 7.2).

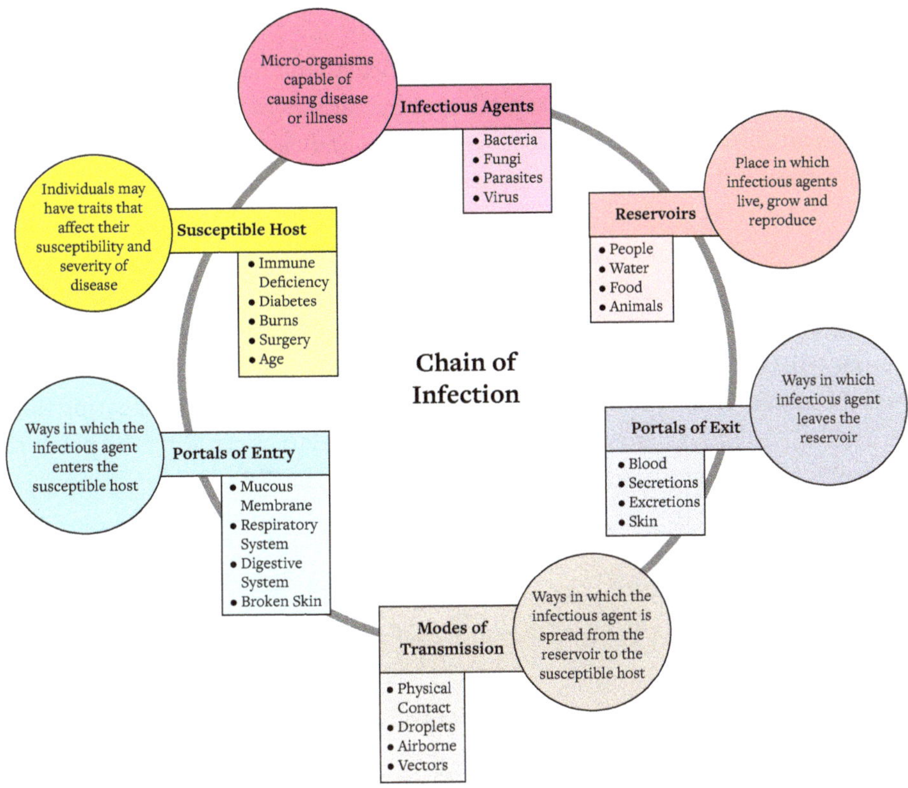

FIGURE 7.1 Six Stages of the Chain of Infection

Type of pathogen	Description	Human diseases caused by pathogens of that type
Bacteria *Escherichia coli*	Single-celled organisms without a nucleus	Strep throat, staph infections, tuberculosis, food poisoning, tetanus, pneumonia, syphilis
Viruses *Herpes simplex*	Thread-like particles that reproduce by taking over living cells	Common cold, flu, genital herpes, cold sores, measles, AIDS, genital warts, chiken pox, small pox
Fungi *Death cap mushroom*	Simple organisms, including mushrooms and yeasts, that grow as single cells or thread like filaments	Ringworm, athlete's foot, tinea, candidiasis, histoplasmosis, mushroom poisoning
Protozoa *Giardia lamblia*	Single-celled organism with a nucleus	Malaria, "traveler's diarrhea" giardiasis, trypanosomiasis ("sleeping sickness")

FIGURE 7.2 Types of Pathogens

Bacteria

Bacteria are single-cell organisms that are critical to maintaining our ecosystem. The human body contains a vast number of bacteria, which are relatively harmless. Harmful bacteria are noted as pathogenic and cause issues in the human body (National Human Genome Research Institute [NHGRI], 2024a). Examples of specific bacteria are *Escherichia coli* O157:H7 (*E. coli*), *Salmonella*, *Staph*, *Strep*, and *H. pylori* (Cleveland Clinic, 2022).

Antibiotics are used for bacterial infections. However, there has been a significant rise in antimicrobial-resistant infections, especially in the community setting (CDC, 2021b). This resistance can spread between people, animals, and food through everyday activities, making identifying, tracking, and treating them hard (CDC, 2021b). Community education is critical to controlling the phenomenon of resistant bacterial infections (CDC, 2021c; Box 7.3).

BOX 7.3 ACTIVE LEARNING REFLECTION ACTIVITY

Educating the Community on Bacteria Resistance Problems

A nursing student is doing a community health rotation at a health department. The community nurse states that there has been a considerable increase in antimicrobial resistance to many diseases in the local community. The nurse asks the student to create a handout for prescribed antibiotics clients. Use the following website and other evidence-based resources to complete the activity: https://www.cdc.gov/drugresistance/communities.html.

First, answer the following proposed questions. Then, create an educational handout for those prescribed antibiotics.

1. What specific details will the nursing student include in the pamphlet? List at least five items.
2. What criteria will the nursing student use to write the pamphlet so that clients can comprehend the education?
3. What population has the highest prevalence of antibiotic resistance?

AACN *Essentials* (2021): Domains: #1; #2; #3; #4; #5; #8

- Competencies: 1.1; 1.2; 1.3; 2.2; 2.5; 2.8; 3.1; 4.2; 5.1; 8.2
- Subcompetencies: 1.1b; 1.2a; 1.3a; 1.3b; 1.3c; 2.2e; 2.5c; 2.5d; 2.8a; 2.8b; 2.8c; 3.1b; 3.1c; 3.1f; 4.2c; 5.1a; 5.1c; 8.2c; 8.2d

Spheres of Care: Wellness/Disease prevention; Chronic disease management

Concepts: Clinical judgment; Evidence-based practice; Communication; SDOH; Diversity, equity and inclusion (DEI)

Source: CDC, 2021c.

Viruses

A *virus* is a microbe consisting of a segment of nucleic acid (either DNA or RNA) that cannot replicate alone. Instead, it must infect cells, use components of the host cell to make copies of itself, and kill the host cell. Viruses include COVID-19, hepatitis, HIV, measles, influenza, and smallpox (NHGRI, 2024b).

Antiviral medications help combat certain viruses that can cause disease. They can also be preventive and protect from getting and spreading the disease. Unlike antibiotics, antiviral drugs work on one type of virus (Cleveland Clinic, 2021).

Fungus

There are millions of types of fungi; however, only a few make an individual sick. Fungi reside outdoors, such as in soil and on plants. They can also be indoors in places such as the air or on surfaces. Fungi can also inhabit an individual's skin and body. Examples of fungi are mold, yeast, and mushrooms (CDC, 2019).

Fungi infections are challenging to treat and manage. Fungal diseases are common in the nails, mouth, skin, and vaginal areas. There are both topical and oral fungal treatments, but oral provides the best avenue to eliminate the issue. Individuals must take the drug for several weeks to months (CDC, 2023g).

Protozoa

Protozoas are one type of parasite that infects the human body. They are one-celled organisms that can be free-living or parasitic. They multiply in humans, permitting them to cause serious infections. The transmission of protozoa that live in a human's intestine to another human could occur through contaminated food or water or person-to-person contact. Protozoa that live in the blood or tissue of humans could be transmitted through the bite of a mosquito or sandfly (CDC, 2022b).

Reservoir

Pathogens must have an environment/habitat where a pathogen can live and multiply. Environmental surfaces/equipment, body fluids (blood, saliva), urine/fecal material, food/water, soil, skin, and respiratory tract are all examples of reservoirs (CDC, 2022a).

Breaking the chain is the key to limiting the spread. Cleaning, disinfecting, and sterilization could help with this issue. Effective infection policies at highly populated places and routine pest control could also help with environment/habitat problems (Association of Professionals in Infection Control and Epidemiology [APIC], n.d.).

BOX 7.4 ACTIVE LEARNING REFLECTION ACTIVITY

Foodborne Education

There has been a steady yearly increase in hospitalization and deaths of younger children in a community regarding foodborne illnesses. Visit the following link: https://www.cdc.gov/foodsafety/keep-food-safe.html. Develop a primary prevention public service announcement for young adult parents regarding the importance of food safety.

AACN *Essentials* (2021): Domains: #1; #2; #3; #8

- Competencies: 1.1; 1.3; 2.2; 2.5; 3.1; 3.5; 3.6; 8.1; 8.3; 8.4
- Subcompetencies: 1.1b; 1.3a; 1.3b; 1.3c; 2.2c; 2.2e; 2.5d; 3.1a; 3.1b; 3.1c; 3.1e; 3.5d; 3.6a; 3.6b; 3.6c; 8.1a; 8.1b; 8.1c; 8.1d; 8.3a; 8.4c

Spheres of Care: Wellness/Disease prevention

Concepts: Evidence-based practice; Communication; Clinical judgment

Sources: CDC, 2023d; 2023e.

The United States has one of the safest drinking water supplies in the world; however, water used for drinking, swimming, and even cooling high-rise buildings could be safer. About 7.2 million Americans become sick yearly from diseases spread through water (CDC, 2023h). Further policy and safety initiatives must be implemented to protect American citizens.

Foodborne diseases are also an issue in the United States. The CDC estimates that 48 million people get sick from these illnesses each year, 128,000 are hospitalized, and 3,000 die in the United States (CDC, 2023d). Unfortunately, some foodborne illnesses are antibiotic-resistant, making them hard to treat. Educating using primary prevention concerning food safety is vital to decreasing hospitalization and death from foodborne diseases (Box 7.4).

Vectors are living organisms that can transmit infectious pathogens between humans or from animals to humans. Mosquitoes, ticks, and fleas are some of the most common vectors. The vector ingests disease-producing microorganisms during a blood meal from an infected host (human or animal) and later transmits them to a new host after the pathogen has replicated. An infected vector can often transmit the pathogen for the rest of its life during each subsequent bite/blood meal (WHO, 2020b).

About 17% of the global infections are vector-borne (WHO, 2020b). Vector-borne diseases can be caused by parasites, viruses, or bacteria (WHO, 2024b). Education about primary or secondary prevention strategies is critical to preventing vector-borne diseases (Figure 7.3).

Preventing Vector Borne Diseases

What are Vector Borne Diseases?

Vector-borne diseases are illnesses spread by vectors, small organisms like:

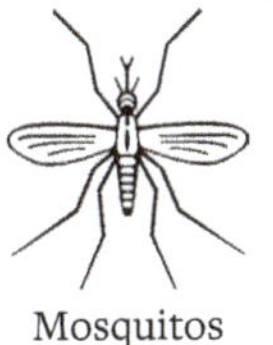

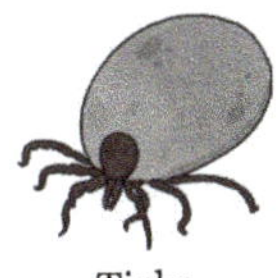

Vector-borne diseases include:

- Malaria
- Lyme disease
- Zika
- West Nile Virus
- Dengue Fever
- Yellow Fever
- Rocky Mountain Spotted Fever

How Can Vector-Borne Disease Be Prevented?

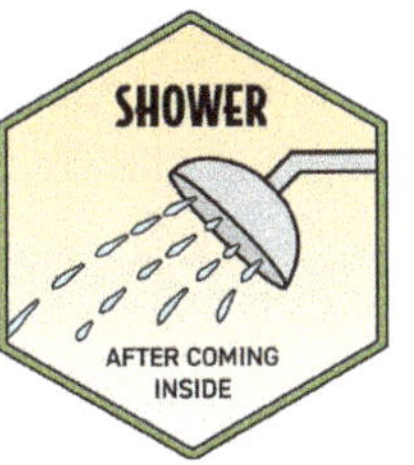

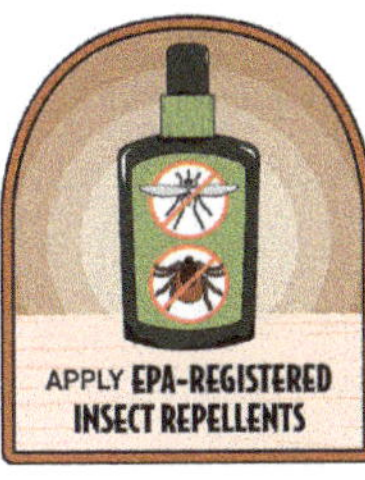

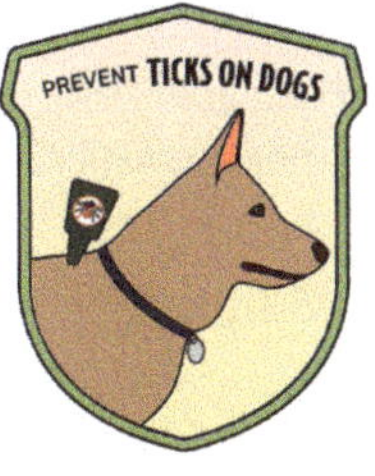

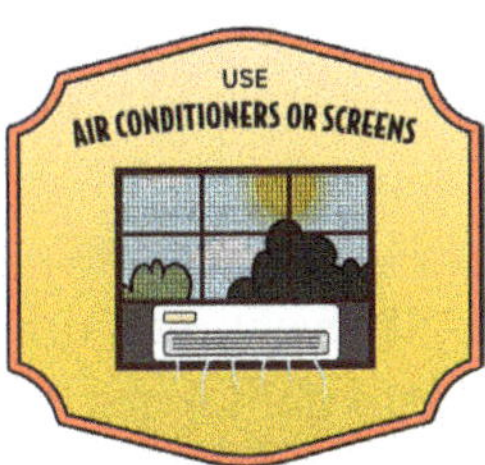

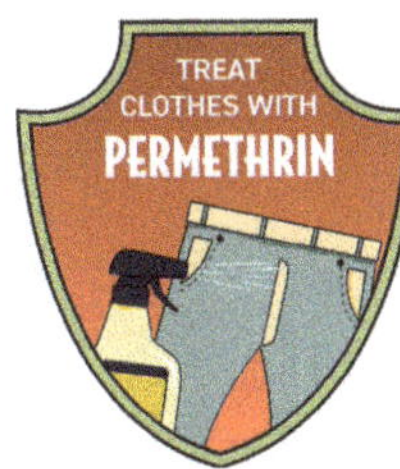

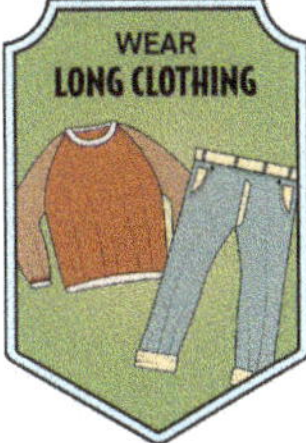

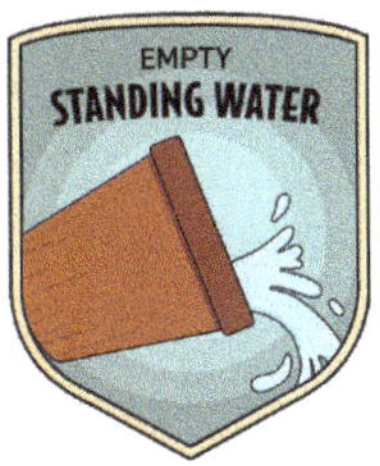

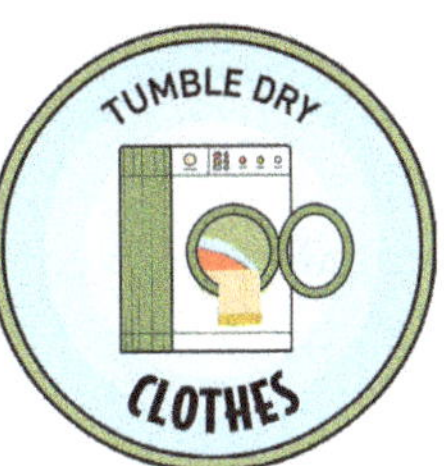

FIGURE 7.3 Vector-Borne Information

Portal of Exit

The *portal of exit* is the route that the pathogen takes to leave its current host. The exit route can include sneezing/coughing, body secretions, and feces (THHS, 2021a). In humans, the leading portals of exit include the alimentary system (vomiting, diarrhea, saliva), genitourinary system (sexual contact), respiratory system (secretions from coughing, sneezing, or talking, and open skin wounds; THHS, 2021a).

There are many ways to decrease a portal of exit: following effective hand hygiene practices, using appropriate personal protective equipment, controlling aerosols and splatters, using suitable respiratory etiquette (sneezing into the arm and not the hand; using a tissue), and properly disposing of contaminated objects (APIC, n.d.). The key is to teach the population adequate ways to manage and break the infectious process.

Mode of Transmission

The *mode of transmission* is how a pathogen is transferred. This can be accomplished through direct contact (e.g., inhaling a droplet containing flu virus), indirect contact (e.g., touching a remote that has *C. difficile* spores attached), or vectors (e.g., ticks transmitting the bacteria responsible for Lyme disease; THHS, 2021a).

Zoonoses

Zoonosis is an infectious disease that has spread from a nonhuman animal to a human. Zoonotic pathogens may be bacterial, viral, or parasitic and can spread to humans through direct contact with food, water, or the environment. Globally, zoonoses are a problem due to animals, agriculture, and the natural environment. Zoonoses can also disrupt the production and trade of animal products for food and other uses (WHO, 2020c).

Prevention is the basis for preventing the spread of zoonosis. Safe and appropriate guidelines for animal care in the agricultural sector help reduce the potential for foodborne zoonotic disease outbreaks through foods (meat, eggs, dairy, or some vegetables). Standards for clean drinking water, waste removal, and surface water protection in the natural environment are also essential and effective. Education campaigns to promote handwashing after contact with animals could reduce a community's spread of zoonotic diseases (WHO, 2020c; Figure 7.4).

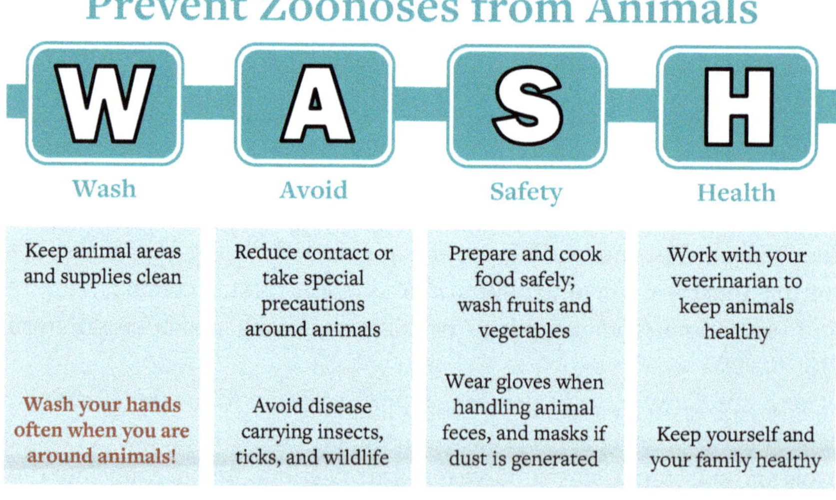

FIGURE 7.4 Zoonoses Prevention

Parasitic Diseases

Protozoa, as discussed earlier, is a type of *parasite disease*. Two other common parasite diseases are helminths and ectoparasites. *Helminth groups* include roundworms, flatworms, and thorny-headed worms. *Ectoparasites* can include blood-sucking arthropods such as mosquitoes. Still, this term is generally used more narrowly to refer to organisms such as ticks, fleas, lice, and mites that attach or burrow into the skin and remain there for extended periods (CDC, 2022b).

Parasites are treated with antiparasitic drugs. The type of parasite determines which medications can be used. Overall health, age, weight, and other factors are considered regarding treatment. A healthcare provider must also consider overall health, age, weight, and other factors. In some areas of the world, different parasites resist one type of treatment (e.g., malaria; Koo, 2023).

Portal of Entry

The *portal of entry* is the pathogen's route to the new host. It is usually through a mucus membrane on the face but can be any route that allows entry inside the body. Pathogens enter the body through a host. This can happen through breathing, blood, contact, food/water, the fecal/oral route, and physical contact (Koo, 2023).

If the pathogen finds a mode of transmission, many precautions and interventions can be implemented to block the portal of entry. Mitigation interventions such as appropriate masks and eye protection can be used. Skin breaks can be covered and cleaned immediately. Removing equipment and items such as catheters and drains/tubes will prevent a more accessible portal of entry (Windsor, 2022).

Susceptible Host

The new host may become infected and continue the cycle again. Many human factors can affect the susceptibility to infection. Those circumstances/persons who are considered more susceptible are:

- The person at risk: client or healthcare worker
- Age: very young or very old
- Health/nutrition: unhealthy, malnourished, poor cough/sneeze reflexes
- Immune system: use of immune-suppressing medications
- Infective dose: nonintact mucous membranes or skin, exposure time/amount (CDC, 2022a; THHS, 2021b)

Interventions for Containment

Keeping infectious and communicable diseases under control involves many steps. Surveillance of outbreaks and identifying where those who are infected is critical. Contact tracing identifies, assesses, and manages people exposed to a disease to prevent onward transmission (WHO, 2024a). Effective contact tracing provides necessary follow-up actions such as diagnostic tests, postexposure prophylaxis, and quarantine (WHO, 2024a). Contact tracing is an effective public health tool. However, additional evidence is needed to inform how, where, and when to deploy this tool most effectively for maximum effect in disease control (Hossain et al., 2022).

Isolation Versus Quarantine

When an infectious disease is present, isolation or quarantine must occur. *Isolation* is used when a contagious/sick individual is moved away from other people who are not ill. *Quarantine* separates and restricts the movement of people exposed to a contagious disease to see if they become sick. These people may have been exposed to an illness and do not know it or may have the condition but do not show symptoms (Department of Health and Human Services, 2022; Box 7.5).

BOX 7.5 ACTIVE LEARNING REFLECTION ACTIVITY

Isolation Versus Quarantine

There has been an increase in COVID-19 outbreaks at the local public health department. As the nursing student assigned to the infectious/communicable disease department, you are asked to develop and present a 10-minute podcast to be posted on the health department website. Create a podcast with appropriate information that is education-specific and culturally appropriate. Focus the podcast on the difference between isolation and quarantine. Discuss three primary prevention strategies. Provide other pertinent information critical for the public.

Use the following video to get started: https://www.hhs.gov/answers/public-health-and-safety/what-is-the-difference-between-isolation-and-quarantine/index.html.

AACN *Essentials* (2021): Domains: #1; #2; #3; #4; #7; #8

- Competencies: 1.1; 2.2; 2.4; 3.1; 4.1; 7.3; 8.1; 8.2; 8.4
- Subcompetencies: 1.1b; 1.1d; 2.2a; 2.2b; 2.2c; 2.2e; 2.4a; 2.4d; 3.1a; 3.1c; 3.1d; 3.1e; 3.1f; 3.1g; 4.1c; 7.3a; 7.3b; 7.3c; 7.3d; 8.1a; 8.1d; 8.2a; 8.2b; 8.2c; 8.2d; 8.4a

Spheres of Care: Wellness/Disease prevention; Chronic disease management

Concepts: Communication; Social determinants of health (SDOH); Diversity, equity, and inclusion (DEI); Evidence-based practice

Source: CDC, 2020.

Emerging and Reemerging Infectious Diseases and Global Trends

According to the National Institute of Allergy and Infectious Diseases, *emerging infectious diseases* are commonly defined as outbreaks of previously unknown diseases (such as COVID-19), known diseases that increase incidence rates, or persistent uncontrolled infectious diseases (2018). Emerging diseases include

BOX 7.6 ACTIVE LEARNING REFLECTION ACTIVITY

Teaching Plan Regarding Immunizations

Immunization rates are decreasing in the community, especially the measles, mumps, and rubella (MMR) vaccine. Develop a teaching pamphlet for parents of a rural area where MMR rates have increased by 5% in the past five years. Address the following points in the pamphlet to provide an evidence-based approach:

1. Note the importance and definition of herd immunity.
2. Note the concept of Ro values for the three communicable diseases.
3. Research the overall characteristics of rural populations to provide a practical educational approach.

Use the following articles to assist with this activity:

- Albers, A. N., Thaker, J., & Newcomer, S. R. (2022). Barriers to and facilitators of early childhood immunization in rural areas of the United States: A systematic review of the literature. *Preventive Medicine Reports*, *27*, 101804. https://doi.org/10.1016/j.pmedr.2022.101804
- Albers, A. N., Wright, E., Thaker, J., Conway, K., Daley, M. F., & Newcomer, S. R. (2023). Childhood vaccination practices and parental hesitancy barriers in rural and urban primary care settings. *Journal of Community Health*, *48*(5), 798–809. https://doi.org/10.1007/s10900-023-01226-4

AACN *Essentials* (2021): Domains: #1; #2; #3; #4; #8

- Competencies: 1.1; 1.2; 1.3; 2.2; 2.8; 3.1; 3.3; 3.4; 3.5; 3.6; 4.2; 8.1; 8.3
- Subcompetencies: 1.1b; 1.1d; 1.2a; 1.3a; 2.2b; 2.2c; 2.2e; 2.8c; 2.8d; 3.1a; 3.1b; 3.1c; 3.1d; 3.1h; 3.3b; 3.4c; 3.5d; 3.6a; 3.6c; 4.2c; 8.1a; 8.3a; 8.3c

Spheres of Care: Wellness/Disease prevention

Concepts: Communication; Evidence-based practice; Clinical judgment; SDOH

Source: Albers et al., 2022; 2023.

HIV infections, SARS, Lyme disease, *E. coli*, hantavirus, dengue fever, West Nile virus, and the Zika virus (Johns Hopkins Medicine, n.d.).

Reemerging diseases reappear after they have been on a significant decline. Returning diseases may happen from reasons such as public health measures that are not intact, new strains, and human behavior issues such as the overuse of antibiotics for problems that do not warrant the usage. Reemerging diseases include malaria, tuberculosis, cholera, pertussis, influenza, pneumococcal disease, and gonorrhea (Johns Hopkins Medicine, n.d.).

Decreasing immunization rates have now caused the reemergence of certain infectious diseases. Disruptions caused by the COVID-19 pandemic have contributed to declining vaccination uptake (Hamson et al., 2023). Low vaccine uptake and/or coverage can have many causes, such as a lack of vaccination policy, political conflicts, parental vaccine refusal, vaccine procurement problems, antivaccination sentiments, vaccine safety concerns, and changes in vaccine schedule. Low vaccination rates have increased the infectious disease burden, particularly in vulnerable populations (Hamson et al., 2023).

Social Determinants of Health and Infectious and Communicable Diseases

An unidisciplinary approach to infectious disease control is no longer sufficient in light of emerging and re-emerging infections and is required. Working with others can identify practical ways to address all the factors in the emergence and persistence of infectious diseases. The significant influence of the SDOH on rates of infectious and noninfectious disease and mortality must be recognized and applied (Butler-Jones & Wong, 2016).

A perfect illustration of the influence of the SDOH on infectious and communicable diseases can be illustrated with tuberculosis and COVID-19. Socioeconomic status, environmental conditions, food insecurity, alcohol consumption, smoking, drug consumption, comorbidities such as AIDS and mental disease, and incarceration seem to predispose people to develop tuberculosis (TB; Duarte et al., 2021). Many SDOHs, such as poverty, physical environment, and racial and ethnic discrimination, can considerably affect COVID-19 outcomes (Duarte et al., 2021; Figure 7.5).

Associated with the SDOH is the issue of health equity and infectious and communicable diseases. Local health departments and officials should focus on addressing this issue. Local health partners should start collecting data on races, ethnicities, genders, health insurance statuses, ZIP codes, primary languages, and disability statuses, as national data reporting does not have fields that address health equity issues (Leach, 2023).

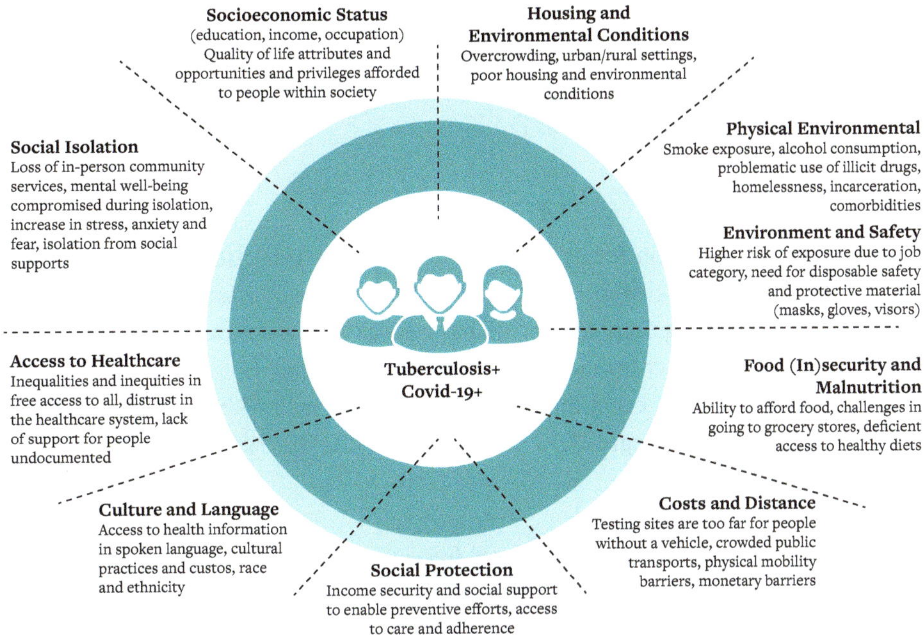

FIGURE 7.5 Social Determinants for TB and COVID-19

Levels of Prevention and Infectious and Communicable Diseases

Applying the levels of prevention, mainly primary and secondary, is critical to containing infection and communicable diseases. Levels of prevention need to occur at all three levels of government (local, state, national, and global). By investing in preventive care and implementing these strategies, healthcare providers can play an essential role in disease prevention and contribute to the well-being of individuals, families, communities, and populations globally (AbdulRaheem, 2023).

Primary

The WHO is invested in global health through infection control programs (ICPs) and has called on all countries around the globe to increase their investment in ICPs to ensure quality of care and clients' and health workers' safety. This will protect their populations, and increased investment in ICPs has also been demonstrated to improve health outcomes and reduce healthcare costs and out-of-pocket expenses (WHO, 2022c). By initiating simple, cost-effective practices such as good hand hygiene, 70% of those infections can be prevented (WHO, 2022c).

Nursing students can provide valuable assistance in the primary prevention of infectious and contagious diseases. Many schools have only part-time nurses or none at all. Academic-community partnerships with schools could assist with increasing the overall education of school-aged individuals regarding hand hygiene. By providing practical education to this population, nursing students can also benefit by increasing their knowledge and application of the subject while becoming better educators (Perry et al., 2021).

Secondary and Tertiary

The primary prevention focus should always be on infectious and communicable diseases. Healthcare providers should use a wide variety of public health approaches. Screening early for the disease is critical to containing its spread to other members of the community, especially susceptible hosts. Early treatment is crucial to preventing complications. Understanding and implementing quarantine or isolation strategies will assist in the wide distribution of the disease (Open University, 2024).

Immunization Schedules for Children and Adults

Each year, the CDC updates immunization schedules for both children and adults. Healthcare providers must use the updated immunization schedule to enhance their knowledge of current immunization practices and provide the best education to populations. Healthcare providers can utilize updated apps for the new schedule that can be added to devices to ensure quick and easy access (CDC, 2024). Current immunization schedules can be found at https://www.cdc.gov/vaccines/schedules/index.html.

Noncommunicable Diseases

Discussion about noncommunicable diseases (NCDs) will be limited in this chapter. The relationship between SDOH factors, social injustice, health inequality, and health disparities lends further to the number of NCDs. NCDs, such as heart disease, cancer, chronic respiratory disease, and diabetes, are the leading cause of death worldwide and represent an emerging global health threat. Deaths from NCDs now exceed all communicable disease deaths combined. NCDs kill 41 million people every year, equivalent to more than seven out of every 10 deaths worldwide. Changing social, economic, and structural factors such as more people moving to cities and the spread of unhealthy lifestyles have fueled the NCD crisis that kills 15 million people prematurely—before age 70—each year. The high burden of NCDs among working-age people leads to high healthcare costs, limited ability to work, and financial insecurity (CDC, 2021a; Figure 7.6).

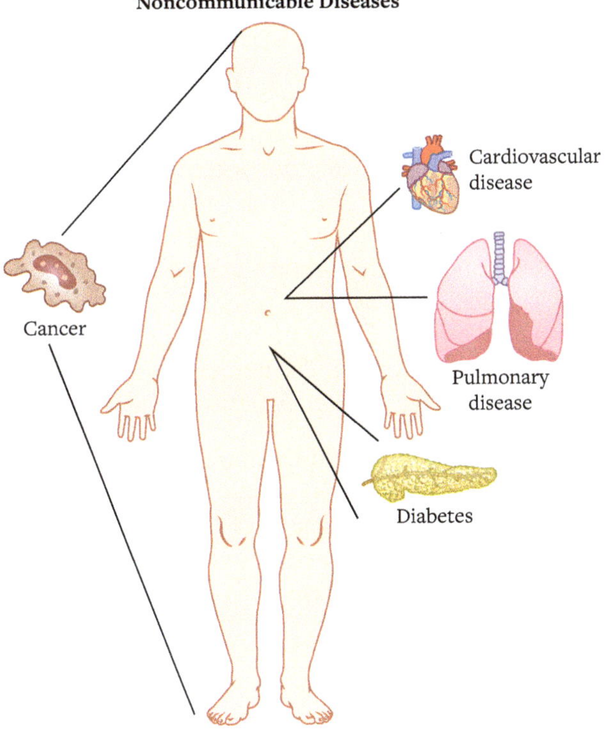

FIGURE 7.6 Examples of Noncommunicable Diseases

Chapter Highlights

- Explanation of the stages of a disease or infection
- Discussion of the chain of infection
- Active learning application of Ro
- Active learning application of types of immunity
- Active learning application of immunization education
- Active learning application of bacteria resistance problems
- Active learning application of foodborne education
- Active learning application of isolation versus quarantine
- Case studies related to intervention wheel, communicable diseases, outbreak investigation, and measles
- Explanation of the difference between communicable and noncommunicable diseases

Active Learning Exercises

Application to Intervention Wheel

Read the following case study and answer the proposed questions. Use the following link to assist with this learning activity: https://www.health.state.mn.us/communities/practice/ta/phnresidency/casestudies/docs/OutbreakInvestigation-Preceptor.pdf.

A nurse at a summer camp for adolescents observed an excessive number of people at the camp seeking help for diarrhea and/or vomiting. Typically, two or three campers per week report to the health office with these symptoms; however, 23 campers and staff sought help in a two-day span. The nurse reported the increased incidence to the camp manager and the local health department, and the camp was closed.

1. What type of education should the nurse provide campers and staff as they go home?
2. What could be some possible causes of the outbreak?
3. What sort of investigation process should take place?
4. What part of the intervention wheel is noted here?

Provide a step-by-step plan for instituting contact tracing and surveillance of the cause of the outbreak, including education for the dismissed campers and their families.

AACN *Essentials* (2021): Domains: #1; #2; #3; #8; #9

- Competencies: 1.1; 1.3; 2.3; 2.9; 3.1; 3.2; 3.6; 8.3; 9.2
- Subcompetencies: 1.1b; 1.3a; 2.3a; 2.3b; 2.9a; 2.9b; 2.9e; 3.1a; 3.1b; 3.1c; 3.1e; 3.1f; 3.2a; 3.2b; 3.6a; 3.6c; 3.6d; 3.6e; 8.3a; 8.3c; 9.2c

Spheres of Care: Wellness/Disease prevention

Concepts: Communication; SDOH; Compassionate care; Clinical judgment

Source: Adapted from Minnesota Department of Health, 2019.

Case Studies

Case Study #1: Application to Communicable/Infectious Diseases: Reverse Case Studies

A nursing student is assigned four communicable diseases to investigate for an assignment. Use the following outline to complete the requirements for the listed communicable diseases. Be specific in your understanding of these diseases.

Once completed, take one communicable disease and write a reverse case study on it. Use the following links to assist with reverse case studies:

- https://evolve.elsevier.com/education/expertise/build-knowledge/using-reverse-case-studies-for-clinical-learning/
- https://www.wolterskluwer.com/en/expert-insights/the-reverse-case-study

AACN *Essentials* (2021): Domains: #1; #3; #4

- Competencies: 1.1; 1.2; 1.3; 3.1; 4.2
- Subcompetencies: 1.1b; 1.2a; 1.3a; 1.3b; 1.3c; 3.1a; 3.1b; 3.1c; 3.1f; 4.2c

Spheres of Care: Wellness/Disease prevention

Concepts: Evidence-based practice; Clinical judgment; Communication

Sources: Silvestri, n.d.; Wolters Kluwer, 2021.

Outline to Use for Case Study #1 Assignment

Communicable Disease	Route of Transmission	S/S (3) (Specific to Disease) Incubation Period	Treatment (1)/Nursing Interventions Specific to Disease (2)	R-Naught Value (if Applicable)	Vaccination Available. If So, When Is It Administered?
Pertussis					
Varicella					
Rotavirus					
Malaria					

Source: Adapted from in-class activity created by authors.

Case Study #2: Solving the Outbreak (CDC)

Understanding how to address infectious and communicable disease outbreaks is critical to preventing further transmission. Go to the following website and solve the outbreak under Level 1, "Birthday Party Gone Bad": https://www.cdc.gov/digital-social-media-tools/mobile/applications/sto/web-app.html.

Reflect on the following questions:

1. What two specific points did you learn about and why?
2. How will you use this activity/case study for your future nursing practice?

AACN *Essentials* (2021): Domains: #1; #3; #4; #8

- Competencies: 1.1; 3.1; 3.6; 4.1c; 8.3
- Subcompetencies: 1.1a; 3.1a; 3.1b; 3.1c; 3.1e; 3.1; 3.6a; 3.6b; 3.6c; 4.2c; 8.3a; 8.3b; 8.3c; 8.3e

Spheres of Care: Wellness/Disease prevention

Concepts: Clinical judgment; Compassionate care; Evidence-based practice; Communication

Source: CDC, n.d.b.

Case Study #3: Application of Infectious Disease: Measles

The community instructor assigns the following article to population health nursing students: Kongthavonsakul, K., Henry, C. H., & Oberdorfer, P. (2012). A 6-year-old boy with fever, rash and severe pneumonia. *BMJ Case Reports*, bcr1220115411. https://doi.org/10.1136/bcr.12.2011.5411

Reflect on the following questions after reading the article:

1. Explain the importance of vaccination history and contact sourcing.
2. Discuss briefly what clinical characteristics and treatments were used.
3. What are two priority points that you learned about and why?
4. How will you use this activity for your future nursing practice?
5. How could information from this article be used today as measles cases are on the rise around the globe?

AACN *Essentials* (2021): Domains: #1; #2; #3; #4; #8; #10

- Competencies: 1.1; 2.2; 3.1; 3.6; 4.2; 8.1; 10.2
- Subcompetencies: 1.1b; 2.2c; 3.1b; 3.1c; 3.1f; 4.2c; 8.1a; 10.2a; 10.2d

Spheres of Care: Wellness/Disease prevention

Concepts: Clinical judgment; SDOH; Communication

Source: Kongthavonsakul et al., 2012.

NCLEX Questions

1. During which stage would the community health nurse first expect to see signs of disease via laboratory testing?
    a. Susceptibility stage
    b. Preclinical stage
    c. Clinical disease stage
    d. Recovery stage

2. Immunizations would be an example of which type of immunity?
    a. Active natural
    b. Active acquired
    c. Passive natural
    d. Passive acquired

References

AbdulRaheem, Y. (2023). Unveiling the significance and challenges of integrating prevention levels in healthcare practice. *Journal of Primary Care and Community Health, 14*, 21501319231186500. https://doi.org/10.1177/21501319231186500

Albers, A. N., Thaker, J., & Newcomer, S. R. (2022). Barriers to and facilitators of early childhood immunization in rural areas of the United States: A systematic review of the literature. *Preventive Medicine Reports, 27,* 101804. https://doi.org/10.1016/j.pmedr.2022.101804

Albers, A. N., Wright, E., Thaker, J., Conway, K., Daley, M. F., & Newcomer, S. R. (2023). Childhood vaccination practices and parental hesitancy barriers in rural and urban primary care settings. *Journal of Community Health,* 48(5), 798–809. https://doi.org/10.1007/s10900-023-01226-4

American Association of Colleges of Nursing. (2021). *The essentials: Core competencies for professional nursing education.* https://www.aacnnursing.org/Essentials

Association of Professionals in Infection Control and Epidemiology. (n.d.). *Break the chain of infection.* https://infectionpreventionandyou.org/protect-your-patients/break-the-chain-of-infection/

Butler-Jones, D., & Wong T. (2016). Infectious disease, social determinants and the need for intersectoral action. *Canadian Communicable Disease Report,* 42(Suppl 1),18–20. https://doi.org/10.14745/ccdr.v42is1a04

Center for Food Security and Public Health. (2024). *Zoonotic diseases.* https://www.cfsph.iastate.edu/zoonoses/

Centers for Disease Control and Prevention. (n.d.a.). *Healthcare- and community-associated infections.* https://arpsp.cdc.gov/profile/infections?tab=eip

Centers for Disease Control and Prevention. (n.d.b.). *Solve the outbreak.* https://www.cdc.gov/digital-social-media-tools/mobile/applications/sto/web-app.html

Centers for Disease Control and Prevention. (2016). *How infections spread.* https://www.cdc.gov/infectioncontrol/spread/index.html

Centers for Disease Control and Prevention. (2019). *About fungal diseases.* https://www.cdc.gov/fungal/about-fungal-diseases.html

Centers for Disease Control and Prevention. (2020). *What's the difference between isolation and quarantine?* YouTube, July 14, 2020. https://www.youtube.com/watch?v=l3s75_X8Xjs

Centers for Disease Control and Prevention. (2021a). *About global NCDs.* https://www.cdc.gov/globalhealth/healthprotection/ncd/global-ncd-overview.html

Centers for Disease Control and Prevention. (2021b). *Immunity types.* https://www.cdc.gov/vaccines/vac-gen/immunity-types.htm

Centers for Disease Control and Prevention. (2021c). *Where resistance spreads: Your community.* https://www.cdc.gov/drugresistance/communities.html

Centers for Disease Control and Prevention. (2022a). *Chain of infection components.* https://www.cdc.gov/niosh/learning/safetyculturehc/module-2/3.html

Centers for Disease Control and Prevention. (2022b). *Parasites.* https://www.cdc.gov/parasites/about.html

Centers for Disease Control and Prevention. (2022c). *Tetanus.* https://www.cdc.gov/tetanus/index.html

Centers for Disease Control and Prevention. (2023a). *2022 outbreak cases and data.* https://www.cdc.gov/poxvirus/mpox/response/2022/index.html

Centers for Disease Control and Prevention. (2023b). *Aircrew safety & health—Communicable diseases.* https://www.cdc.gov/niosh/topics/aircrew/communicablediseases.html

Centers for Disease Control and Prevention. (2023c). *CDC museum COVID-19 timeline.* https://www.cdc.gov/museum/timeline/covid19.html

Centers for Disease Control and Prevention. (2023d). *Food-borne germs and illnesses.* https://www.cdc.gov/foodsafety/foodborne-germs.html

Centers for Disease Control and Prevention. (2023e). *Four steps to food safety.* https://www.cdc.gov/foodsafety/keep-food-safe.html

Centers for Disease Control and Prevention. (2023f). *How it spreads/Monkeypox.* https://www.cdc.gov/poxvirus/mpox/if-sick/transmission.html

Centers for Disease Control and Prevention. (2023g). *Types of fungal diseases.* https://www.cdc.gov/fungal/diseases/index.html

Centers for Disease Control and Prevention. (2023h). *Waterborne disease in the United States.* https://www.cdc.gov/healthywater/surveillance/burden/index.html

Centers for Disease Control and Prevention. (2024). *Immunization schedules*. https://www.cdc.gov/vaccines/schedules/index.html

Cheung, J. (2024). *Nosocomial infection: What is it, prevention, and more*. https://www.osmosis.org/answers/nosocomial-infection#

CK-12. (2024). *Infectious diseases*. https://www.ck12.org/book/ck-12-life-science-for-middle-school/section/21.1/

Cleveland Clinic. (2021). *Antivirals*. https://my.clevelandclinic.org/health/drugs/21531-antivirals

Cleveland Clinic. (2022). *Bacteria*. https://my.clevelandclinic.org/health/articles/24494-bacteria

Correll, R. (2023). *Differences between communicable and infectious diseases: It's more than just semantics*. https://www.verywellhealth.com/the-difference-between-communicable-and-infectious-diseases-4151985

Department of Health and Human Services. (2022). *What is the difference between isolation and quarantine?* https://www.hhs.gov/answers/public-health-and-safety/what-is-the-difference-between-isolation-and-quarantine/index.html

Dr. Matt and Dr. Mike. (2019). *Four types of immunity*. YouTube, February 21, 2019. https://www.youtube.com/watch?v=yvKENnMUxLA

Duarte, R., Aguiar, A., Pinto, M., Furtado, I., Tiberi, S., Lönnroth, K., & Migliori, G. (2021). Different disease, same challenges: Social determinants of tuberculosis and COVID-19. *Pulmonology, 27*(4), 338–344. https://doi.org/10.1016/j.pulmoe.2021.02.002

Frontier Nursing University. (2022). *Epidemiology and biostatistics*. https://library.frontier.edu/c.php?g=1248178&p=9135211

Geography of Transport Systems. (2023). *Basic reproduction number (R0) of major infectious diseases*. https://transportgeography.org/contents/applications/transportation-pandemics/basic-reproduction-number-r0-of-major-infectious-diseases/

Gunderson, A., & Woskie, L. (2023). *Understanding predictions: What is R-naught?* https://globalhealth.harvard.edu/understanding-predictions-what-is-r-naught/

Hamson, E., Forbes, C., Wittkopf, P., Pandey, A., Mendes, D., Kowalik, J., Czudek, C., & Mugwagwa, T. (2023). Impact of pandemics and disruptions to vaccination on infectious diseases epidemiology past and present. *Human Vaccines and Immunotherapeutics, 19*(2), 2219577. https://doi.org/10.1080/21645515.2023.2219577

Hossain, A. D., Jarolimova, J., Elnaiem, A., Huang, C. X., Richterman, A., & Ivers, L. C. (2022). Effectiveness of contact tracing in the control of infectious diseases: A systematic review. *Lancet Public Health, 7*(3), e259–e273. https://doi.org/10.1016/s2468-2667(22)00001-9

Indus Health Plus. (2024). *NCD—Non-communicable diseases*. https://www.indushealthplus.com/ncds-non-communicable-diseases.html

Johns Hopkins Bloomberg School of Public Health. (2022). *Global health now*. https://mailchi.mp/14a7cca69053/global-health-now-measles-exploits-vaccination-gaps-malnutritions-fingerprints-and-polio-free-at-last?e=b347c358fc

Johns Hopkins Medicine. (n.d.). *Emerging infectious diseases*. https://www.hopkinsmedicine.org/health/conditions-and-diseases/emerging-infectious-diseases

Karimizadeh, Z., Dowran, R., Mokhtari-azad, T., & Shafiei-Jandaghi, N. (2023). The reproduction rate of severe acute respiratory syndrome coronavirus 2 different variants recently circulated in human: A narrative review. *European Journal of Medical Research, 28*(94), 1–10. https://doi.org/10.1186/s40001-023-01047-0

Kongthavonsakul, K., Henry, C. H., & Oberdorfer, P. (2012). A 6-year-old boy with fever, rash and severe pneumonia. *BMJ Case Reports*, bcr1220115411. https://doi.org/10.1136/bcr.12.2011.5411

Koo, I. (2023). *What are pathogens?* https://www.verywellhealth.com/what-is-a-pathogen-1958836

Leach, R. (2023). Health equity and the impact on infectious disease. *Contagion, 8*(1). https://www.contagionlive.com/view/health-equity-and-the-impact-on-infectious-disease

Medical News Today. (2023). *Everything you need to know about communicable diseases.* https://www.medicalnewstoday.com/articles/communicable-diseases

Merriam-Webster. (n.d.a.). *Immunity definition.* https://www.merriam-webster.com/dictionary/immunity

Merriam-Webster. (n.d.b.). *Isolation definition.* https://www.merriam-webster.com/dictionary/isolation

Merriam-Webster. (n.d.c.). *Quarantine definition.* https://www.merriam-webster.com/dictionary/quarantine.

Merriam-Webster. (n.d.d.). *Susceptibility definition.* https://www.merriam-webster.com/dictionary/susceptibility.

Merriam-Webster. (n.d.e.). *Transmission definition.* https://www.merriam-webste.r.com/dictionary/transmission

Minnesota Department of Health. (2019). *Case study: Outbreak investigation.* https://www.health.state.mn.us/communities/practice/ta/phnresidency/casestudies/docs/OutbreakInvestigation-Preceptor.pdf

Monegro, A., Muppidi, V., & Regunath, H. (2023). *Hospital-acquired infections.* StatPearls. https://www.ncbi.nlm.nih.gov/books/NBK441857/

Moore, S. (2021). *History of infectious diseases.* https://www.news-medical.net/health/History-of-Infectious-Diseases.aspx#

National Human Genome Research Institute. (2024a). *Bacteria.* https://www.genome.gov/genetics-glossary/Bacteria

National Human Genome Research Institute. (2024b). *Virus.* https://www.genome.gov/genetics-glossary/Virus

National Institute of Allergy and Infectious Diseases. (2018). *NIAID emerging infectious diseases/pathogens.* https://www.niaid.nih.gov/research/emerging-infectious-diseases-pathogens

Open University. (2024). *Public health approaches to infectious disease: 3.2 Secondary prevention strategies.* https://www.open.edu/openlearn/science-maths-technology/public-health-approaches-infectious-disease/content-section-3.2

Perry, J., McClure, N., Palmer, R., & Neal, J. (2021). Utilizing academic–community partnerships with nursing students to improve hand hygiene in elementary students to reduce transmission of COVID-19. *NASN School Nurse, 36*(6), 333–338. https://doi.org/10.1177/1942602X20986958

Silvestri, L. (n.d.). *Using reverse case studies for clinical learning.* https://evolve.elsevier.com/education/expertise/build-knowledge/using-reverse-case-studies-for-clinical-learning/

SingHealth. (2021). *Community acquired infections.* https://www.singhealth.com.sg/patient-care/conditions-treatments/Community-acquired-infections

Texas Health and Human Services. (2021a). *Nurse aide Infection Control Module: Modes of transmission.* https://apps.hhs.texas.gov/providers/NF/credentialing/cna/infection-control/module2/Module_2_Chain_of_Infection_print.html

Texas Health and Human Services. (2021b). *Nurse aide infection control module: Susceptible host.* https://apps.hhs.texas.gov/providers/NF/credentialing/cna/infection-control/module2/Module_2_Chain_of_Infection18.html

Windsor, M. (2022). *An infection prevention expert explains how to avoid COVID, flu—and the next pandemic.* https://www.uab.edu/reporter/resources/be-healthy/item/9796-an-infection-prevention-expert-explains-how-to-avoid-covid-flu-and-the-next-pandemic

Wolters Kluwer. (2021). *The reverse case study: An innovative approach to develop critical thinking skills.* https://www.wolterskluwer.com/en/expert-insights/the-reverse-case-study

World Health Organization. (2014). *Vector-borne diseases: World Health Day.* https://staging.afro.who.int/pt/node/4602

World Health Organization. (2020a). *Coronavirus disease (COVID-19): Herd immunity, lockdowns and COVID-19.* https://www.who.int/news-room/questions-and-answers/item/herd-immunity-lockdowns-and-covid-19

World Health Organization. (2020b). *Vector-borne diseases.* https://www.who.int/news-room/fact-sheets/detail/vector-borne-diseases

World Health Organization. (2020c). *Zoonoses.* https://www.who.int/news-room/fact-sheets/detail/zoonoses

World Health Organization. (2022a). *Vaccine-preventable disease outbreaks on the rise in Africa.* https://www.afro.who.int/news/vaccine-preventable-disease-outbreaks-rise-africa

World Health Organization. (2022b). *UNICEF and WHO warn of perfect storm of conditions for measles outbreaks, affecting children.* https://www.who.int/news/item/27-04-2022-unicef-and-who-warn-of--perfect-storm--of-conditions-for-measles-outbreaks--affecting-children#

World Health Organization. (2022c). *WHO launches first ever global on infection prevention and control.* https://www.who.int/news/item/06-05-2022-who-launches-first-ever-global-report-on-infection-prevention-and-control

World Health Organization. (2023). *Infectious diseases.* https://www.emro.who.int/health-topics/infectious-diseases/index.html

World Health Organization. (2024a). *Coronavirus disease (COVID-19): Contacttracing.* https://www.who.int/news-room/questions-and-answers/item/coronavirus-disease-covid-19-contact-tracing

World Health Organization. (2024b). *COVID-19 vaccines.* https://www.who.int/emergencies/diseases/novel-coronavirus-2019/covid-19-vaccines

Credits

CHAPTER 8

Disaster Preparedness

"By failing to prepare, you are preparing to fail."

—Benjamin Franklin

Learning Outcomes

After reading this chapter, students should be able to:

1. Understand the difference between natural and humanmade disasters
2. Apply examples of the four stages of disasters
3. Define the terms *multiple-casualty* and *mass-casualty*
4. Understand the structure of the U.S. federal disaster management system as well as state and local emergency preparedness

Keywords and Concepts

Department of Homeland Security (DHS), Federal Emergency Management Agency (FEMA), humanmade disaster, mass-casualty, multiple-casualty, National Incident Management System (NIMS), natural disaster, phases of disasters, triage

Definitions of the Keywords

DHS: A U.S. government department that focuses on emergency responses to aviation and border security, cybersecurity, and chemical inspections (DHS, 2024)

Disaster: A sudden calamitous event bringing significant damage, loss, or destruction (Merriam-Webster Dictionary, 2024a)

FEMA: Works to assist in preparation for, during, and in response to disasters (FEMA, 2023a)

Humanmade disasters: Traumatic disasters that involve the loss of life or property but do not occur naturally (Substance Abuse and Mental Health Services Administration [SAMHSA], 2023b)

Mass-casualty incident: Event that overwhelms the local healthcare system in which the number of casualties vastly exceeds the local resources and capabilities in a short time (Lincoln et al., 2023)

Multiple-casualty incident: Any event causing injury and/or death of many clients beyond what an emergency medical services (EMS) system is routinely capable of handling; however, full resources can be brought to bear on each client (County of Santa Clara Emergency Medical Services, 2019)

Natural disasters: Innate disasters, often without warning, that include severe weather-related incidents that may cause considerable damage to human life, property, infrastructure, and homeland security (DHS, n.d.)

Phases of disasters: The four phases of disasters, which are prevention (mitigation), preparedness, response, and recovery (Klein & Irizarry, 2023)

NIMS: A comprehensive method to assist all levels of governmental, nongovernmental organizations (NGOs), and the private sector, allowing a community approach to prevent, protect, mitigate, respond, and recover the effects of disasters (FEMA Emergency Management Institute, 2018)

Triage: The sorting of and allocation of treatment to patients, especially disaster victims, according to a system of priorities designed to maximize the number of survivors (Merriam-Webster Dictionary, 2024b)

Introduction

In the world today, the United States and international groups are affected increasingly by humanmade and natural forms of disasters and wars. The primary concerns are the unknowns and risks that may be present to individuals, families, communities, and populations globally. Studying and preparing for such events is required to deal with the meeting and protect individuals and properties effectively. By doing so, the National Preparedness Goal developed through FEMA includes a definition for the entire involved community to be prepared for various disasters and other emergencies. The goal states that "a secure and resilient nation with the capabilities required across the whole community to prevent, protect against, mitigate, respond to, and recover from the threats and hazards that pose the greatest risk" (FEMA, 2023b, para 2).

The International Federation of Red Cross and Red Crescent Societies (IFRC), functioning as the world's largest humanitarian network, developed Strategy 2030. This strategy is designed to build on the past 100 years of humanitarianism to meet the issues and problems that the 21st century brings. By providing a more comprehensive global network of organizations, this strategy will meet the needs of all communities (IFRC, 2024b). The IFRC is looking at the change in what may be a part of the world and how individuals and communities will function to the best of their abilities (IFRC, 2024b).

Many agencies focus on providing disaster education and training for individuals in various disciplines, especially those in healthcare and service organizations. These include FEMA, the American Red Cross (ARC), DHS, and NIMS. Throughout this chapter, disaster information will be presented using the guidelines for the phases of disasters, types of disasters, responses best used for each phase, and emergency response agencies.

Background of the Concepts

The International Disaster Database Centre for Research on the Epidemiology of Disasters (CRED; 2024) is the global database for comprehensive disaster data. From 1900 to the present, it has identified more than 26,000 disasters gathered by the United Nations (UN) and NGOs, insurance companies, research institutes, and press agencies.

The National Centers for Environmental Information (NCEI), an agency used to summarize global and U.S. information related to historical precipitation and temperature trends, has identified that the United States has had climate disasters that cost more than $18 billion in the past five years (NCEI, 2024). The latest report from FEMA identified that the disasters have resulted in a significant need for long-term housing, relocation assistance, and community sheltering for those affected (FEMA, 2023c).

Overall, the effects of the disasters have made individuals more aware of the need to consider that disasters may occur in any state or country, some with warnings and others without any. Tracking disasters and their effects historically and developing practical plans to deal with what occurs are essential. Numerous organizations must come together to share resources and support the needs of those requiring assistance (FEMA, 2023b).

The American Association of Colleges of Nursing (AACN) essentials emphasize the need for better preparation for future nurses due to increased disasters and emergencies. Domain #3, population health, notes that nurses are critical in advocating for, developing, and implementing policies that affect population health globally and locally. In addition, nurses respond to crises and provide care during emergencies, disasters, epidemics, and pandemics. Even though every disaster or emergency is different and requires different competencies, nurses must prepare to respond to the events effectively (AACN, 2021).

Disaster Management, Planning, and Agencies

Several federal and private disaster management agencies manage, educate, and respond to relief efforts worldwide. Whether locally, statewide, nationally, or internationally, all focus on the need for an effective plan to ensure public safety. Plans include the organization of mock drills to allow for modifications as needed. With continued practice, individuals may remember their role during the disaster and can provide effective interventions (Chartoff et al., 2023; FEMA, 2023d).

U.S. Department of Homeland Security

The DHS is an organization that focuses on improving security in the United States. This department includes customs, border control, immigration, emergency response to natural and humanmade disasters, human trafficking, antiterrorism work, and cybersecurity (USA.gov, n.d.).

The DHS was developed by combining more than 22 federal departments and agencies into one cohesive and effective department to respond strongly to various threats (DHS, 2023). The creation of a more defined avenue to prepare and respond to emergencies and disasters in the United States was due to the 9/11 terrorist attacks (DHS, 2023). The DHS has presented a specific focus and policies to meet the goals and needs against potential threats. These issues include the need for preparedness for any catastrophic events; transportation for assisting people and obtaining supplies; enhancing and enforcing border security and immigration processes; promoting effective communication with other agencies; and identifying the means for financial management, human resource procedures, information technology, and methods to boost overall organizational performance (DHS, 2022c).

Federal Emergency Management Agency

FEMA was initially created in 1979 and is now part of DHS. FEMA is the leading agency for response and recovery from disasters. Its strategic plan focuses on three significant goals: dealing with equity for emergency management, collaborating with community climate resilience efforts, and promoting and sustaining national emergency preparedness (FEMA, 2023a).

The mission of FEMA focuses on assisting individuals before, during, and after a disaster. The period before a disaster occurs is the national preparedness phase, according to FEMA. The primary focus in this phase is to practice the community's actions in preparing individuals through training and educational sessions. Understanding the risks, such as living in a flood plain, is essential for preparing for this disaster. The next phase instills the needs during a disaster. Here, communities must understand how a disaster is declared and what governmental agencies will do to control the functioning and direction of individuals affected (FEMA, 2024b).

Using the Robert T. Stafford Disaster Relief and Emergency Assistance Act, the president of the United States can announce a disaster as a major disaster or an emergency declaration that will direct which resources will be used for each. A mobile app is additionally available to the community for assistance as needed. The last phase is that of recovery. Here, the community resources are made available to those needing help. The timeliness of response can be significant, especially with disasters related to healthcare needs, electricity and power, housing, and communication. Another aspect of this phase is to review the actions provided for the current disaster and determine how to make revisions for future situations (FEMA, 2024b; Box 8.1).

BOX 8.1 ACTIVE LEARNING REFLECTION ACTIVITY

Education About FEMA and Using the FEMA App

A community group contacted your university school of nursing and asked for education on using technology to prepare for an emergency/disaster. The community faculty instructs the community nursing students to design a 10-minute presentation on components of FEMA and on downloading and using its app. Use the following website to assist with the presentation: https://www.fema.gov/about/news-multimedia/mobile-products#download.

AACN *Essentials* (2021): Domains: #1; #2; #3; #8

- Competencies: 1.1; 2.2; 3.6; 8.1; 8.3
- Subcompetencies: 1.1b; 2.2c; 2.2e; 3.6a; 3.6c; 8.1a; 8.1b; 8.1c; 8.1d; 8.3a; 8.3c; 8.3d; 8.3e

Spheres of Care: Wellness/Disease prevention

Concepts: Clinical judgment; Communication; Evidence-based practice

Source: FEMA, 2024a.

National Incident Management System

Guidance through NIMS works with all governmental, nongovernmental, and private areas for disasters (FEMA, 2024c). A specific vocabulary for describing all activities is necessary to succeed with follow-through in the system and in the processes to intervene and guide personnel working, as defined by the National Preparedness System (NPS; FEMA, 2023d).

All phases of the disaster process are a function and provide the necessary needs from prevention to recovery. Through the use of the NPS, NIMS has studied previous disasters. Looking at the contributing factors, both new and old, identifies the challenges that need to be considered. A gathering of experts to assist with managing areas of concern is sought. Recently, concerns about climate control have become apparent with the fluctuations between cold and heat that have manifested in hurricanes, droughts, and wildfires. The current preparedness report reflects disasters from 2022 and has identified four specific areas: fire management and suppression; logistics and supply chain management; public health, healthcare, and EMS; and long-term vulnerability reduction (FEMA, 2023c, p. 1). Continuous review and updating of procedures and adding other partners to contribute and assist in providing their knowledge and services are undertaken. Challenges are always present, but overall, they can effectively make the best decisions for many as the world looks at ensuring every possibility is considered and planned before, during, and after disasters (FEMA, 2023c).

The joint field office will organize the responses (Department of the Interior [DOI], n.d.). During this time, information and communication must include the following with reporting as to the type of disaster or emergency (biological, environmental, nuclear, radiation, infectious agent), location, number of victims, protection needed for first responders, specific departments needing to be notified (Centers for Disease Control and Prevention [CDC], Federal Bureau of Investigation [FBI], local health department), immediate resources required and where to obtain, what agency is in charge, and what to share with the media (FEMA, 2024b).

Molassiotis et al. (2021), through a 30-year review of disaster nursing research, identified that this field has significant development to fulfill the growth of disasters. The need to continue to analyze disaster management along with inclusion in interacting with international agencies is essential. By networking with national and international agencies, nurses must be more involved in this profession from the perspectives of administration, education, patient care, policy, and procedure development (Molassiotis et al., 2021).

American Red Cross

The ARC, established by Clara Barton in 1881, dedicates itself to assisting those in the armed service, veterans, and their families while providing the United States and the world with various forms of disaster relief. As a nonprofit organization, volunteers focus on the mission to help set up shelters, feed people, and comfort those affected by disasters (ARC, 2024). The ARC Global Foundation has identified areas to support, including humanity and reducing human suffering through interaction with others, effective communication and friendships, and promoting peace. Impartiality includes prohibiting discrimination, especially regarding race, religious beliefs, and political opinions. The need for neutrality may exist when affected by hostilities or any other types of controversies. Independence and guidance to follow the mission and visions of the ARC through the use of volunteers to assist victims. Unity with services to assist in all forms of humanitarian efforts in all areas of the world and universality, meaning that all individuals are to be viewed as equal in their status, responsibilities, and duties (ARC, 2024).

Military

Since 1959, the U.S. military has assisted in foreign and domestic disasters (Irwin, 2022). Depending on the type of need, service members can participate in such areas as meeting basic needs of food, water, shelter, medical care, and other resources. When the severity of a crisis demands it, the Robert T. Stafford Disaster Relief and Emergency Assistance Act authorizes the president to deploy military forces to U.S. states and territories to provide additional assistance (Cheatham et al., 2023; Irwin, 2022).

Medical Reserve Corps

The Medical Reserve Corps are medical and public health professionals who volunteer in the United States and donate their time and knowledge to assist with recruitment training and activate those in the medical field when emergencies occur. Community members who do not have expertise in healthcare can help in many other ways to care for their communities. Some examples of MRC activities include such interventions as emergency shelter operations and medical care; dispensing of medications, water, and other supplies; disease testing and surveillance; vaccination clinics; veterinary care; communication services; search and rescue; cleanup resources; and administrative support (Administration for Strategic Preparedness and Response, n.d.).

Community Emergency Response Team

The Community Emergency Response Team (CERT) program offers a consistent, nationwide approach to volunteer training and organization on which professional responders can rely during a disaster (FEMA, n.d.). Preparing for emergencies and disasters is critical to prompt response, recovery, and preventing life-threatening issues (FEMA, n.d.; Box 8.2).

BOX 8.2 ACTIVE LEARNING REFLECTION ACTIVITY

What Is CERT?

Complete the online training module titled *IS-317.A: Introduction to Community Emergency Response Team (CERTs)* at the FEMA Emergency Management Institute at https://training.fema.gov/is/courseoverview.aspx?code=IS-317.a&lang=en.

Create a profile, complete the course, and download the certificate. Reflect on the following question:

1. Name three ways you will use what you learned from the online CERT course in your future nursing practice.

AACN *Essentials* (2021): Domains: #1; #3; #4; #6; #9

- Competencies: 1.1; 3.2; 3.6; 4.2; 6.2; 9.3
- Subcompetencies: 1.1b; 3.2a; 3.2b; 3.6a; 4.2c; 6.2a; 6.2b; 6.2c; 6.2d; 9.3a

Spheres of Care: Wellness/Disease prevention; Regenerative/Restorative care

Concepts: Clinical judgment; Communication; Evidence-based practice

Source: FEMA Emergency Management Institute, 2020.

Disasters

When a disaster occurs, these disruptions can significantly affect the community involved and how the community members function with the resources present. The means to analyze situations may influence the community's vulnerability (IFRC, 2024a).

Types of Disasters

The term *disaster* includes two types: natural and humanmade. *Natural disasters* often occur without warning and can consist of loss of life and damage to property, technology, and infrastructure (DHS, n.d.). *Humanmade disasters* may also involve a loss of life or property (SAMHSA, 2023b). Due to the unpredictable nature of these events, the effects on those affected not only lead to suffering and possible loss of life but also possible long-term emotional and mental concerns (DHS, n.d.; SAMHSA, 2023a).

Natural Disasters

Winter storms, floods, tornadoes, mudslides, droughts, tidal waves, and hurricanes are natural disasters (DHS, n.d.). Each type of natural disaster has its forms of destruction and different means for prevention, preparation, mitigation, response, recovery, and rehabilitative needs (Amatya & Khan, 2023). With natural disasters, agencies have been able to use technology such as early warning systems, methods to monitor the activities of the disasters, and specific techniques to communicate the effects and needs for the methods to respond in real time (Krichen et al., 2024; Figure 8.1).

Humanmade Disasters

Examples of humanmade disasters include industrial accidents, shootings, acts of terrorism, and incidents of mass violence. As with natural disasters, these traumatic events may also cause loss of life and property. They may also prompt evacuations from certain areas and overwhelm health resources in the affected communities (SAMHSA, 2023b; Figure 8.2).

Common Natural Disasters
Earthquakes
Volcanoes
Tsunami
Landslides
Hurricane
Tornadoes
Blizzards
Dust storms
Floods
Droughts

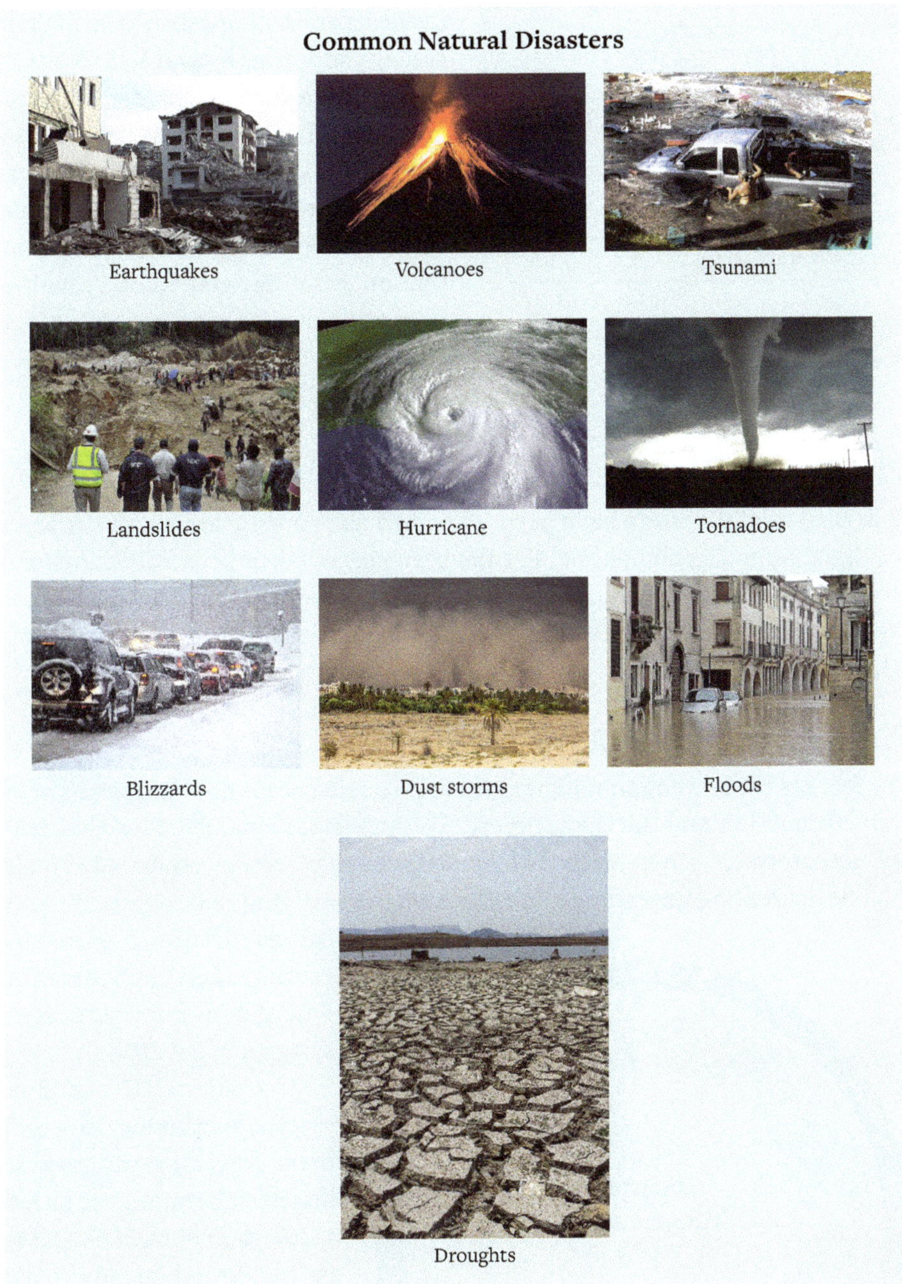

FIGURE 8.1 Natural Disaster Examples

Multiple-/Mass-Casualty Incidents

Having available resources to meet all needs is vital to addressing a disaster. Large numbers of victims may need triage, stabilization, and evacuation. The safety of the rescuers must also be of concern, especially in a mass-casualty event. Mass-casualty incidents are distinguished from multiple casualty situations by available resources: with mass casualties, resources for each client are limited, whereas, as with multiple casualties, full resources can be brought to bear on each client. Mass-casualty triage begins with recognizing that an event has generated casualties exceeding available resources (Alpert & Kohn, 2023; American Roentgen Ray Society, n.d.).

1.	Car, bus, train, boat and plane crashes
2.	Non-natural wildfires
3.	Chemical spills, leaks or contamination from industrial locations
4.	Critical failures of buildings, bridges and other manmade structures
5.	Acts of warfare or terror

FIGURE 8.2 Examples of Humanmade Disasters

Phases of Disasters

Four phases of disasters have been identified as being a framework known as the disaster management cycle. The first two phases occur before the disaster or emergency (primary prevention). In comparison, the last two phases arise after the event (secondary and tertiary prevention; Center for Disaster Philanthropy [CDP], 2024a; Figure 8.3).

Prevention/Mitigation Phase

The focus of the prevention/mitigation phase is on the means to limit any loss of life and/or properties and the environment. This process is conducted by developing policies, procedures, and methods to enhance public sector awareness. Examples include decreasing greenhouse gas emissions, identifying floodplains, building infrastructure to withstand earthquakes, and installing emergency communication systems (CDP, 2024a).

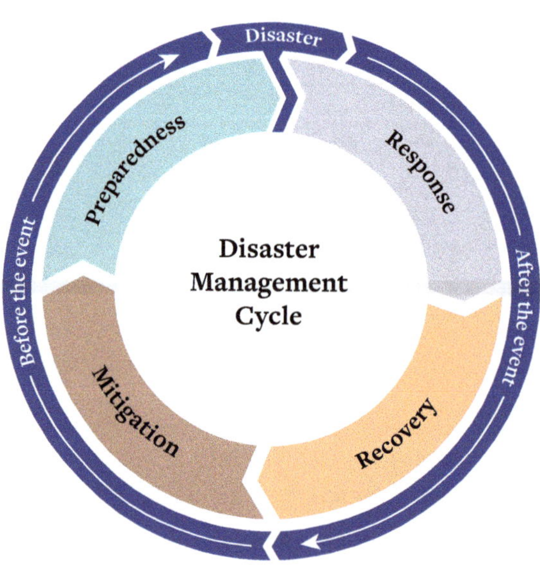

FIGURE 8.3 Phases of Disaster

As the CDP (2024a) reports, humans may have a role in the prevention/mitigation of disasters. Examples can include methods to prevent flood risks by building dams and barriers; enforcing building codes to withstand high winds, tsunamis, and earthquakes; and developing specific immunizations for disease prevention. Chai and Wu (2023) address natural disasters with an emphasis on climate changes affecting extreme weather situations. The use of methods to implement prevention activities and practical strategies to provide early prediction and warning systems are needed to be put into disaster plans to assist with limiting the damage that occurs. Additionally, enhanced field monitoring, artificial intelligence technology, and multi-criteria decision-making can be identified for early assessment of upcoming potential risks and hazards.

Specific analyses of the disasters are conducted through risk identification, mapping, and warning of areas that may be affected and their severity, how immediate communication to individuals and groups will occur, and the rescue organization timeline. Continuation of analysis after the disaster should address the positive and the harmful activities and how to update and revise the plans for future situations (Oshiro et al., 2022).

Here, the importance of putting in place the policies and procedures developed and having mock practices for various disaster events. Sharing knowledge from potential upcoming and past disasters from local, national, and international situations is put into plans. Through continuous review, anticipating what may occur assists with the knowledge and preparation to meet the needs of all organizations and communities. Examples of this phase may include installing smoke detectors, securing supplies and equipment, practicing mock disaster drills, learning cardiopulmonary resuscitation, preparing a home disaster supply kit, and identifying safe places in the home, school, and community settings (CDP, 2024a).

Preparedness

Preparedness is vital to the needs of disaster knowledge and disaster activities. As disasters are often not planned but occur at random, the importance of taking the initiative and possibly preventing a disaster must be thought out thoroughly. The CDP notes that disasters result from humans' actions and decisions. Humans can alter a disaster (CDP, 2024a).

Disasters often include communities and countries but can also focus on individuals. With this in mind, there is a need to plan for this disaster at this level. Some examples of this may be a house fire, a tornado affecting the home, and a flood of the home and surrounding land. The importance here is to plan for those in the home, and a different approach may be needed. Adequate communication with family members to discuss, prepare, and conduct a plan is vital. Gathering all individuals to develop the plan for several types of emergencies, especially those that commonly may affect your areas, and how the team will work is essential. Practice sessions will enhance the process after the plan or plans are finalized. Factors to consider include how to evacuate, where the resources and supplies are kept, how communications will be managed, where emergency contact information is maintained, and how one will oversee pets in the home (Ready.gov, 2024; Figure 8.4; Box 8.3).

Being prepared helps achieve goals and avoid possible adverse outcomes. Technology and innovative techniques are valuable in all disaster phases to be

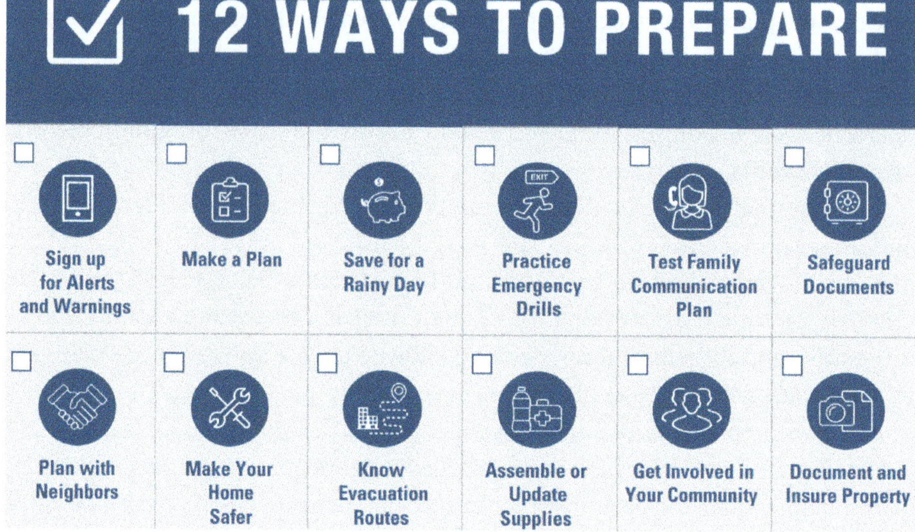

FIGURE 8.4 Preparing for a Disaster/Emergency

BOX 8.3 ACTIVE LEARNING REFLECTION ACTIVITY

Making a Personal Tornado Disaster Plan

While visiting an older couple on a home visit, the community nurse assesses whether the couple has an emergency plan. Since tornadoes are typical for the area, the nurse focuses on preparation for this type of disaster. The couple state that they do not have a plan. Using the website Ready.gov, assist the couple in making a tornado plan. The following ARC website could also be helpful: https://www.redcross.org/get-help/how-to-prepare-for-emergencies/make-a-plan.html.

Reflect on the following questions:

1. What three priority concepts were noted in the tornado plan?
2. How did you feel about this activity?
3. What did you learn from this activity that you will use in future nursing practice?

AACN *Essentials* (2021): Domains: #1; #3; #4; #8; #9

- Competencies: 1.3; 3.6; 4.2; 8.1; 8.3; 9.3
- Subcompetencies: 1.3a; 3.6a; 3.6b; 4.2c; 8.1a; 8.3a; 8.3d; 9.3a

Spheres of Care: Wellness/Disease prevention

Concepts: Communication; Evidence-based practice; Clinical judgment

Sources: ARC, 2024; Ready.gov, 2024.

initiative-taking and predict financial needs. In practice, preparedness can consist of early warning systems, contingency planning, stockpiling equipment and supplies, and creating a coordination plan (CDP, 2024a).

Response

A disaster has occurred. So, now what happens? Communication and how it is conducted is critical to success. Key personnel who specialize in being effective in the specific type of disaster and the level of emergency management need to be notified. When a disaster is declared, the federal government, led by FEMA, responds to the request of and in support of any state, tribes, territories, and local jurisdictions affected by a disaster. Response actions are organized under the National Disaster Recovery Framework (NDRF). FEMA appoints a federal coordinating officer to establish a joint field office and lead the response (DOI, n.d.).

Incident Command

The NIMS guides all levels of government, NGOs, and the private sector to work together to prevent, protect against, mitigate, respond to, and recover from incidents (FEMA, 2024c). The NIMS directs the management of the medical section with disasters. Effective uses of medical resources such as triage procedures, interventions performed, and transport of victims are assigned, and communications are provided for all responders. Proper organizational methods include general operations, plan development, logistics, and financial needs. Several other roles are implemented, such as the medical director, triage officer, treatment officer, medical supply officer, and morgue officer (Lincoln et al., 2023).

Triage

The critical goal in triage is saving as many as possible and providing immediate care to those with the best chance of survival. Response and triage are also based on the available resources, including the type of event. Treatment during triage is minimal and counterintuitive to move clients away from the incident and toward more comprehensive care resources (Clarkson & Williams, 2023).

Clarkson and Williams (2023) concurred on revising the nurses' educational practices and actions to significantly improve triage understanding and proficiency. Simple triage and rapid treatment (START) triage method is commonly used in the United States, whereas several different algorithms are used in other areas worldwide. Overall, following an organized process and pretraining staff are vital in assisting with immediate lifesaving measures and adequate usage of resources (Lincoln et al., 2023). When using the START format, first responders assign how the injured individuals are placed into a specific area by using colored tags depicting the severity of the injuries (Figure 8.5).

START Triage
Assess, *Treat, (use bystanders)*
When you have a color
STOP - TAG - MOVE ON

Minor — ***- Move Walking Wounded***

Deceased — - No RESPIRATIONS after *head tilt*

Immediate:
- **Breathing** but UNCONSCIOUS
- **Respirations** - over 30
- **Perfusion** Capillary refill > 2 or NO RADIAL PULSE *Control bleeding*
- **Mental Status** Unable to follow simple commands

Delayed — - Otherwise

REMEMBER:

Respirations - 30
Perfusion - 2
Mental Status - Can Do

FIGURE 8.5 SMART Triage

Black
Deceased/expectant: Injuries incompatible with life or without spontaneous respiration; should not be moved forward to the collection point
Red
Immediate: Severe injuries but high potential for survival with treatment; taken to collection point first
Yellow
Delayed: Serious injuries but not immediately life-threatening
Green
Walking wounded: Minor injuries

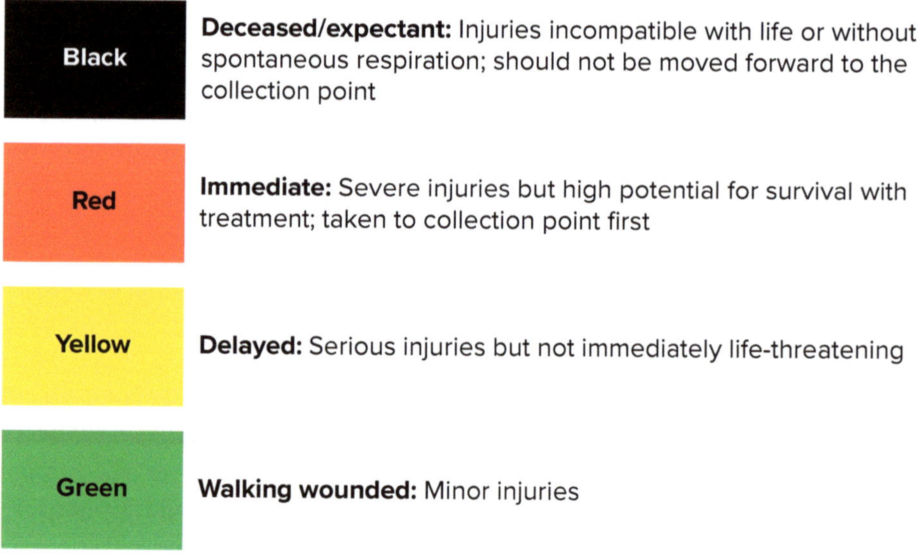

FIGURE 8.6 Colored Tag System

The colored tag system allows for quick triaging with minimal intervention. If the condition declines or improves, the injured can be moved to other colored areas (Clarkson & Williams, 2023; Figure 8.6; Box 8.4).

BOX 8.4 ACTIVE LEARNING REFLECTION ACTIVITY

Who Should Be Triaged First?

Four clients have been involved in a car wreck in a small rural area. EMS consist of volunteers in the community, and the nearest emergency department is more than 20 miles away. Only one ambulance and two volunteers are available. One police officer is also available. You happen upon the scene and engage in making priority triage decisions. Based on the information on the following four clients:

Client 1: A woman who is seven months pregnant was able to walk around but is reporting severe pain in her abdomen. Her previous child was born prematurely at 34 weeks.
Client 2: A young child who is wearing a medical bracelet stating she has type 1 diabetes. She can walk but doesn't know where she is or what happened.
Client 3: An older obese adult is lying on the ground. There is bleeding from the forehead and a firm abdomen, and they are unresponsive.
Client 4: A younger adult is trapped on the car's driver's side. They are unresponsive, and an open compound fracture is noted on the right leg.

1. How would you triage/tag each client and provide rationales?
2. Would there be other assessment data or information for each client that would assist in better identification of how to triage and prioritize the care?
3. With limited resources, who would use the ambulance first? Provide your rationale.

AACN *Essentials* (2021): Domains: #1; #2; #3; #4; #6; #7; #9

- Competencies: 1.1; 1.3; 2.3; 2.5; 3.6; 4.2; 6.1; 6.2; 6.4; 7.2; 9.2; 9.4b
- Subcompetencies: 1.1b; 1.3b; 2.3e; 2.5c; 2.5d; 2.5e; 3.6a; 3.6c; 4.2c; 6.1a; 6.1c; 6.1e; 6.2c; 6.4 d; 7.2b; 9.2b; 9.2f; 9.4b

Spheres of Care: Regenerative/Restorative care

Concepts: Compassionate care; Clinical judgment; Evidence-based care; Social determinants of health (SDOH)

Source: Clarkson & Williams, 2023.

Recovery/Rehabilitation

In this phase, the focus on resilience is vital. It is essential to meet the needs of the individual, family, and community to recover the damaged environment. Systems and concerns such as power, search and rescue, temporary shelters, debris clearance, medical needs, job assistance, and food and water must be addressed by those most vulnerable. Additional needs include economic, mental, emotional, and spiritual aspects. The value of surveying the damage left by the disaster and looking at these concerns is vital. Gathering information on the degree of damage and a needs assessment is essential to ascertain what resources are currently available and those that need to be acquired (CDP, 2024a).

The recovery/rehabilitation part of the disaster emergency response process begins when the disaster occurs and continues for several days to several years (Brown et al., 2010). The DOI interacts in areas that can restore, redevelop, and revitalize the affected community. Through the use of the NDRF, work is done to assist with the following six specific areas: community planning and capacity-building, housing, economics, infrastructure systems, health, and natural and cultural resources through solving problems, resource access, and coordination of governmental and nongovernmental agencies (Firouzkouhi et al., 2021; DOI, 2024).

As nurses are active participants before, during, and following disasters, their involvement has led to significant numbers of survivors and decreased mortalities. Those recovering present various types of injuries and disabilities depending on the kind of disaster sustained. The injuries may be temporary or permanent and can present as related to such conditions as musculoskeletal, traumatic brain injury, and burns (Amatya et al., 2023).

Additional conditions nurses face are the prevention of disabilities and infectious diseases, the provision of psychological and mental health support, the organization of shelters, and the continuation of nursing care. Disasters produce a prevalence of victims with exacerbations of noncommunicable diseases such as cardiac, cancer, respiratory diseases, diabetes, depression, and other mental disorders. As seen in a disaster, the difficulties in obtaining access to specific healthcare and specialties, disruption of services, financial issues, transportation, and illiteracy of the injured are common (Ngaruiya et al., 2022). Tsuji et al. (2017) reduced depressive symptoms after the Great East Japan Earthquake in older survivors through group exercise participation, regular walking, rehabilitation, caring for chronic conditions, and overall evaluation of disaster response actions. Collaborating with multidisciplinary teams that offer specialized services is critical to facilitating rehabilitation (Ching & Lazaro, 2019).

Meeting the needs of individuals, families, and entire communities is vital to recovery, as this may require making several adjustments or even assisting in starting a new life. Whatever the need, the nurse's role is essential to providing crisis intervention during all stages of disasters (Firouzkouhi et al., 2021).

Although disasters affect everyone, they often spotlight longstanding disparities and inequities experienced by people from racial and ethnic minority groups and low-income people. These groups are also disproportionately affected by disasters due to decades of systemic and environmental injustices. Communities with less power and access to resources also experience inequities during disaster response and recovery (SAMHSA, 2024; Box 8.5).

BOX 8.5 ACTIVE LEARNING REFLECTION ACTIVITY

Postrecovery Case

The CDP provides recovery assistance for those met with a disaster. Proceed to the following website: https://disasterphilanthropy.org/resources/disaster-phases/. Watch the video on the Van Buren Missouri 2017 flood disaster.

You are in charge of helping the town recover. Determine three priority long-term recovery strategies for the city and provide a brief plan for accomplishing these strategies.

Please use the CDP website and the disaster philanthropy playbook to help with the plan.

AACN *Essentials* (2021): Domains: #1; #3; #6; #9

- Competencies: 1.1; 1.3; 3.1; 3.2; 3.3; 3.5; 3.6; 6.1; 9.2; 9.3
- Subcompetencies: 1.1b; 1.3a; 3.1a; 3.1b; 3.1c; 3.1e; 3.1f; 3.2a; 3.2b; 3.3a; 3.3b; 3.5a; 3.6a; 3.5c; 3.5d; 3.6c; 6.1c; 9.2b; 9.3a

Spheres of Care: Regenerative/Restorative care

Concepts: Compassionate care; SDOH; Clinical judgment

Sources: CDP, 2024a; Critical Disaster Playbook, 2024.

Rehabilitation practices in disasters involve a significant number of individuals and situations. Amatya and Khan (2023) reported that this area of care needs to be better prioritized than the importance of initial stabilization of the injured. There is evidence that improving the interventions for rehabilitation helps minimize mortality and disabilities. The inclusion of rehabilitation algorithms continues to be developed and implemented both nationally and internationally for all levels of responders.

It is important to remember that despite nurses' role in disasters to assist with various activities, nurses also need time to physically rest and mentally deal with what has occurred. Perhaps they have had members of their own family or community involved with injury or loss of life. Diversity and cultural needs are also vital to disasters but may be challenging to meet. Overcoming these obstacles may be daunting, but meeting nurses and other first responders must come into plans when a disaster occurs (Solikhah & Aditya, 2022).

Other Aspects of Emergency Disasters

Healthcare providers must understand that emergencies and disasters come in many forms and types, depending on location and geography. Regardless, communities must plan and prepare to respond to various emergencies and disasters (Rural Health Information Hub, 2024).

TABLE 8.1 Possible Bioweapons

Name of Disease	Type of Organism	Mode of Trans- mission	Signs/Symptoms/ Treatment/ Vaccine	Areas Found
Anthrax (CDC, 2020)	Gram-positive, rod-shaped bacteria, *Bacillus anthracis*	Occurs in soil; contact with infected animals or contaminated animal products	Cutaneous: blisters, swelling, sores; inhalation: cough, shortness of breath, fever and chills, nausea/ vomiting, bloody stools, abdominal pain; vaccine available	It is found on most continents; rare in the United States
Ebola (CDC, 2024b)	Ebolaviruses	Contact with an infected animal (bat or nonhuman primate) or a sick or dead person infected with the Ebola virus	Begins with "dry" symptoms: fever, aches/pains, and fatigue; progresses to "wet" symptoms: diarrhea/vomiting; vaccine available	Found in sub-Saharan Africa
Smallpox (CDC, 2016)	Variola virus	Direct face-to-face contact results in mouth and throat sores caused by coughing and sneezing; the sores continued to be contagious until the last scab was gone	Fever, progressive skin rash; vaccination available	Eradicated in 1977 due to vaccine
Plague (CDC, 2024c; WHO, 2022)	Caused by bacterium Yersinia pestis	Bite from infected fleas or by managing infected rodents Types: Bubonic (most common) and Pneumonic (most virulent)	Bubonic-painful swollen lymph nodes, or buboes Pneumonic-lung-based plague; transmitted via droplets The WHO does not recommend vaccination in high-risk groups such as laboratory or healthcare workers	Occur in rural areas in the western United States and are significantly present in parts of Africa and Asia

Cholera (WHO, 2023)	Infection of the intestines with the bacterium *Vibrio cholerae*	Found in water or foods contaminated by feces from an infected person	Watery diarrhea, vomiting, and leg cramps or no symptoms Vaccine: oral Vaxchora for those traveling to an area with active cholera transmission	Cholera occurs in places with inadequate water treatment, poor sanitation, and inadequate hygiene; raw shellfish are a source of infection

Sources: CDC, 2020; CDC, 2024a; CDC, 2024b; WHO, 2022; WHO, 2023.

Terrorism

The FBI defines *terrorism* as being international, such as significant criminal actions by foreign organizations or nations. In contrast, *domestic terrorism* is those criminal acts related to areas of political, religious, social, racial, or environmental topics that involve individuals or groups. The FBI collaborates closely with its partners to neutralize terrorist cells and operatives here in the United States, help dismantle extremist networks worldwide, and cut off financing and other forms of support provided to foreign terrorist organizations (FBI, n.d.).

During a terror event, the reactions of those affected are presented with mass hysteria. Although expected, these perceptions must allow healthcare professionals to exhibit a sense of calm to best manage the needs of those requiring attention. Training and preparation in terrorist situations are essential for all to provide the most practical needs for the type of terrorism setting (Williams et al., 2023).

Bioweapons

The World Health Organization (WHO) defines *bioweapons* as toxic substances that present as viruses, bacteria, or fungi, causing diseases or death in people, along with animals and plants in the environment. Several biological agents, such as anthrax, Ebola, smallpox, plague, and cholera, can potentiate significant health issues, including epidemics. Unconventional weapons, also known as *weapons of mass destruction*, include chemical, nuclear, and radiological weapons. Statistics from the WHO have found that terrorist attacks using bioweapons have increased (UN, n.d.; WHO, 2024a).

In these situations, the WHO works closely with the affected local, state, and governmental agencies, the UN, and international groups. Activities include the cause, scope, and situational influence of those involved. Laboratory assistance is needed to isolate the organism and take proper precautions, work with those infected, and provide vaccines or cures (WHO, 2024a; Table 8.1).

Radiological and Nuclear Terrorism

Nuclear agents are found in many areas of the environment to which individuals are exposed, such as intense light, heat, soil, water, and food. To understand nuclear weapons, the degree of energy given off consists of a blast wave, intense light, heat, and radiation from the explosion (CDC, 2019). Fallout of the materials is radioactive and contaminates the areas where it is deposited (CDC, 2024a). World War II ended after the use of the nuclear bomb by the United States (Williams et al., 2023).

The International Criminal Police Organization (INTERPOL) was developed to assist in protecting the world. This group works with 196 global police groups to strive for world safety. The countries work as a team by using a secure network to communicate with each other for support in handling fugitives. Through INTERPOL, the primary areas of concern include fighting crimes of terrorism, cybercrime, organized crime and financial crime, and corruption (INTERPOL, n.d.).

Chemical Warfare

Terrorist attacks using deadly chemical agents are a significant concern. When reviewing chemical warfare, the use of toxic chemicals in the form of vapors, gases, liquids, or aerosols is identified. Depending on the chemical, the effects can be related to skin, blood, lungs, gastrointestinal, and central and peripheral nervous system injury. Chemical warfare has not been used since World War I when, in 1925, the Geneva Protocol prohibited usage. In recent years, some chemical incidents included Iraqi forces in 1987–1988 and in Syria in 2017 (Amend et al., 2020; DHS, 2022b; Mphuthi et al., 2023; Williams et al., 2023).

The need to identify the chemical agent and provide the most effective intervention is recognized. Overall, the importance focuses on adequately preparing and initiating proper response training. The use of governmental agencies and their expertise is essential for providing for current events and the means to prepare for future events (Tin & Ciottone, 2022).

Infectious Diseases

Infectious disease outbreaks can be transmitted through many avenues. Person-to-person contact, animal-to-person contact, environmental, and exposure to chemicals or radioactive materials are transmission methods (WHO, 2024b).

Various forms of disasters cause various effects on the environment and people. That said, resulting hazards such as infectious disease may be the cause or can develop from the event. Globally, the vulnerable populations in critical positions during the disaster can be severely affected, leading to significant outbreaks that cause morbidity and mortality. The UN Sendai Framework for Disaster Risk Reduction is the first global policy framework representing a step toward coherence with explicit reference to health, development, and climate change. The specifics of this framework are to assist globally with disaster risk management in health, human rights, development, and climate change (Aitsi-Selmi et al., 2015). Disasters that affect humans through outbreaks of infectious diseases are specifically addressed (Charnley et al., 2020).

War and natural disasters have significant and devastating impacts on the presentation of infectious diseases. The disasters may affect healthcare systems and the environment, allowing for the presentation of various exposures to health risks and emergence of infectious diseases. Such events tend to cause population movements such as floods, hurricanes, and tornadoes, leading to vector-borne diseases (Topluoglu et al., 2023). Depending on the type of disaster, infectious conditions can be especially detrimental to those with compromised immune systems, older adults, and children (Gray-Miceli et al., 2023).

SDOH and Emergency Preparedness

Public health emergencies can highlight the problems of existing health disparities. At all levels of emergency planning, public health and its partners must be accountable to populations with existing inequities, which requires a conceptual shift toward using SDOH data. Changes in disaster preparedness require a shift in emergency activities toward interventions that target the SDOH to adequately address long-standing systemic health disparities and socioeconomic inequities in the United States (Levine & Jansson, 2021). Identification and accounting for other factors, such as location and poverty, must be used rather than relying on chronic conditions alone (McQueen et al., 2022).

Levels of Prevention and Emergency Preparedness

Unfortunately, public health prevention budgets have decreased. The CDC's Public Health Emergency Preparedness (PHEP) funding has been reduced by 30% over the past two decades. The PHEP is the primary source of federal funding for state public health and emergency response. Funding should increase as emergencies and disasters increase (Sen-Crowe et al., 2020).

The first two stages of disaster are primary prevention in nature. These two stages occur before the disaster or emergency has occurred. Secondary and tertiary prevention steps are key once a disaster or emergency occurs. In the response phase, actions relate to the immediate needs of those affected. By working to save lives and promote public safety, this phase considers the disaster plans that have been developed. Looking at the current disaster and considering planning assists with preparation before the next disaster may occur (CDP, 2024b).

Healthy People 2030 and Emergency Preparedness

Emergency preparedness is essential to Healthy People (HP) 2030, which aims to improve emergency preparedness and response by building community resilience (Office of Disease Prevention and Health Promotion, n.d.). There are many objectives, and the number of adults with an emergency plan and the number of globally important public health events tracked and reported are just two in the developmental stage. HP 2030 ensures that individuals, communities, and organizations are prepared for disasters, disease outbreaks, and medical emergencies.

Chapter Highlights

- Discussion and application of the four stages of disaster
- Discussion about significant emergency/disaster planning organizations
- Application of active learning reflection activity for postrecovery care
- Application of active learning reflection activity for CERTs
- Application of active learning reflection activity for triage/priority emergency management
- Application of active learning reflection activity understanding FEMA
- Application of active learning reflection activity developing a personal tornado disaster plan

Active Learning Exercises

Application to Intervention Wheel

Please use the yellow wedge section of https://www.health.state.mn.us/communities/practice/research/phncouncil/docs/PHInterventions.pdf to address the following story. Watch the video/story regarding public health preparedness in a particular county in Minnesota.

Lia Roberts is a public health nurse (PHN) and the public health preparedness coordinator for Dakota County in Minnesota. To learn about her work in emergency preparedness, watch the video at https://www.youtube.com/watch?v=qTUHoztIFYY (Dakota County, 2018).

Consider this example of pandemic flu planning. Consider how the yellow wedge interventions of advocacy, social marketing, and policy development and enforcement occur when conducting emergency preparedness activities for the pandemic flu.

1. Apply two interventions from each section (advocacy, social marketing, and policy development and enforcement) to the overall planning of an emergency or a disaster of your choice other than the pandemic flu. Think about a disaster or emergency that could occur in your community.

You can also use the DHS website at https://www.dhs.gov/topics/disasters, which contains many resources for emergency preparedness planning to analyze effective advocacy, social marketing, and policy development/enforcement interventions. PHNs can access these resources at Ready.gov.

AACN *Essentials* (2021): Domains: #1; #3; #4; #5; #6; #7; #8

- Competencies: 1.2; 1.3; 3.2; 3.4; 3.5; 3.6; 4.2; 5.2; 6.3; 7.2; 8.1
- Subcompetencies: 1.2e; 1.3a; 1.3b; 1.3c; 3.2a; 3.2b; 3.4a; 3.4b; 3.4c; 3.5c; 3.5d; 3.5e; 3.6a; 3.6c; 4.2c; 5.2a; 5.2c; 6.3a; 6.3c; 7.2c; 8.1c; 8.1d; 8.1e

Spheres of Care: Wellness/Disease prevention

Concepts: Clinical judgment; SDOH; Evidence-based practice; Health policy

Sources: DHS, 2022b; Minnesota Department of Health, 2019; Ready.gov, 2024; Dakota County Videos, 2018.

Case Studies

Case Study #1

It is a Sunday at 3 p.m. The city's professional sports team is playing, filling the covered stadium (55,000 people). The EMS personnel on site have called to report that they have seen 32 people exhibiting symptoms of watery eyes, coughing, dyspnea, fever, hypotension, and extreme weakness. Those who accompanied the victims to the event have begun to talk with other spectators, and the people have begun to respond to the news of a possible biological release. Fans started rushing from the stadium. A triage area has been set up in a nearby facility. You are part of a response team and arrive at the facility.

1. What is the first thing you should do?
2. Describe the appropriate emergency response plan.
3. Who is in charge of the response?
4. Which government response units are needed?
5. What challenges could be encountered with fans rushing from the stadium in this scenario?
6. Describe the psychosocial assistance you would offer victims and their families.
7. How would an event like this affect the community?
8. What role would the nurse play in developing management plans?

AACN *Essentials* (2021): Domains: #1; #2; #3; #4; #6; #7; #8; #9

- Competencies: 1.2; 1.3; 2.1; 2.2; 2.3; 2.4; 3.6; 4.2; 6.1; 6.2; 6.4; 7.1; 8.3; 9.1; 9.2; 9.4
- Subcompetencies: 1.2e; 1.3a; 1.3b; 2.1b; 2.2c; 2.3a; 2.3c; 2.3g; 2.4c; 3.6a; 3.6c; 3.6e; 4.2c; 6.1a; 6.1b; 6.2a; 6.2c; 6.4d; 7.1d; 8.3a; 9.1a; 9.1c; 9.2b; 9.4b

Spheres of Care: Regenerative/Restorative care

Concepts: Clinical judgment; Communication; Evidence-based practice; Ethics; Compassionate care

Sources: Developed by authors.

Case Study #2

A family consisting of parents ages 34 with two children, ages 8 and 6, have asked for assistance in building a kit and planning for a disaster. Using the steps outlined in this chapter and the following other websites, assist them in this activity. To determine the type of disaster, review which disaster may be a common situation—a flood, tornado, chemical spill—you may experience, according to where you live, learn, work, and play. Use the website Ready.com or https://www.ready.gov/kids/games/data/bak-english/index.html to assist with the activity.

What are the three most essential priorities/steps the family should complete first?

Step 1:
Step 2:
Step 3:

Reflect on what three things you learned from this case study that you could use as a future nurse.

AACN *Essentials* (2021): Domains: #1; #2; #3; #4; #8

- Competencies: 1.3; 2.2; 3.1; 3.6; 4.2; 8.1
- Subcompetencies: 1.3a; 1.3c; 2.2a; 2.2e; 3.1a; 3.1c; 3.1f; 3.6a; 3.6c; 3.6d; 4.2c: 8.1a; 8.1e

Spheres of Care: Wellness/Disease prevention

Concepts: Evidence-based practice; Communication; Clinical judgment

Sources: Ready.gov, n.d.a.; 2024.

Case Study #3

A nursing student collaborates with a middle school nurse in a community clinical rotation. The school nurse has been asked to present ideas about how to teach sixth graders about the concept of disaster prevention and preparation. Use the Ready.gov website to develop a plan as well as the game noted on the website https://www.ready.gov/kids/games/data/dm-english/index.html.

1. Develop two specific objectives/SMART goals (discussed in depth in Chapter 4) regarding the Disaster Master game.
2. How will you instruct the students on accessing and completing the game?

3. What kind of reward or follow-up could you provide to evaluate whether the students met the objectives?

AACN *Essentials* (2021): Domains: #1; #2; #3; #4; #5; #8; #9

- Competencies: 1.3; 2.2; 3.1; 3.6; 4.2; 5.2; 8.1; 8.3: 9.3
- Subcompetencies: 1.3a; 1.3b; 2.2c; 2.2e; 3.1a; 3.1c; 3.6a; 3.6e; 4.2c; 5.2a; 8.1d; 8.3a; 9.3a

Spheres of Care: Wellness/Disease prevention

Concepts: Communication; Evidence-based practice; Clinical judgment

Sources: Ready.gov, n.d.b.; 2024.

NCLEX Questions

1. Nurses need to be knowledgeable about disaster issues. Which three statements relate to disaster management? **Select all that apply.**
   a. Nurses must be assessed for disasters during annual competency exams.
   b. Nurses are commonly asked by family, neighbors, friends, and communities for health care information and advice.
   c. Nurses are responsible for teaching emergency service workers.
   d. Nurses commonly respond to the needs of society in times of disaster.
   e. Nurses are essential in assisting with developing disaster policies and procedures.

2. Which statements does disaster preparedness include? **Select all that apply.**
   a. Disaster preparation needs to be reviewed monthly.
   b. Disaster plans need to be adjusted to individual and community needs.
   c. Disaster plans are dynamic and change as community needs shift.
   d. A lack of understanding of disaster plans could negatively affect the actions of the community members.
   e. A multidisciplinary team is most effective in defining the roles of others for an effective disaster plan.

References

Administration for Strategic Preparedness and Response. (n.d.). *The Medical Reserve Corp.* https://aspr.hhs.gov/MRC/Pages/index.aspx

Aitsi-Selmi, A., Egawa, S., Sasaki, H., Wannous, C., & Murray, V. (2015). The Sendai Framework for Disaster Risk Reduction: Renewing the global commitment to people's resilience, health, and well-being. *International Journal of Disaster Risk Science*, *6*, 164–176. https://doi.org/10.1007/s13753-015-0050-9

Alpert, E., & Kohn, M. (2023). *EMS mass casualty response.* StatPearls. https://www.ncbi.nlm.nih.gov/books/NBK536972/

Amatya, B., & Khan, F. (2023). Disaster response and management: The integral role of rehabilitation. *Annual Rehabilitation Medicine, 47*(4), 237–260. https://doi.org/10.5535/arm.23071

Amend, N., Niessen, K., Seeger, T., Wille, T., Worek, F., & Thiermann, H. (2020). Diagnostics and treatment of nerve agent poisoning-current status and future developments. *Annals of the New York Academy of Science, 1479*(1), 13–28. https://doi.org/10.1111/nyas.14336

American Association of Colleges of Nursing. (2021). *The essentials: Core competencies for professional nursing education.* https://www.aacnnursing.org/Essentials

American Red Cross. (2024). *Disaster preparedness plan.* https://www.redcross.org/get-help/how-to-prepare-for-emergencies/make-a-plan.html

American Roentgen Ray Society. (n.d.). *Mass casualty incidents: An introduction for imagers.* https://arrs.org/ARRSLIVE/Education/InPractice/Winter_2020/radiology-imaging-mass-casualty-incidents.aspx#

Brown, L. M., Hickling, E. J., & Frahm, K. (2010). Emergencies, disasters, and catastrophic events: The role of rehabilitation nurses in preparedness, response, and recovery. *Rehabilitation Nursing, 35*(6), 236–241. https://doi.org/10.1002/j.2048-7940.2010.tb00053.x

Center for Disaster Philanthropy. (2024a). *Disaster phases.* https://disasterphilanthropy.org/resources/disaster-phases/

Center for Disaster Philanthropy. (2024b). *Empowering rural communities.* https://disasterphilanthropy.org/resources/empowering-rural-communities/

Centers for Disease Control and Prevention. (2016). *What is smallpox?* https://www.cdc.gov/smallpox/about/index.html

Centers for Disease Control and Prevention. (2019). *Nuclear weapons.* https://www.cdc.gov/nceh/multimedia/infographics/nuclear_weapon.html

Centers for Disease Control and Prevention. (2020). *Anthrax.* https://www.cdc.gov/anthrax/symptoms/index.html

Centers for Disease Control and Prevention. (2024a). *CDC's response to nuclear or radiological emergencies.* https://www.cdc.gov/radiation-emergencies/programs/index.html#

Centers for Disease Control and Prevention. (2024b). *Ebola disease basics.* https://www.cdc.gov/ebola/about/index.html

Centers for Disease Control and Prevention. (2024c). *Plague.* https://www.cdc.gov/plague/about/index.html

Chai, J., & Wu, H. (2023). Prevention/mitigation of natural disasters in urban areas. *Smart Construction and Sustainable Cities*, 1, 4. https://doi.org/10.1007/s44268-023-00002-6

Charnley, G., Kelman, I., Gaythorpe, K., & Murray, K. (2020). Understanding the risks for post-disaster contagious disease outbreaks: a systematic review protocol. *BMJ Open, 10*(9), e039608. https://bmjopen.bmj.com/content/10/9/e039608

Chartoff, S., Kropp, A., & Roman, P. (2023). *Disaster planning.* StatPearls [Internet]. https://www.ncbi.nlm.nih.gov/books/NBK470570/

Cheatham, A., Roy, D., & Labrador, R. (2023). *US disaster relief at home and abroad.* https://www.cfr.org/backgrounder/us-disaster-relief-home-and-abroad

Ching, P., & Lazaro, R. (2019). Preparation, roles, and responsibilities of Filipino occupational therapists in disaster preparedness, response, and recovery. *Disability and Rehabilitation, 43*(9), 1333–1340. https://doi.org/10.1080/09638288.2019.1663945

Clarkson, L., & Williams, M. (2023). *EMS mass casualty triage.* StatPearls [Internet]. https://www.ncbi.nlm.nih.gov/books/NBK459369/

County of Santa Clara Emergency Medical Services. (2019). *Multiple casualty incident plan.* https://emsagency.sccgov.org/sites/g/files/exjcpb266/files/General/811MCI.pdf

Critical Disaster Playbook. (2024). *Disaster philanthropy playbook.* https://disasterphilanthropy.org/disaster-philanthropy-playbook/

Dakota County Videos. (2018). *Dakota County public health emergency preparedness.* YouTube, May 18, 2018. https://www.youtube.com/watch?v=qTUHoztIFYY

Department of Homeland Security. (n.d.). *Natural disasters.* https://www.dhs.gov/natural-disasters

Department of Homeland Security. (2022a). *Chemical attack fact sheet.* https://www.dhs.gov/publication/chemical-attack-fact-sheet

Department of Homeland Security. (2022b). *Department six-point agenda.* https://www.dhs.gov/department-six-point-agenda

Department of Homeland Security. (2022c). *Disasters.* https://www.dhs.gov/topics/disasters

Department of Homeland Security. (2023). *Creation of the Department of Homeland Security.* https://www.dhs.gov/creation-department-homeland-security

Department of Homeland Security. (2024). *About DHS.* https://www.dhs.gov/about-dhs

Department of the Interior. (n.d.). *Natural disaster response and recovery.* https://www.doi.gov/recovery

Federal Bureau of Investigation. (n.d.). *Terrorism.* https://www.fbi.gov/investigate/terrorism

Federal Emergency Management Agency. (n.d.). *Getting involved with CERT.* https://community.fema.gov/PreparednessCommunity/s/welcome-to-cert?language=en_US

Federal Emergency Management Agency. (2023a). *About.* https://www.fema.gov/about

Federal Emergency Management Agency. (2023b). *National preparedness goal.* https://www.fema.gov/emergency-managers/national-preparedness/goal

Federal Emergency Management Agency. (2023c). *National preparedness report.* https://www.fema.gov/sites/default/files/documents/fema_2023-npr.pdf

Federal Emergency Management Agency. (2023d). *Training and education.* https://www.fema.gov/emergency-managers/national-preparedness/training

Federal Emergency Management Agency. (2024a). *FEMA mobile products.* https://www.fema.gov/about/news-multimedia/mobile-products#download

Federal Emergency Management Agency. (2024b). *How FEMA works.* https://www.fema.gov/about/how-fema-works#FEMA

Federal Emergency Management Agency. (2024c). *National Incident Management System.* https://www.fema.gov/emergency-managers/nims

FEMA Emergency Management Institute. (2018). *IS-700.B: An introduction to the National Incident Management System.* https://training.fema.gov/is/courseoverview.aspx?code=is-700.b&lang=en

FEMA Emergency Management Institute. (2020). *IS-317.A: Introduction to community emergency response team (CERTs).* https://training.fema.gov/is/courseoverview.aspx?code=IS-317.a&lang=en

Firouzkouhi, M., Kako, M., Abdollahimohammad, A., Balouchi, A., & Farzi, J. (2021). Nurses' roles in nursing disaster model: A systematic scoping review. *Iranian Journal of Public Health, 50*(5), 879–887. https://doi.org/10.18502/ijph.v50i5.6105

Future Learn. (n.d.). *Preparedness and the disaster cycle.* https://www.futurelearn.com/info/courses/humanitarian-action-response-relief/0/steps/60986

Gray-Miceli, D., Gray, K., Sorenson, M., & Holtzclaw, B. J. (2023). Immunosenescence and infectious disease risk among aging adults: Management strategies for FNPs to identify those at greatest risk. *Advances in Family Practice Nursing, 5*(1), 27–40. http://dx.doi.org/10.1016/j.yfpn.2022.11.004

International Criminal Police Organization. (n.d.). *What is INTERPOL?* https://www.interpol.int/en/Who-we-are/What-is-INTERPOL

International Disaster Database Centre for Research on the Epidemiology of Disasters. (2024). *EM-DAT and the CRED.* https://doc.emdat.be/docs/about/emdat-and-the-cred/

International Federation of Red Cross and Red Crescent Societies. (2024a). *Disasters, climates, and crises.* (https://www.ifrc.org/our-work/disasters-climate-and-crises/what-disaster

International Federation of Red Cross and Red Crescent Societies. (2024b). *Strategy 2030.* https://www.ifrc.org/who-we-are/about-ifrc/strategy-2030

Irwin, J. F. (2022). The emergency service: Evaluating the role of militaries in humanitarian operations, disaster relief, and other nonconflict crises. *Journal of Advanced Military Studies, 13*(1), 5–13. https://www.muse.jhu.edu/article/857228

Klein, T., & Irizarry, L. (2023). *EMS disaster response.* StatPearls [Internet]. https://www.ncbi.nlm.nih.gov/books/NBK560710/

Krichen, M., Abdalzaher, M., Elwekeil, M., & Fouda, M. (2024). Managing natural disasters: An analysis of technological advancements, opportunities, and challenges. *Internet of Things and Cyber-Physical Systems, 4,* 99–109. https://doi.org/10.1016/j.iotcps.2023.09.002

Levine, C. A., & Jansson, D. R. (2021). Concepts and terms for addressing disparities in public health emergencies: Accounting for the COVID-19 pandemic and the social determinants of health in the United States. *Disaster Medicine and Public Health Preparedness,* 1–7. https://doi.org/10.1017/dmp.2021.181

Lincoln, E., Freeman, C., & Strecker-McGraw, M. (2023). *EMS incident command.* StatPearls [Internet]. StatPearls Publishing. https://www.ncbi.nlm.nih.gov/books/NBK534800

McQueen, A., Charles, C., Staten, J., Broussard, D. J., Smith, R. E., Verdecias, N., & Kreuter, M. W. (2022). Social needs are associated with greater anticipated needs during an emergency and desire for help in emergency preparedness planning. *Disaster Medicine and Public Health Preparedness, 17,* e279. https://doi.org/10.1017/dmp.2022.208

MedicTests. (2024). *START triage.* https://medictests.com/units/start-triage

Medium. (2023). *Natural disasters that are man-made.* https://medium.com/@jabonetakevin/natural-disasters-that-are-man-made-251d54f2ec91

Merriam-Webster Dictionary. (2024a). *Disaster.* https://www.merriam-webster.com/disctionary/disaster.

Merriam-Webster Dictionary. (2024b). *Triage.* https://www.merriam-webster.com/dictionary/triage

Minnesota Department of Health. (2019). *Public health interventions: Applications for public health nursing practice* (2nd ed.). https://www.health.state.mn.us/communities/practice/research/phncouncil/docs/PHInterventions.pdf

Molassiotis, A., Guo, C., Abu-Odah, H., West, C., & Yuen Loke, A. (2021). Evolution of disaster nursing research in the past 30 years (1990–2019): A bibliometric and mapping analysis. *International Journal of Disaster Risk Reduction, 58,* 102230. https://doi.org/10.1016/j.ijdrr.2021.102230

Mphuthi, N., Jijana, A., Mhlanga, N., Muchindu, M., Nyembe, S., Mwakikunga, B., Gebhu, N., Sikhwivhilu, L. (2023). Chapter 1: Chemical warfare agents: An outlook on past and present technologies. In S. Das, S. Thomas, & P. Pratim (Eds.), *Sensing of deadly toxic chemical warfare agents, nerve agent simulants, and their toxicological aspects* (pp. 3–31).

National Centers for Environmental Information. (2024). *U.S. billion-dollar weather and climate disasters.* https://www.ncei.noaa.gov/access/billions/

Ngaruiya, C., Bernstein, R., Leff, R., Wallace, L., Agrawal, P., Selvam, A., Hersey, D., & Hayward, A. (2022). Systematic review on chronic non-communicable disease in disaster settings. *BMC Public Health, 22,* 1234. https://doi.org/10.1186/s12889-022-13399-z

Office of Disease Prevention and Health Promotion. (n.d.). *Emergency preparedness.* Healthy People 2030. https://health.gov/healthypeople/objectives-and-data/browse-objectives/emergency-preparedness

Oshiro, K., Tanioka, Y. Schweizer, J., Zafren, K. Brugger, H., & Paal, P. (2022). Prevention of hypothermia in the aftermath of natural disasters in areas at risk of avalanches, earthquakes, tsunamis and floods. *International Journal of Environmental Research and Public Health, 19*(3), 1098. https://doi.org/10.3390/ijerph19031098

Ready.gov. (n.d.a.). *Build a kit.* https://www.ready.gov/kids/games/data/bak-english/index.html

Ready.gov. (n.d.b.) *Disaster master.* https://www.ready.gov/kids/games/data/dm-english/index.html

Ready.gov. (2024). *Plan ahead for disasters.* https://www.ready.gov/

Rural Health Information Hub. (2024). *Module 4: Types of public health emergencies and disasters.* https://www.ruralhealthinfo.org/toolkits/emergency-preparedness/4/types-of-emergencies-and-disasters

Sen-Crowe, B., McKenney, M., & Elkbuli, A. (2020). Public health prevention and emergency preparedness funding in the United States: Are we ready for the next pandemic? *Annals of Medicine and Surgery, 59,* 242–244. https://doi.org/10.1016/j.amsu.2020.10.007

Singamator the Educator. (2020). *Disaster part 2 (Man-made disasters and effects of disasters).* YouTube, September 1, 2020. https://www.youtube.com/watch?v=rQKJyj-15-0

Solikhah, F. K., & Aditya, R. A. (2022). Healing in nurses after assignment in natural disasters. *Folia Medica Indonesiana, 58*(4), 377–382. https://doi.org/10.20473/fmi.v58i4.37410

Substance Abuse and Mental Health Services Administration. (2023a). *Incidents of mass violence.* https://www.samhsa.gov/find-help/disaster-distress-helpline/disaster-types/incidents-mass-violence

Substance Abuse and Mental Health Services Administration. (2023b). *Types of disasters.* https://www.samhsa.gov/find-help/disaster-distress-helpline/disaster-types

Substance Abuse and Mental Health Services Administration. (2024). *Diversity, equity, and inclusion in disaster planning and response.* https://www.samhsa.gov/dtac/disaster-planners/diversity-equity-inclusion

Tin, D., & Ciottone, G. R. (2022). Chemical agent use in terrorist events: A gathering storm requiring enhanced civilian preparedness. *Prehospital and Disaster Medicine, 37*(3), 327–332. https://doi.org/10.1017/s1049023x22000528

Topluoglu, S., Taylan-Ozkan, A., & Alp, E. (2023). Impact of wars and natural disasters on emerging and re-emerging infectious diseases. *Frontiers in Public Health, 11,* 1215929. https://doi.org/10.3389/fpubh.2023.1215929

Tsuji, T., Sasaki, Y., Matsuyama, Y., Sato, Y., Aida, J., Kondo, K., & Kawachi, I. (2017). Reducing depressive symptoms after the Great East Japan Earthquake in older survivors through group exercise participation and regular walking: a prospective observational study. *BMJ Open, 7,* e013706. https://doi.org/10.1136/bmjopen-2016-013706

United Nations. (n.d.). *What are biological weapons?* https://disarmament.unoda.org/biological-weapons/about/what-are-biological-weapons/

USA.gov. (n.d.). *U.S. Department of Homeland Security (DHS).* https://www.usa.gov/agencies/u-s-department-of-homeland-security

Williams, M., Armstrong, L., & Sizemore, D. (2023). *Biologic, chemical, and radiation terrorism review.* StatPearls [Internet]. https://www.ncbi.nlm.nih.gov/books/NBK493217/

World Health Organization. (2022). *Plague.* https://www.who.int/news-room/fact-sheets/detail/plague

World Health Organization. (2023). *Cholera*. https://www.who.int/news-room/fact-sheets/detail/cholera

World Health Organization. (2024a). *Biological weapons*. https://www.who.int/health-topics/biological-weapons#tab=tab_1

World Health Organization. (2024b). *Environment, climate change and health*. https://www.who.int/teams/environment-climate-change-and-health/emergencies/disease-outbreaks

Credits

Fig. 8.1: Adapted from source: https://medium.com/@jabonetakevin/natural-disasters-that-are-man-made-251d54f2ec91.

Fig. 8.1a: Copyright © 2023 Depositphotos/CanerArican.

Fig. 8.1b: Copyright © 2012 Depositphotos/pxhidalgo.

Fig. 8.1c: Copyright © 2005 by Khao Lak Ausflüge (CC BY-SA 4.0) at https://commons.wikimedia.org/wiki/File:Tsunami_Khao_Lak_2004.jpg.

Fig. 8.1d: Copyright © 2012 by Department of Foreign Affairs and Trade (CC BY 2.0) at https://commons.wikimedia.org/wiki/File:Landslide_in_the_southern_highlands_of_PNG,_2012._Photo-_AusAID_(10707798284).jpg.

Fig. 8.1e: Copyright © 2005 Depositphotos/alancrosthwaite.

Fig. 8.1f: Copyright © 2007 by Justin Hobson (CC BY-SA 3.0) at https://commons.wikimedia.org/wiki/File:F5_tornado_Elie_Manitoba_2007.jpg.

Fig. 8.1g: Copyright © 2014 Depositphotos/weyo.

Fig. 8.1h: Copyright © 2014 Depositphotos/perszing1982.

Fig. 8.1i: Copyright © 2013 Depositphotos/ChiccoDodiFC.

Fig. 8.1j: Copyright © 2023 Depositphotos/algifs.

Fig. 8.2: Singamator the Educator, Screenshot from "DISASTER PART 2 (MAN MADE DISASTERS AND EFFECTS OF DISASTERS)," https://www.youtube.com/watch?v=rQKJyj-15-0. Copyright © 2021 by Singamator the Educator.

Fig. 8.3: Copyright © 2022 Depositphotos/FPCreativeStock.

Fig. 8.4: U.S. Department of Homeland Security, https://www.fema.gov/about/how-fema-works#FEMA, 2024.

Fig. 8.5: Medic Tests, https://medictests.com/units/start-triage. Copyright © 2024 by Medic Tests.

CHAPTER 9

Environmental

"We won't have a society if we destroy the environment."

—Margaret Mead

Learning Outcomes

After reading this chapter, students should be able to:

1. Understand the effects of environmental health on health outcomes
2. Understand the meaning of the I PREPARE mnemonic
3. Discuss elements of the natural, built, and social environments affecting population health
4. Apply the educational role of the nurse to significant global environmental health concerns
5. Understand the roles of government and public agencies in assisting with issues associated with environmental health

Keywords and Concepts

American Public Health Association (APHA); built environment; climate change; ecology; environmental health; Environmental Protection Agency (EPA)

Definitions of the Keywords

APHA: Serves as a facilitator, catalyst and advocate to build capacity in the public health community (APHA, 2024a)

Built environment: Humanmade or modified structures that provide people with living, working, and recreational spaces (EPA, 2024c)

Climate change: Shifting of temperatures and weather patterns over a long period of time (United Nations [UN], n.d.e.)

Ecology: A branch of science concerned with the interrelationship of organisms and their environments (Merriam-Webster, n.d.)

Environmental health: Focus on the environment and the health of the individuals who live and work there (APHA, 2024d)

EPA: A federal agency whose mission is to protect human health and the environment (EPA, 2024h)

Introduction

The environment and how it affects the world are vital concerns for everyone. It is essential to consider how the relationship to the environment contributes to human health. Healthcare professionals use research data to guide the planning and revising goals to determine environmental health needs. More than 12 million people globally are living or working in unhealthy settings, leading to their deaths (Prüss-Ustün et al., 2016).

The need for appropriate settings to work, live, learn, play, and worship must be safe and provide protection. Considering how and what humans do that affect the environment, the continued proliferation of the world may be protected. Many organizations, researchers, and scientists focus on the environment to prevent, plan, develop, and evaluate strategies to address appropriate functioning for current and future needs. Identifying the current concerns and improving environmental functioning will be vital to the global environment. Clean air, stable climate, adequate water, sanitation and hygiene, safe use of chemicals, protection from radiation, healthy and safe workplaces, sound agricultural practices, health-supportive cities and built environments, and a preserved nature are all prerequisites for good health (World Health Organization [WHO], 2024e).

Current environmental facts include several significant findings that must be addressed. Some issues noted are the following: Globally, temperatures rose in 2022 and were found to be higher than before 2015; the identification that in 2022, nine states had unusually higher-than-average temperatures above the 20th-century averages; in 2022, weather and climate disasters cost more than $1 billion and wildfires damaging 7.6 million acres; and there was governmental spending of $31.2 billion on resources for the environment (USAFacts.org, 2024). By acquiring reporting, analyzing, and researching events, those knowledgeable can assist with adequate planning and intervening in what can best assist in keeping the environment healthy and the well-being of the individuals living in it (USAFacts.org, 2024). This chapter will discuss environmental health issues, proper environmental health assessment, and major environmental health concerns.

Background of the Concepts

Significant concerns have become evident in the environment today. Without attention to the present damage and how to best deal with further environmental conditions, the world may be in great danger in future years. Such hazards as air pollution, toxins in surfaces and groundwater, including lead, car emissions, and pesticides, could lead to the development of severe health conditions such as heart disease, cancer, and dementia and therefore should be investigated (Centers for Disease Control and Prevention [CDC], 2024e).

Currently, the importance of meeting the needs for an environment that is viable for sustained development and usage for all people is emphasized. Through a sound ecosystem, the role of plants, animals, and biological agents; the weather and climate; terrains such as rivers and oceans; and natural resources, including air, water, and fuels, are considered in the natural environment. While some benefit humans, some may be identified as detrimental, such as acting as a poison and disease-causing. A nonlinear analysis of the impacts of natural resources, such as green energy and education on environmental quality, is critical for the future (Liu et al., 2022).

The social environment, which consists of various resources, communities, neighborhood economic status, social cohesion, societal norms and policies (nonsmoking housing), water protection, pollution reduction, energy consumption, and waste management, must be considered. The Agency for Healthcare Research and Quality (2022) discusses the framework for agencies to assess problems and identify progress using initiatives and interventions. The following assessment areas include care with performance of safety, providing practical services without negative intentions, offering patient-centered care respecting the needs and values of each client, using timely use to delay care, being aware of misuse of resources and supplies, and including special equitable needs for all regarding gender, ethnic backgrounds, area living, and their socioeconomic status (Romanello et al., 2022).

Tobin et al. (2022) include walkability with the environment. The research studied defining the concept of walkability and identification to active living environments. The definition of *walkability* involves the built and social environment and how it affects populations related to physical activity, energy balance, and health. The actual conceptual definition needs to be formulated. These researchers, after communicating with many different groups, presented this concept termed *Active Living Environments* (ALEs), developing a more concise meaning for ALEs as "emergent natural, built, and social properties of neighborhoods that promote physical activity and health and allow for equitable access to health-enhancing resources." (p. 5). Overall, it was concluded that this definition would be a comprehensive form to include improving aspects of health for all populations (Tobin et al., 2022).

Rodriguez and Wilson (2022) researched that through the Data Modernization Initiative, a method to incorporate data, technology, and workforce use. They suggest that by doing so, those in public health leadership positions will provide intensive surveillance, research, and critical decision-making. By doing so, the initiative will assist the CDC in being more responsible for providing information to be effective with their actions and directions to others and provide effective environmental health measures (CDC, 2024d).

This chapter will investigate environmental factors that could cause diseases and exacerbations of chronic illnesses. Discussion about practical environmental health assessments and specific nursing-focused interventions with application through active learning reflection activities are noted.

Environmental Health

Environmental health is the health of those individuals who live, work, play, and learn in that setting (APHA, 2024d). The description also includes that the environment may be modified or manipulated to assist with decreasing disease risks while not affecting the ecosystem. The APHA plays a significant role in bringing national attention to environmental health issues, focusing on environmental justice, lead contamination, water equity, and climate change (APHA, 2024a). The APHA includes such concerns as air pollution and lead-based drinking water, which can cause diseases such as heart disease, cancer, and dementia. In poverty-stricken areas, the APHA addresses any inequalities affecting their health and overall care (APHA, 2024d; APHA, 2024e).

The WHO is instrumental in global environmental health. A healthy environment attribute includes clean air, proper sanitation and hygiene, healthy and nonviolent workplaces, sufficient water supplies, healthy living environments, and safe food resources (WHO, 2024b). When the death rates relate to the many environmental risks, that can, overall, be risks that can be changed to promote health instead of death. The WHO has identified one in four global deaths fits this category. Preventing diseases, including noncommunicable conditions, tends to be a component of the environment that produces damaging diseases and poor client health outcomes (WHO, 2024b).

The WHO's specialization in assisting in healthy environments is critical to improving health. By networking with others worldwide, the WHO can provide the means to share technology and methods to decrease global insecurities and promote enhanced abilities to use good practices, perform research, and develop policies and procedures to review and evaluate current environmental practices effectively. The identification of processing assessments, setting goals, conducting interventions, and, finally, evaluating assist with meeting the needs of all (WHO, 2024b; 2024c).

Purpose

All communities should be concerned about environmental and climate change care. There are several purposes related to environmental health, including ensuring sufficient human health conditions that lead to healthy settings where individuals can live, work, worship, learn, and play. To secure this for all communities, agencies must ensure that a risk assessment is performed and policies and procedures are formulated for preventative measures and interventions to put into action (APHA, 2024d; 2024e).

Ecology

A healthy relationship between plants, animals, ecosystems, and resources is necessary for the environment's current status and future generations' needs (Ecology Society of America [ESA], 2024). Public health considers the actual environment and how it relates to people's health and safety. Environmental health professionals focus on areas that review the possibilities of harmful exposures and develop and enforcing policies to prevent injury or disease development (ESA, 2024).

Ecologists study and work with various organisms and their many environments. Participation in environmental health programs allows ecologists to gather data, inspect environments, award violations or close facilities as needed, award permits or licenses, and respond to public complaints. Without the timely work of environmental inspectors, populations may be negatively affected. Safety measures are vital and can be identified by following evidence-based practice guidelines (Rodriguez & Wilson, 2022).

Effective environmental health must protect all people from environmental hazards. Some of these have been known to affect individuals with cancer, respiratory, and cardiac conditions. Diverse ethical and cultural groups often need help to maintain good health practices. They tend to reside in poor communities, burdened with poverty and structural limitations. These negative connotations must be decreased so that safety is present for all (APHA, 2024d; 2024e).

Environmental Protection Agency

Nationally, the EPA is the keeper of the environment. The EPA's mission and focus is to protect human health and the environment. They ensure clean air, land, and water; reduce environmental risks based on EBP; ensure federal laws that protect human health and the environment are administered and enforced relatively; educate communities, individuals, businesses, and state, local, and tribal governments regarding accurate information sufficient to effectively participate in managing human health and environmental risks; monitor/oversee contaminated lands and toxic sites, ensuring that they are cleaned up; and ensure that chemicals in the marketplace are reviewed for safety (EPA, 2024e; 2024h).

Educating the public is critical to ensuring that negative effects on the environment do not affect community health. The EPA provides extensive information and education on many environmental topics, such as greener living, health risk information, and the science of environmental problems (EPA, 2024g). The EPA website provides lesson plans, science fair topics, and community service projects. Interactive activities are noted for younger children to learn about the importance of environmental factors (EPA, 2024g).

American Public Health Association

The APHA brings national attention to environmental health issues, focusing on environmental justice through policies that promote community health. The APHA also focuses on climate change issues and works with many other organizations to ensure the future of our environment. They strongly advocate against environmental racism, where those of Black, Brown, Indigenous, and low-wealth communities continue to experience disproportionate exposures and cumulative impacts from environmental health justice issues (APHA, 2024e).

Concepts and Theories

Environmental health approaches can be viewed by several means. The significance is the correlation with humans, their health, and their connection with other forms of organisms (Badash et al., 2017). Taking an upstream approach to the environment is a crucial concept. This approach encourages taking action to prevent illness and injury, protect people, promote environments that foster good health, and, importantly, address social injustice (Pacific Public Health Foundation [PPHF], 2020).

Upstream Focus on the Environment

An upstream approach identifies the root causes of disease and manufacturers of illness, considering socioeconomic factors and the environmental origins of disease and health problems. Public health nurses are often involved in disease surveillance, detecting unusual illness patterns, and responding to environmental emergencies in work and community settings (PPHF, 2020; Figure 9.1; Box 9.1).

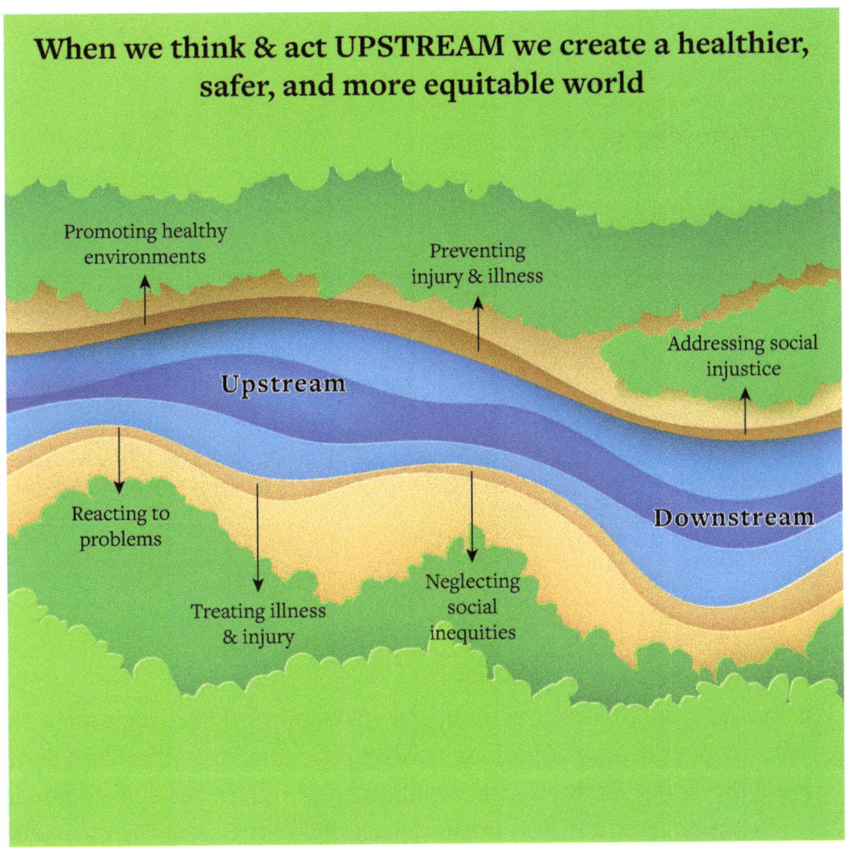

FIGURE 9.1 Upstream Approach: Promoting Healthier Environments

BOX 9.1 ACTIVE LEARNING REFLECTION ACTIVITY

Applying the Upstream Approach to the Environment

How could a nurse take a more active upstream approach to providing a better environment, leading to better health and improved health outcomes? Watch the following video and answer the following reflection questions: https://www.ted.com/talks/shweta_narayan_it_s_impossible_to_have_healthy_people_on_a_sick_planet?language=en&subtitle=en.

1. What are two ways you could apply an upstream approach for improving a community's health about housing where homes were built before 1978?
2. Name three evidence-based resources related to an adequate housing environment.

3. Name two ways you will utilize what you have learned about the upstream approach and its application to your future nursing practice.
4. Develop a public service announcement (PSA) outline for educating adolescents and assisting with an upstream approach to better environmental health.

American Association of Colleges of Nursing (AACN) *Essentials* (2021): Domains: #1; #2; #3; #4; #8; #9

- Competencies: 1.1; 1.2; 1.3; 2.2; 3.1; 4.2; 8.3; 9.3
- Subcompetencies: 1.1b; 1.2a; 1.2c; 1.3a; 2.2e; 3.1c; 3.1f; 4.2c; 8.3a; 8.3c; 9.3a

Spheres of Care: Wellness/Disease prevention

Concepts: Communication; Clinical judgment; Evidence-based practice

Source: Narayan, 2021.

Critical Theory Approach

The critical theory approach uses an upstream framework for thinking. It raises questions about oppressive situations, involves community members in defining and solving problems, facilitates interventions that reduce the health-damaging effects of environments, and asks critical questions about clients' work and home environments to help discern the contributions of specific hazards to health (APHA, 2024d; 2024e).

An application of this type of approach is the critical race theory of environmental disaster associated with the Flint, Michigan, water crisis. In 2014, Flint was considered a socioeconomically depressed area with state and local involvement. A city emergency manager instituted cost-saving water infrastructure measures without public or city knowledge, which led to the city developing lead issues. The theory incorporates interpretations of the causes and consequences of environmental disasters, which are instrumental in creating social understandings of and experiences with environmental disasters and the importance of environmental justice (Ezell & Chase, 2022).

Precautionary Principle

The *precautionary principle* states that when an activity raises threats of harm to human health or the environment, precautionary measures should be taken if some cause-and-effect relationships are not fully established scientifically (International Institute for Sustainable Development, 2020). This principle has been used in international law for many years. Recently, several countries used the principle during the COVID-19 crisis as early interventions and precautionary measures, including travel restrictions, mandatory lockdowns, and quarantines, and therefore saw fewer severe cases and deaths (Pinto-Bazurco, 2020).

One Health Conceptual Framework

The WHO defines *One Health* as an "approach to designing and implementing programs, policies, legislation, and research in which multiple sectors communicate and work together to achieve better public health outcomes" (2024f, para. 1). This framework is a method in which to use research findings to support humans, animals, and the environment by looking at identified problems and developing positive interventions. Although this process can be complex, the framework helps the researchers to design and analyze the findings. Using multidisciplinary experts to follow the research process from global areas, the wealth of knowledge contains significant challenges and obstacles. As many of the participants involved in the research have varying views, the importance of collaboration is promoted significantly when the environments, laws, cultures, and populations vary greatly. Ogunseitan (2022) supports the realization that the translation of the different health, wildlife, and environmental ministries, food and drug administrations, and local environmental community involvement may vary significantly, leading to differences in perspectives of the actual needs. Health conditions related to humans and animals and how they interact are different.

Environmental Health Assessment

As with any form of planning, an assessment is the first step. An environmental assessment focuses on observing the environment and noting any issues that could affect health outcomes (CDC, 2019). The EPA has The Center for Public Health and Environmental Assessment (CPHEA), which provides science that notes the interrelationship between people and nature in support of assessments and policies to protect human health and ecological integrity. The CPHEA provides and monitors for gaps in research and data needed to adequately assess all aspects of the environment to preserve favorable health outcomes (EPA, 2024b).

I PREPARE

In 2005, a team of nurses devised a framework, called *I PREPARE*, for conducting individual environmental health assessments and an action plan. *I PREPARE* is a mnemonic that allows for easy reconstruction of environmental assessment areas (Paranzino et al., 2005).

As a significant reference for identifying the facets of environmental history, I PREPARE has been used to contain specific references to focus on for healthcare providers. Paranzino et al. (2005) found that this simple tool helped significantly improve the quality of information and findings to assist with healthcare needs. This mnemonic can follow specific health history questions. I PREPARE stands for the following: *I*nvestigate potential exposures; ask questions related to *p*resent work, *r*esidence, *e*nvironmental concerns, *p*ast work, *a*ctivities; provide *r*eferrals and resources; and *e*ducate the individual through a checklist. The interviewer could obtain the information and offer educational content and resources using specific questions (Parazino et al., 2005). This will allow for a thorough environmental assessment in any nursing setting (Table 9.1).

TABLE 9.1 I PREPARE

	Explanation	Examples of Nursing Actions
I	**Investigate potential exposures:** Ask questions to uncover possible sources of exposure to environmental hazards.	Ask about feeling ill after handling chemicals or toxic substances.
P	**Present work:** Inquire about the person's current occupation and potential workplace hazards.	Ask the client to describe their current job, industry, and any hazardous substances they manage.
R	**Residence:** Assess potential residential exposures. Ask about their built community.	Ask about the age and type of dwelling, water source, and indoor hazards.
E	**Environmental concerns:** Encourage clients to discuss environmental problems in their neighborhood.	Ask if they live near landfills, lakes, rivers, farms, or factories.
P	**Past work:** Inquire about past occupations or exposures that may have exposed the client to hazardous materials.	Ask if they have ever worked on a farm or in a factory, coal mine, or construction site or used solvents or other chemicals.
A	**Activities:** Assess the client's activities that may have exposed them to environmental hazards.	Ask about hobbies, outdoor recreation, smoking, and diet.
R	**Referrals and Resources:** Provide information about relevant resources, referrals, or organizations that can help the individual address their environmental health concerns.	Provide information on government sites such as the CDC, EPA, or Occupational Safety and Health Administration (OSHA).
E	**Educate:** Share information about the client's potential environmental health risks and provide guidance on preventing or reducing exposure to protect their health.	If they may have been exposed to lead in their drinking water, provide information about testing and mitigation from local, state, and federal resources.

Sources: Parazino et al., 2005; adapted from Mager & Cornelius, 2019.

TABLE 9.2 Examples of Environmental Health Guiding Documents and Organizations

Organization	Guiding Documents
American Nurses Association's (ANA) *Principles of Environmental Health for Nursing Practice with Implementation Strategies*	Guide environmentally safe nursing care (ANA, 2007)
ANA Nursing: Scope and Standards of Practice; Standard 17: Environmental Health	Provision 17. Environmental Health: The registered nurse practices in an environmentally safe and healthy manner (ANA, 2022)
Healthy People 2030 initiatives	Create social, physical, and economic environments that promote attaining the full potential for health and well-being for all (Office of Disease Prevention and Health Promotion [ODPHP], n.d.a.; n.d.b.)
Core functions of public health	Enable optimal health for all and seek to remove systemic and structural barriers that have resulted in health inequities (CDC, 2024a; 2024b)

Sources: ANA, 2007; ANA, 2022; CDC, 2024a; CDC, 2024b; ODPHP, n.d.a.; ODPHP, n.d.b.

Tracking of Environmental Health Data

The CDC (2023) tracks national, state, and local environmental issues through the National Environmental Public Health Tracking Network (NEPHTN). The network contains data and information on environments and hazards, health effects, and population health. Data can be obtained nationally, by state, and, in some cases, by county regarding subjects such as congenital disabilities, chronic obstructive pulmonary disease, and asthma concerning environmental effects. Many other vital documents, guidelines, and organizations assist in understanding the impact of environmental issues (Table 9.2; Box 9.2).

BOX 9.2 APPLICATION OF NATIONAL ENVIRONMENT PUBLIC HEALTH TRACKING NETWORK

The NEPHTN is a resource to investigate environmental data. Go to https://ephtracking.cdc.gov/ and perform the following steps. Analyze the results by answering the following questions. Click on the "Explore Data" tab.

Step 1: Under the "Select Content" area, choose "Built Environment." Under "Select Indicator," choose "Age of Housing." Under "Select Measure," choose "Percentage of Housing Units by Year Structure."
Step 2: Choose "Nation by County."
Step 3: Choose "All Counties."

Step 4: Choose the latest year.
Step 5: Pick "Before 1980" and then hit the green "Go" button.

Answer the following reflection questions:

1. Name three states with the highest number of houses built before 1980.
2. Provide evidence-based research on why houses built before 1980 could be environmental issues and what would be two environmental concerns.
3. Name three nursing interventions that include educating the population of those areas that live in housing before 1980.
4. Discuss two referrals/agencies that could assist the population.

AACN *Essentials* (2021): Domains: #2; #3; #4; #7; #8

- Competencies: 2.4; 3.1; 3.3; 4.2; 7.2; 8.3
- Subcompetencies: 2.4b; 3.1a; 3.1b; 3.1c; 3.1d; 3.3b; 4.2c; 7.2b; 8.3c; 8.3e

Spheres of Care: Wellness/Disease prevention; Chronic disease management

Concepts: Communication; Clinical judgment; Evidence-based practice; Social determinants of health (SDOH)

Source: CDC, 2023.

Alliance of Nurses for Healthy Environments

The Alliance of Nurses for Healthy Environments (ANHE) is a national nursing organization that reflects on how health and the environment interact. It aims to provide education to lead nurses through evidence-based practice and research to develop policies dealing with health disparities and facilitate what will be needed (ANHE, n.d.).

The ANHE has a vast number of environmental resources. Its website presents tools related to community, home, hospital, general, pediatrics, schools, and women. English and Spanish versions are available for healthcare providers who need assessment tools in a particular area and language (ANHE, n.d.).

Major Global Environmental Concerns

The WHO has data supporting that without the scrutiny of adequate living settings, prevention of health conditions may have been able to be decreased globally. The WHO addresses significant areas that must be a part of the crucial needs of all environments. The WHO's global concerns include clean air, a stable climate, adequate water, sanitation and hygiene, safe use of chemicals, healthy and safe workplaces, sound agricultural practices, and health-supportive cities. The experiences with the

COVID-19 pandemic are an example that allowed the world to view the significance of the relationship between people and the planet (WHO, 2024b; 2024e).

One organization, Earth.org, is dedicated to sharing information about the crucial issues affecting the planet (Earth.org, n.d.). As some countries do not have the capabilities to oversee public health concerns, including disease monitoring, surveillance use, and appropriate laboratory systems for testing and reporting, an association with other agencies is most helpful. It is associated with the identification, training, education, and evaluation processes, including communication with global members (Earth.org, n.d.).

Earth.org (2024) has listed its most significant global concerns for 2024, which include global warming from fossil fuels, poor governance, food waste, biodiversity loss, plastic pollution, deforestation, air pollution, melting ice caps and sea level rise, ocean acidification, food and water insecurity, fast fashion and textile waste, overfishing, cobalt mining, and soil degradation. Earth.org (n.d.) has a mission in which human society develops the maturity to manage itself, the planet, its natural resources, and global commons for multigenerational benefit and equity, and a vision to assist in a societal change for a sustainable planet.

Overpopulation

Overpopulation today affects the ability of our ecosystem to support itself and acquire additional resources. Exceeding the population continues when people migrate to other ecosystems to preserve their current standard of living (Center for Biological Diversity [CBD], n.d.; Earth.org, 2023). Scott (2022) notes that the increase in global population will mean that available resources will not catch up with the increased population, leading to food insecurities, water shortages, famine, depletion of other vital resources, and epidemics.

Some solutions to overpopulation are controversial depending on cultural concerns, religious beliefs, personal values, and convictions. The need to teach about birth spacing, preventing high-risk pregnancies, preventing the growing epidemic of HIV/AIDS, providing family planning education, and providing prenatal care can assist with the extended population numbers (CBD, n.d.; Earth.org, 2023).

Air Pollution

Today's world is filled with air contaminants that cause changes in the atmosphere, both internal and external. One of the most hazardous sources is chemical contamination, which has adverse effects that include costs to property, productivity, and quality of life. Some geographic regions are more susceptible to adverse impacts due to the weather or physical terrain. Examples of contaminants can vary and include combustible chemicals, automobiles, industrial businesses, forest fires, carbon monoxide, dust, gases, ozone, carbon monoxide, radon, volcanic ash, and acid precipitation. These irritants can be detrimental, especially to individuals with cardiac and respiratory diseases, and most affected are people from low- to middle-income countries (EPA, 2023b; WHO, 2024a).

Nurses can play a huge role in educating the population about the risks and dangers of air pollution. It is critical to educate the population on the importance of monitoring daily air quality before proceeding outdoors and its effect on particular health problems. Indoor air quality education is also essential for those with chronic respiratory diseases. Nurses can function as a force for change in supporting healthy communities and challenging local, regional, and national policy and practice, especially for health equity (Waterall et al., 2021).

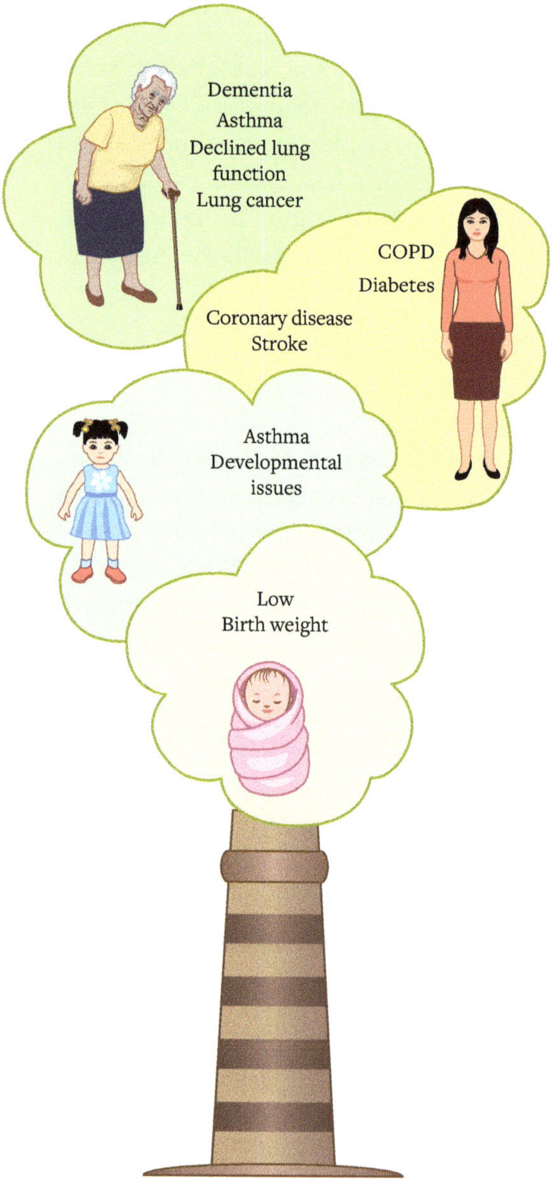

FIGURE 9.2 Air Pollution Affects Across the Lifespan

Ozone Depletion and Global Warming

The ozone layer has become a vital area of communication in recent years as it is becoming depleted. This results in the earth having less protection from exposure to the sun and increased exposure to radiation by ultraviolet B (UVB) rays. UVB rays affect the skin primarily by causing skin burning, whereas ultraviolet A rays focus on skin aging. There are increased risks for people to develop skin cancer and cataracts, indirectly damaging the food chain, increasing exposure to vector-borne diseases, rising ocean levels, mutations of marine ecosystems, causing increases in certain atmospheric gasses such as carbon monoxide and carbonyl sulfide, and negative impact on crop production (Skin Cancer Foundation, 2022). Nurses can help the community through education about protection from increased skin cancer risks. Lobbying for appropriate legislation regarding ozone depletion, including reducing greenhouse gases, is also vital to assist with ozone layer depletion (EPA, 2023a; National Aeronautics and Space Administration, 2024).

Deforestation, Wetlands Destruction, and Desertification

Deforestation occurs when forests are removed to provide land for agricultural areas and manufacturing and building resources, including road construction. The ecosystem becomes ineffective and contributes to ozone depletion, geographic changes occur, and the development of landslides, drought, famine, and starvation results. Deforestation may also affect biodiversity. This process causes harm to valuable animal and plant species, leading to their extinction. Erosion also depletes the forests as the trees are removed, leading to the vulnerability of forest fires. To assist with conservation, leaders can be vocal at all governmental levels and work to promote efforts to replenish forests (National Geographic, n.d.a.; UN, n.d.a.).

Desertification relates to when fertile land becomes desert. When this occurs, diseases develop and spread, especially respiratory conditions, food production decreases, causing malnutrition, and reducing water sources leads to hygiene and self-care limitations. This desertification encourages people to move to more accessible environments (WHO, 2020). Methods to assist include planting trees in forests and practical water management actions, including collecting rainwater, fertilizing soil, and mulching to decrease evaporation and retain water (UN, n.d.a.).

One solution is Sustainable Development Goal #15, life on land, which is devoted to protecting and returning the ecosystem to provide effective means for biodiversity conservation. Education and advocating for recycling activities are beneficial in addressing this condition. Additional interventions can focus on leaving wildlife in their habitats and promoting a healthy ecosystem (Global Goals, n.d.; UN, 2024).

Wetlands provide several ecological, economic, and social benefits, citing fish habitats for wildlife and plants. Flood waters and melted snow can be released slowly to help facilitate available groundwater, filter contaminants, and provide salt and freshwater for marine life and recreation opportunities. These resources can assist with climate change and biodiversity by delivering interventions in the wetlands. If fewer wetlands are available to filter pollutants from surface waters, those pollutants could become more concentrated in the remaining wetlands. Wetland loss can also decrease habitat, landscape diversity, and connectivity among aquatic resources. For example, converting from one wetland type to another by cutting down trees in forested wetlands can have a significant ecological impact by changing habitat types and community structure (EPA, 2024f).

Lawton (2023) noted that preserving wetlands is crucial to combating the health effects of impending climate change. Advocating to protect these wetlands is critical to combating droughts, absorbing pollutants, and storing much-needed carbon to maintain the ecosystem if left undisturbed. Nurses can be at the forefront of educating the population and political leaders on the importance of wetlands.

Water Pollution

Water pollution can significantly affect human health and the environment. It has many causes, including agricultural/farm runoff, sewage, radioactive substances, stormwater runoff, and oil pollution. Many at-risk live close to pollution sites, leaving contaminated drinking water (Natural Resources Defense Council, 2017). Diseases from polluted drinking water are cholera, giardia, and typhoid. Education for methods for decreasing water pollution include practicing recycling of plastics; correct disposal of chemical cleaners; proper car care of motor oil, antifreeze, and coolants; using approved nontoxic pesticides; discarding unneeded medications in appropriate containers; performing care of storm sewers, maintenance of septic systems, and routine community water quality testing; and identifying increased incidences of water-related diseases (National Defense Resource Center, 2023; EPA, n.d.; EPA, 2024f).

Energy Depletion

Energy depletion occurs when natural resources become exhausted and cannot be replaced naturally at the speed of consumption. Today, the energy sources used are primarily nonrenewable and include fossil fuels, oil, natural gas, coal, and nuclear energy. Burning fossil fuels harm the environment by releasing particles into the air, water, and land, causing pollution (National Geographic, n.d.b.).

Constant energy utilization globally has resulted from the development of various industries and people moving into more densely populated areas. Carbon dioxide emissions and the growth of the world's economy have contributed to the underrated growth of natural resources, while energy depletion has increased them. Meeting the needs of those who need access to sufficient energy is essential. Xu and Zhao (2023) researched those that were underexploited and suggested some recommendations that could assist with this concern, which may be enhanced by technologies focused on environmental and healthcare matters. The development and implementation of sustainable energy systems will be the role of governmental policymakers through policies, technological means, and even alternatives to the current energy uses. The challenges are in planning for the future with the current alignment of natural resources.

Nurses can be involved with education about energy conservation and alternative energy sources. The encouragement to assist others in becoming interested in and knowledgeable about potential energy depletion will help increase public awareness of the concern while offering information to individuals, communities, and other populations (Xu & Zhao, 2023).

Unhealthy and Contaminated Food

Access to safe and healthy foods is vital for the population's health and sustenance. The WHO has estimated that more than 600 million individuals become ill after eating food that is contaminated, and an additional 420,000 die (WHO, 2024d). Some foods are spoiled due to contamination, primarily affecting those in low to middle-income countries. Foodborne disease conditions produce bacteria, viruses, parasites, and chemicals relating to various diseases and malnutrition. Some conditions that may develop include salmonella, listeria, norovirus, tapeworms, mad cow disease, lead poisoning, and mercury poisoning (WHO, 2024d).

The U.S. Department of Agriculture (USDA) assists Americans with food insecurity. Worldwide, more than 870 million people experience insufficient safe and nutritious food (USDA, n.d.c.). The USDA emphasizes that children and those with low incomes should be able to increase healthy food resources, decrease hunger, and provide educational means (USDA, n.d.a.).

As the United States is a global leader in agriculture, it deals with how the economy is growing due to climate change and food insecurity. Researching the needs of farmers and progressing with the food that populations eat produces challenges. Illnesses that affect communities worldwide impact many, resulting in the importance of proper food cleaning, storage, and preparation. Continual evaluation of current methods in agriculture needs to be improved to help all populations along with adequate population education (USDA, n.d.b.; n.d.d.).

Waste Disposal

With the growth of the world's population, the need for and use of specific products such as plastics, paper, and aluminum are being extensively used. Practices must be implemented using the best possible means to manage, collect, store, and recycle these items as concerns relate to adverse environmental and public health effects. Damage affects the ecosystem through uncontrolled dumping, open-air incinerators, land degradation, climate change, air and water pollution, and landfills cause contamination of the rivers, lakes, and oceans. The impacts associated with public health costs must be considered and reviewed, especially for individuals who reside in marginalized areas (Abubakar et al., 2022; Ritchie, 2023).

The world must consider the proper policies and procedures for disposal through recycling to decrease the use of these items. As waste disposal significantly impacts areas with inadequate waste management systems, governments must promote active community members to become involved through campaigns encouraging proper waste disposal activities such as littering and recycling. Education of the public and lobbying for legislation, avoiding using aerosol sprays, plastics, and other non-recyclable items. By improving waste management systems, monitoring, enforcing, and practices, the world will also see decreased raw materials created for materializing products and compliance (Abubakar et al., 2022; Ritchie, 2023; Box 9.3).

BOX 9.3 ACTIVE LEARNING REFLECTION ACTIVITY

Microplastics and Environmental Harm

Watch the following video about microplastics: https://x.com/todayshow/status/1385923933388648452?s=12.

Reflect on the following questions:

1. How can you take this information and reinforce the presentation to a group of older adults who are not concerned with the effects of climate change and who do not understand what and how this is affecting life currently and will continue to do so in the future?
2. Develop a list of what recycling would do if everyone participated in this process. Give examples of effective recycling materials.
3. How can they volunteer to help their communities and teach the upcoming generation about the importance of this?

Further develop a one-page fact sheet on microplastics for children ages 5 to 8.

AACN *Essentials* (2021): Domains: #1; #3; #4; #7; #8

- Competencies: 1.2; 1.3; 3.2; 3.3; 3.4; 3.6; 4.2; 7.2; 8.1
- Subcompetencies: 1.2a; 1.3a; 3.1a; 3.1c; 3.1e; 3.2c; 3.3b; 3.4c; 3.4d; 3.6a; 3.6b; 4.2c; 7.2b; 7.2d; 8.1a

Spheres of Care: Wellness/Disease prevention; Chronic disease management

Concepts: Ethics: Evidence-based practice; Health policy; SDOH; Communication

Source: Today Show, 2021.

Insect and Rodent Control

Rodents and insects affect humans and animals worldwide by causing health-related conditions and interfering with food and animal feed. Public representatives and health professionals' function by working together to manage the impact on humans as well as animals. Researching knowledge about insects and rodents will help decrease the threats predicted in the future. Identifying this information will assist in looking at insect/rodent health conditions and how they affect food security, the food chain, use of control, care of insects, and incorporation of pest control programs (Belluco et al., 2023).

The National Pest Management Association (NPMA) helps preserve food, properties, and public health. Its goals focus on insects/rodents disrupting consumers through pest control to protect people, homes, land, and businesses from related health conditions. Through support from NPMA, professionals are educated and made knowledgeable and able to network, provide leadership in many areas, and are made profitable by being proactive in pest management and the means to share information with owners of homes and businesses (NPMA, 2024).

Pesticides could control the health concerns of insects/rodents. Mosquitoes, cockroaches, rats/mice, lice, ticks, chipmunks, and fleas can cause conditions such as the Zika virus, Lyme disease, and rabies (EPA, 2024a; 2024d). The importance of education related to identifying the presence of and how to prevent infestations is the primary focus of education as disease spreads readily from insects/rodents to humans. Removal of food, water sources, and sites may be a form of shelter for the vectors (CDC, 2024c).

Safety in the Home, at the Worksite, and in the Community

Safety concerns for the home, work sites, and community must be addressed to protect the population's health. Such exposures include toxic chemicals, radiation, noise pollution, biological pollutants, injury, and psychological hazards (ODPHP, n.d.c.).

Since the home is where most populations spend their time, safety is vital. *U.S. News and World Report* (2024) offers significant tips to follow to keep homes safe, such as installing a home security system, acquiring home/renters insurance, securing storage of hazardous substances, properly disposing of expired/unused medications, removing flammable and dry leaves and brush from around the house, evaluating water lines for cracks and nonworking parts, providing adequate lighting inside and outside of the home, adding security cameras, installing smoke and carbon monoxide detectors, and networking with neighbors. Developing and practicing for unexpected events for the home's occupants is essential, especially with such events as fires, gas emissions, water breaks, and electrical mishaps.

Providing safety for all ages is additionally essential. Special needs are required for children, older adults, and even pets. The National Council on Aging (NCOA) *Advisor* (2023) offers several suggestions for older people that can apply to all ages. Preventing falls, poisonings, and accidents can be addressed by following a home safety checklist. By evaluating each room and modifying it, home occupants can be more protected (Box 9.4).

The workplace is an essential area for proper safety measures. The OSHA reports that violence in the workplace is where not just physical harm can occur but bullying, sexual harassment, frustration, intimidation, homicides, and other forms of disruptive behaviors. Yearly, at least two million individuals can be involved in nonviolent situations, with 1,000 that are considered violent homicides (U.S. Department of Labor [DOL], n.d.).

Nursing is often affected by workplace violence in medical facilities as well as by being employed in home healthcare and community settings. Despite the setting,

BOX 9.4 ACTIVE LEARNING REFLECTION ACTIVITY

Home Safety Checklist

Review the following website. Find an older adult and utilize the checklist to determine the safety in their home. Document the necessary changes and how they can be made safely: https://www.ncoa.org/adviser/sleep/home-safety-older-adults/.

Answer the following reflective questions:

1. Name three specific education interventions completed after the assessment.
2. What education methods were used for teaching and providing evidence-based rationale?

AACN *Essentials* (2021): Domains: #1; #2; #3; #4; #5

- Competencies: 1.3; 2.5; 2.8; 2.9; 3.1; 4.2; 5.2
- Subcompetencies: 1.3a; 1.3b; 2.5d; 2.5g; 2.8e; 2.9c; 3.1c; 3.1f; 4.2c; 5.2c

Spheres of Care: Wellness/Disease prevention

Concepts: Communication; Evidence-based practice; Clinical judgment

Source: NOCA Advisor, 2023.

there is a need to have leaders who educate about and discuss with employees potential threats that can affect the workplace. Some recommendations are strategies and practice educational sessions to counteract episodes, provide security services, and assess and provide early awareness of developing employee conduct concerns. Developing specific policies, planning, and practicing how to interact if violence may occur are essential tools to implement (DOL, n.d.).

OSHA focuses on recommending methods to prevent workplace concerns involving illnesses, injuries, and deaths. By being proactive, employers can analyze potential episodes and practice safety techniques while not just being reactive after a situation occurs. A specific safety plan for workers working with certain items, such as chemicals and machines, should prevent or decrease any adverse effects. OSHA strives to educate others by preventing injuries and illnesses, improving compliance with laws and regulations, reducing costs, engaging workers, enhancing their social responsibility goals, and increasing productivity and overall business operations (OSHA, n.d.).

Climate Change

Climate change can occur from natural changes, but recently, they have been due to the effects of humans. Humans are the primary source of burning fossil fuels,

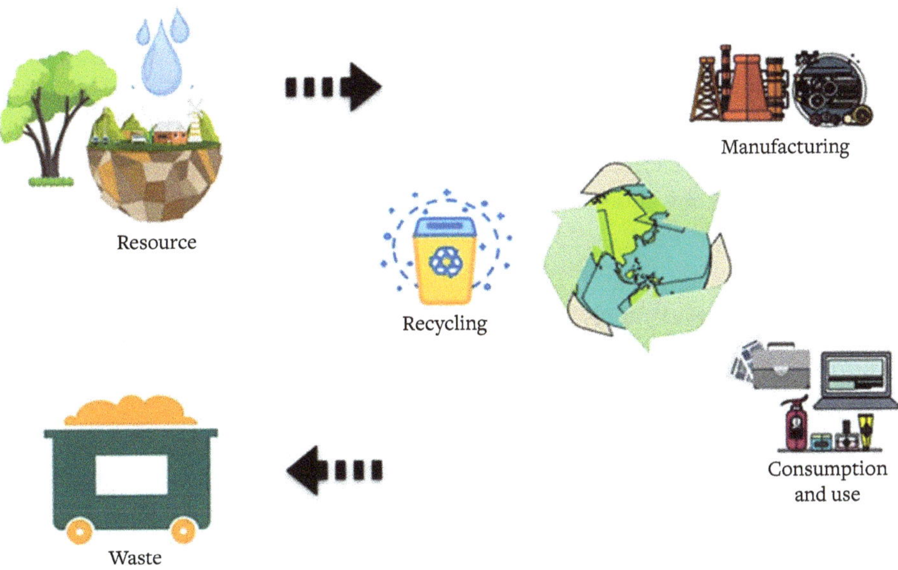

FIGURE 9.3 Circular Strategy for Combating Climate Change

including coal, oil, and gas (UN, n.d.d.). Changes have been suggested to affect the ecosystems, including increasing oceanic acidification and the high amounts of carbon dioxide in the atmosphere. The Royal Society (2020) addressed some of the upcoming challenges for the 21st century and how best to research and provide implementations to maintain resilient and opportunistic effects for future climate change (Malhi et al., 2020). Svarstad et al. (2023) researched how critical the current climate conditions are and strongly emphasized the need for intense attention to further research, education, and implementation of changes that need to be made rapidly (Figure 9.3).

Some causes of climate change would include greenhouse gas emissions-generating power through burning fossil fuels, which contributes to global emissions, manufacturing goods, use of cars, ships, trucks, and planes, deforestation for agriculture growth and manufacturing, power for buildings, and use of too much energy for homes and businesses (UN, n.d.c.). The earth is experiencing hotter temperatures due to greenhouse emissions that are causing significant forest fires and loss of properties; storms are becoming more severe and destructive, resulting in cyclones, hurricanes, and typhoons; droughts; warming, causing the oceans to expand and rise; loss of species in oceans and forests; and damage to crops, limiting food sources, leading to health risks, malnutrition, and poverty (UN, n.d.c.). Scientists are convinced that renewable energy will decrease emissions by almost half by 2030 and reach net zero by 2050. The approach is to use alternative types of energy that are clean, accessible, affordable, sustainable, and dependable (APHA, 2024b).

The long-range problems for climate control in the future are significant. Scientists encourage communities, governments, and organizations to make immediate changes (Ripple et al., 2023). Offering the extensive condition of global temperatures caused by the release of greenhouse gases by humans into the atmosphere is detrimental. Without active strategies to control human actions, changes will continue and worsen, leading to significant crises that have not been seen before (Ripple et al., 2023).

SDOH and Environmental Health

The importance of studying the environment and its relationship with the SDOH is significant. The APHA provides methods for health equity to improve environmental health through the National Council for Environmental Health and Equity. Currently, the primary objectives are to assist with educating communities and those in power to practice environmental health, including environmental justice concerns where everyone should be able to live in a safe and healthy environment, especially in the area of environmental racism; providing equality for all; and using methods to handle any environmental challenges (APHA, 2024d; 2024e).

When discussing environmental justice, the EPA states there is a need for fair treatment and meaningful involvement of all people, regardless of race, color, national origin, or income, concerning the development, implementation, and enforcement of environmental laws, regulations, and policies. Including diverse people, providing equity and health policies reflective of others globally, and meeting all the SDOH criteria are vital to the environmental justice goals (APHA, 2024d).

Collaborating with marginalized communities that are exposed to many risks leads to health issues and complicates the results. It is significant to incorporate solutions through the cooperation of several global governmental agencies to focus on SDOH topics and share innovative findings to grow and gain knowledge. Agencies can positively use appropriate resources to supply safe working conditions, adequate housing, water, and sanitation (APHA, 2024d; 2024e).

The *built environment*, described as homes, schools, highways, parks and recreational areas, waste management systems, and rural, urban, and residential areas, encompasses the land by which we are surrounded. The EPA researches how the environment and health are connected. Three significant topics the EPA studies with the environment are related to the use of land and land development and transportation; surveying the built environment; the usage and safety of the air, water, land, those living in the habitat, and human health; and the benefits that humans view in the land and methods of transportation. Experts can study and improve or reduce the apparent negative impacts by looking at these areas (EPA, 2021).

Climate change worsens health, increases healthcare costs, disproportionately affects vulnerable communities, and exacerbates the effects of other SDOHs.

Research has revealed that the changing climate is inextricably linked to poorer health. The child health impacts are numerous and include worsening asthma and allergies; physical trauma from disasters; mental health symptoms, including posttraumatic stress disorder after disasters; increased exposure to infectious diseases; and lack of access to adequate food and clean water. Addressing climate change could help control healthcare expenditures while promoting child health and well-being (Ragavan et al., 2020).

Health Inequities and Environmental Health

Even though environmental inequalities occur in many countries, the WHO has found that this deficit has increased significantly in the European Region (ER). The safety of water resources and waste disposal have developed as significant concerns. In the environments associated with poverty levels and low-income populations, exposure to toxic substances contributes to health conditions. The environment and living conditions contribute to 29% of health inequalities self-reported in the ER. The WHO explains that at least 90% of the cases are associated with unsafe living conditions, overcrowding, sanitation, and air pollution, which support environmental inequities. With the assistance of governmental organizations that understand the cultures and ethical ways of the group, they will be able to follow through to support the improvement of these environmental health issues (APHA, 2024c; WHO, 2024c; Box 9.5).

BOX 9.5 ACTIVE LEARNING REFLECTION ACTIVITY

Climate Change/Health/Equity

Review the following website: https://www.apha.org/Topics-and-Issues/Climate-Health-and-Equity/Education.

Prepare and present an educational PowerPoint using the toolkit to high school–age students. Submit the PowerPoint to your assigned faculty.

Provide a brief reflection on two aspects learned from doing this assignment.

AACN *Essentials* (2021): Domains: #1; #2; #3, #4; #9

- Competencies: 1.1; 1.2; 1.3; 2.2; 3.1; 3.3; 4.2; 9.3
- Subcompetencies: 1.1b; 1.2a; 1.3a; 2.2a; 2.2c; 3.1c; 3.1f; 3.3b: 4.2c; 9.3a

Spheres of Care: Wellness/Disease prevention

Concepts: Communication; Evidence-based practice; Clinical judgment

Sources: APHA, 2024b; 2024c.

Levels of Prevention and Environmental Health

Incorporating levels of prevention associated with environmental health is vital for everyone. The means to prevent diseases or conditions precipitating additional health conditions can be assessed by starting with the primary level. Basic primary environmental health needs include clean water, safe, nonviolent living conditions, and nutritious foods. Specific guidelines can most benefit health promotion and disease prevention related to one's environment. Organizations, community, and state agencies, and stakeholders can initiate policies to promote health, including no smoking areas, selecting healthy foods in public places, taxing unhealthy foods, maintaining safety in public places, continually reviewing needs, and updating policies to enhance and promote health, including incorporating diversity, cultures, and ethical practices to involve everyone in the communities. Technological interventions can be additionally implemented along with educational programs for safe training for any equipment that may be utilized (Rural Health Information Hub [RHIhub], 2024).

Focusing on environmental changes may include financial means, but it can also be a significant way to promote health. Development and construction of parks, walking trails, adequate signage for safe pedestrians and bike lanes, providing fresh and healthy food in schools and restaurants, free educational measures and activities for prevention and early identification of signs and symptoms of health conditions through health information classes, screenings, support for tobacco cessation and weight loss, medication education and cost savings support, mental health counseling, free dental assessments, community/church/school gardens, food pantries, and uninsured workers clinics can be developed and implemented. Being able to elicit the participation of community members in volunteer services is a significant support for these programs. Keeping a community healthy is vital to keeping the population healthy (RHIhub, 2024).

Chapter Highlights

- Discussion and application of environmental health on health outcomes and primary prevention
- Application of the meaning of the I PREPARE mnemonic
- Application of active learning reflection activities in response to climate control
- Application of active learning to promote exercise in a nursing home environment
- Application of active learning to plan educational activities for a community event
- Application of an active learning activity to educate on radon exposure in the home environment

- Discussion of the upstream focus on the environment for community support
- Case studies on environmental data tracking, built community, climate change, and hazards of radon

Active Learning Exercises

Application to Intervention Wheel

The CDC's Health Environmental Public Health Tracking Network uses climate change and health data to assess the vulnerabilities and disease burden associated with heat, air quality, asthma, and acute myocardial infarction hospitalizations.

Red wedge/surveillance: https://www.health.state.mn.us/communities/practice/
research/phncouncil/docs/PHInterventions.pdf

Use the following website to obtain data about asthma for surveillance data: https://ephtracking.cdc.gov/

Step 1: Access the "Explore data" tab.
Step 2: Choose under "Content:" "Asthma."
Step 3: Under "Select indicator," choose "Prevalence of Asthma in Children."
Step 4: Finally choose "Select measure" "Crude prevalence less than 17 who have ever had asthma."
Step 5: Pick "National by state."
Step 6: Pick the last reported year.
Step 7: Pick "Female" and then change and pick "Male."

Reflect on your findings:

1. Was there a difference in gender rates for the states with the highest percentages?
2. Pick one of the states with the highest percentage and find evidence on why it might have such an issue with asthma in children.
3. Construct a worksheet on your findings and list three specific interventions for education and health policy changes.

AACN *Essentials* (2021): Domains: #1; #2; #3; #4; #8; #9

- Competencies: 1.2; 1.3; 2.4; 3.1; 3.3; 3.4; 4.2; 8.3; 9.4
- Subcompetencies: 1.2a; 1.3a; 1.3b; 1.3c; 2.4b; 3.1a; 3.1b; 3.1c; 3.1d; 3.3b; 3.4c; 4.2c; 8.3c; 8.3e; 9.4a

Spheres of Care: Wellness/Disease prevention; Chronic disease management

Concepts: Communication; Clinical judgment; Evidence-based practice; SDOH; Health policy

Sources: CDC, 2023; Minnesota Department of Health, 2019.

Case Studies

Case Study #1

The activities coordinator for a local urban nursing home is planning exercise activities for a group of assisted living residents. During the initial session, some residents are diaphoretic and dyspneic despite frequent small breaks to rest and hydrate. Consider this situation and assess how you could direct the activities coordinator to assist the residents in better participating in the exercises.

1. What hazards are identified in this natural, built, and social environment?
2. What could be contributing to potential health hazards?
3. Name three specific interventions that would assist the residents.

Helpful information: https://www.ncoa.org/article/evidence-based-program-active-living-every-day

AACN *Essentials* (2021): Domains: #1; #2; #3; #4; #6; #9

- Competencies: 1.1; 1.2; 1.3; 2.1; 2.2; 2.3; 2.4; 3.1; 3.6; 4.2; 6.1; 9.2
- Subcompetencies: 1.1b; 1.2a; 1.3a; 1.3b; 2.1c; 2.2a; 2.3e; 2.4b; 3.1a; 3.1c; 3.6a; 4.2c; 6.1b; 9.2b

Spheres of Care: Wellness/Disease prevention; Chronic disease management

Concepts: Clinical judgment; Communication; Compassionate care; Evidence-based practice

Source: National Council on Aging, 2024.

Case Study #2

A nursing faculty presents a fact sheet on climate and health to the community/public health class.

Use the following site as the basis for the assignment: https://www.un.org/sites/un2.un.org/files/2021/08/fastfacts-health.pdf

The assignment is to prepare a one-minute PSA for the school television station regarding how climate affects health.

AACN *Essentials* (2021): Domains: #1; #2; #3; #4; #6; #8

- Competencies: 1.1; 1.2; 1.3; 2.1; 2.2; 2.5; 3.1; 3.6; 4.2; 6.1; 8.1
- Subcompetencies: 1.1b; 1.2a; 1.3a; 2.1c; 2.2a; 2.5a; 2.5f; 3.1c; 3.6b; 4.2c; 6.1b; 8.1a; 8.1e

Spheres of Care: Wellness/Disease prevention

Concepts: Communication; Clinical judgment; Evidence-based practice

Source: UN, n.d.b.

Case Study #3

The local health department has asked the college community nursing class to assist with home inspections. Radon levels are high in the area and can be deadly in the home environment. Radon can be a big concern for all communities.

Visit the following EPA website: https://www.epa.gov/radon.

1. What exactly is radon? Discuss how radon is detected.
2. What environmental factors (name at least two) that contribute to radon?
3. What two primary prevention and two secondary prevention activities could be used regarding radon?
4. Provide two local resources (you can use your own area) that would benefit the county citizens.
5. Investigate the local (you can use your own area) health policies regarding radon.
6. What SDOH principles could affect this issue?

AACN *Essentials* (2021): Domains: #1; #2; #3; #4; #7; #8; #9

- Competencies: 1.1; 1.2; 1.3; 2.1; 3.1; 3.4; 3.6: 4.2; 7.2; 8.3; 9.4
- Subcompetencies: 1.1a; 1.2a; 1.3a; 1.3c; 2.1b; 3.1a; 3.1c; 3.1f; 3.4b; 3.4c; 3.6a; 4.2c: 7.2b; 8.3a; 9.4a

Spheres of Care: Wellness/Disease prevention; Chronic disease management

Concepts: Clinical judgment; Communication; Evidence-based practice; Health policy; SDOH

Sources: Developed by authors; EPA, 2024i.

NCLEX Questions

1. Which process is an effective way to assess the environmental factors that relate to a population's health?

   a. Use the I PREPARE mnemonic.
   b. Look at the population and ask questions you want to know about their environment.
   c. Use the nursing process to assess the population's needs.
   d. Assess the environmental needs by reviewing the population's health department records.

2. What is the primary purpose for nurses to know about environmental health?

   a. It is a common cause of climate control.
   b. Substances are often found in the air and water.
   c. Chronic illnesses are usually linked to the environment
   d. Nurses are exposed to environmental concerns daily.

References

Abubakar, I., Maniruzzaman, K. M., Dano, U. L., AlShihri, F. S., AlShammari, M. S., Ahmed, S. M. S., Al-Gehlani, W. A. G., & Alrawaf, T. I. (2022). Environmental sustainability impacts of solid waste management practices in the global South. *International Journal of Environmental Research and Public Health, 19*(19), 12717. https://doi.org/10.3390/ijerph191912717

Agency for Healthcare Research and Quality. (2022). *Six domains of healthcare quality.* https://www.ahrq.gov/talkingquality/measures/six-domains.html

Alliance of Nurses for Healthy Environments. (n.d.). *Who we are.* https://envirn.org/

American Association of Colleges of Nursing. (2021). *The essentials: Core competencies for professional nursing education.* https://www.aacnnursing.org/Essentials

American Nursing Association. (2007). *ANA's principles of environmental health for nursing practice with implementation strategies.* https://www.nursingworld.org/~4af4f2/globalassets/docs/ana/ethics/principles-of-environmental-health-online_final.pdf

American Nursing Association. (2022). *ANA's scope and standards of practice: Provision 17* (4th ed.).

American Public Health Association. (2024a). *About APHA.* https://www.apha.org/About-APHA

American Public Health Association. (2024b). *Climate and health youth education toolkit.* https://www.apha.org/Topics-and-Issues/Climate-Health-and-Equity/Education

American Public Health Association. (2024c). *Climate, health and equity.* https://www.apha.org/Topics-and-Issues/Climate-Health-and-Equity

American Public Health Association. (2024d). *Environmental health.* https://www.apha.org/topics-and-issues/environmental-health

American Public Health Association. (2024e). *Environmental justice.* https://www.apha.org/Topics-and-Issues/Environmental-Health/Environmental-Justice

Badash, I., Kleinman, N. P., Barr, S., Jang, J., Rahman, S., & Wu, B. W. (2017) Redefining health: The evolution of health ideas from antiquity to the era of value-based care. *Cureus, 9*(2), e1018. https://doi.org/10.7759/cureus.1018

Belluco, S., Bertola, M., Montarsi, F., Di Martino, G., Granato, A., Stella, R., Martinello, M., Bordin, F., & Mutinelli, F. (2023). Insects and public health: An overview. *Insects, 14*(3), 240. https://doi.org/10.3390/insects14030240

Center for Biological Diversity. (n.d.). *Tackling population pressure.* https://www.biologicaldiversity.org/programs/population_and_sustainability/population/

Centers for Disease Control and Prevention. (2019). *Environmental assessment.* https://www.cdc.gov/workplacehealthpromotion/model/assessment/environmental.html

Centers for Disease Control and Prevention. (2023). *National Environmental Public Health Tracking Network.* https://ephtracking.cdc.gov/

Centers for Disease Control and Prevention. (2024a). *10 essential public health services.* https://www.cdc.gov/public-health-gateway/php/about/index.html

Centers for Disease Control and Prevention. (2024b). *About environmental health services.* https://www.cdc.gov/environmental-health-services/php/about/index.html

Centers for Disease Control and Prevention. (2024c). *Controlling wild rodent infestations.* https://www.cdc.gov/healthy-pets/rodent-control/

Centers for Disease Control and Prevention. (2024d). *Data modernization initiative.* https://www.cdc.gov/surveillance/data-modernization/index.html

Centers for Disease Control and Prevention. (2024e). *Investigate health problems and hazards.* https://www.cdc.gov/environmental-health-services/php/10-essential-services/2-investigate.html

Earth.org. (n.d.). *About.* https://earth.org/mission-statement/

Earth.org. (2023). *How does overpopulation affect sustainability? Challenges and solutions.* https://earth.org/overpopulation-sustainability/

Earth.org. (2024). *15 biggest environmental problems of 2024.* https://earth.org/the-biggest-environmental-problems-of-our-lifetime/

Ecology Society of America. (2024). *What is ecology?* https://www.esa.org/about/what-does-ecology-have-to-do-with-me/

Environmental Protection Agency. (n.d.). *Water topics.* https://www.epa.gov/environmental-topics/water-topics

Environmental Protection Agency. (2021). *Our built and natural environments.* https://www.epa.gov/smartgrowth/our-built-and-natural-environments

Environmental Protection Agency. (2023a). *Air topics.* https://www.epa.gov/environmental-topics/air-topics

Environmental Protection Agency. (2023b). *Health and environmental effects of ozone layer depletion.* https://www.epa.gov/ozone-layer-protection/health-and-environmental-effects-ozone-layer-depletion

Environmental Protection Agency. (2024a). *About rats and mice.* https://www.epa.gov/rodenticides/about-rats-and-mice

Environmental Protection Agency. (2024b). *About the Center for Public Health and Environment Assessment (CPHEA).* https://www.epa.gov/aboutepa/about-center-public-health-and-environmental-assessment-cphea#what

Environmental Protection Agency. (2024c). *Basic information about the built environment.* https://www.epa.gov/smm/basic-information-about-built-environment

Environmental Protection Agency. (2024d). *Controlling rodents and regulating rodenticides.* https://www.epa.gov/rodenticides

Environmental Protection Agency. (2024e). *Environmental topics.* https://www.epa.gov/environmental-topics

Environmental Protection Agency. (2024f). *How can you help protect source water?* https://www.epa.gov/sourcewaterprotection/how-can-you-help-protect-source-water

Environmental Protection Agency. (2024g). *Learning and teaching about the environment.* https://www.epa.gov/students

Environmental Protection Agency. (2024h). *Our mission and what we do.* https://www.epa.gov/aboutepa/our-mission-and-what-we-do

Environmental Protection Agency. (2024i). *Radon.* https://www.epa.gov/radon

Ezell, J., & Chase, E. (2022). Forming a critical race theory of environmental disaster: Understanding social meanings and health threat perception in the Flint water crisis. *Journal of Environmental Management, 320,* 115886. https://doi.org/10.1016/j.jenvman.2022.115886

Global Goals. (n.d.). *Goal 15: Life on land.* https://www.globalgoals.org/goals/15-life-on-land/

International Institute for Sustainable Development. (2020). *The precautionary principles.* https://www.iisd.org/articles/deep-dive/precautionary-principle

Lawton, B. (2023). *Wetlands essential to combatting the health effects of climate change are at risk.* https://www.networkforphl.org/news-insights/wetlands-essential-to-combatting-the-health-effects-of-climate-change-are-at-risk/

Liu, H., Alharthi, A., Atil, A., Wasif Zafar, M., & Khan, I. (2022). A non-linear analysis of the impacts of natural resources and education on environmental quality: Green energy and its role in the future. *Resources Policy, 79,* 102940. https://doi.org/10.1016/j.resourpol.2022.102940

Mager, D., & Cornelius, J. (2019). *Population health for nurses: Improving community outcomes* (1st ed.). Springer. https://openstax.org/books/population-health/pages/14-3-environmental-health-assessment#table-00001

Malhi, Y., Franklin, J., Seddon, N., Solan, M., Turner, M., Field, C., & Knowlton, N. (2020). Climate change and ecosystems: Threats, opportunities and solutions. *Philosophical Transactions of the Royal Society B,* 37520190104. http://dx.doi.org/10.1098/rstb.2019.0104

Merriam-Webster. (n.d.). *Ecology definition.* https://www.merriam-webster.com/dictionary/ecology

Minnesota Department of Health. (2019). *Public health interventions: Application for nursing practice* (2nd ed.). www.health.state.mn.us/communities/practice/research/phncouncil/docs/PHInterventions.pdf

Narayan, Shweta. (2021). *It's impossible to have healthy people on a sick planet.* TED, October 2021. https://www.ted.com/talks/shweta_narayan_it_s_impossible_to_have_healthy_people_on_a_sick_planet?language=en&subtitle=en&delay=5s

National Aeronautics and Space Administration. (2024). *Is the ozone hole causing climate change?* https://science.nasa.gov/climate-change/faq/is-the-ozone-hole-causing-climate-change/

National Council on Aging. (2024). *Evidence-based program: Active Living Every Day.* https://www.ncoa.org/article/evidence-based-program-active-living-every-day

National Council on Aging Advisor. (2023). *Home safety for older adults: A comprehensive guide 2024.* https://www.ncoa.org/adviser/sleep/home-safety-older-adults/

National Defense Resource Center. (2023). *Water pollution: Everything you need to know.* https://www.nrdc.org/stories/water-pollution-everything-you-need-know#whatis

National Geographic. (n.d.a.). *Deforestation.* https://education.nationalgeographic.org/resource/deforestation/

National Geographic. (n.d.b.). *Nonrenewable energy.* https://education.nationalgeographic.org/resource/non-renewable-energy/

National Pest Management Association. (2024). *Our story.* https://www.npmapestworld.org/about-npma/our-story/

Natural Resources Defense Council. (2017). *Safe drinking water.* https://www.nrdc.org/stories/whats-your-drinking-water

Occupational Safety and Health Administration. (n.d.). *Recommended practices for safety and health programs: A safe workplace is sound business.* https://www.osha.gov/safety-management/

Office of Disease Prevention and Health Promotion. (n.d.a.). *Environmental health.* Healthy People 2030. https://health.gov/healthypeople/objectives-and-data/browse-objectives/environmental-health

Office of Disease Prevention and Health Promotion. (n.d.b.). *Healthy People 2030 framework.* Healthy People 2030. https://health.gov/healthypeople/about/healthy-people-2030-framework

Office of Disease Prevention and Health Promotion. (n.d.c.). *Neighborhood and built environment.* Healthy People 2030. https://health.gov/healthypeople/objectives-and-data/browse-objectives/neighborhood-and-built-environment

Ogunseitan, O. (2022). One Health and the environment: From conceptual framework to implementation science. *Environment: Science and Policy for Sustainable Development, 64*(2), 11–21. https://doi.org/10.1080/00139157.2022.2021792

Pacific Public Health Foundation. (2020). *Upstream 101: Decoding public health.* https://pacific-publichealth.ca/resources/upstream-101-decoding-public-health/

Paranzino, G., Butterfield, P., Nastoff, T., & Ranger, C. (2005). I PREPARE: Development and clinical utility of an environmental exposure history mnemonic. *American Association of Occupational Health Nurses, 53*(1), 37–42. https://pubmed.ncbi.nlm.nih.gov/15675156/

Pinto-Bazurco, J. (2020). *The precautionary principle.* https://www.iisd.org/system/files/2020-10/still-one-earth-precautionary-principle.pdf

Prüss-Ustün, A., Wolf, J., Corvalán, C., Bos, R., & Neira, M. (2016). *Preventing disease through healthy environments: A global assessment of the burden of disease from environmental risks.* https://iris.who.int/bitstream/handle/10665/204585/9789241565196_eng.pdf

Ragavan, M. I., Marcil, L. W., & Garg, A. (2020). Climate change as a social determinant of health. *Pediatrics, 145*(5), e20193169. https://doi.org/10.1542/peds.2019-3169

Ripple, W., Wolf, C., Gregg, J., Rockström, J., Newsome, T., Law, B., Marques, L., Lenton, T., Xu, C., & Huq, S., Simons, L., & King, D. A. (2023). The 2023 state of the climate report: Entering uncharted territory. *BioScience, 73*(12), 841–850. https://doi.org/10.1093/biosci/biad080

Ritchie, H. (2023). *Waste management.* https://ourworldindata.org/waste-management

Rodriguez, L., & Wilson, H. (2022). Data modernization: Making environmental health services data more accessible. *Journal of Environmental Health, 84*(8), 34–36. https://go.gale.com/ps/i.do?p=AONE&u=anon~2cec4b22&id=GALE|A697556884&v=2.1&it=r&sid=googleScholar&asid=d184f885

Romanello, M., Di Napoli, C., Drummond, P., Green, C., Kennard, H., Lampard, P., Scamman, D., Arnell, N., Ayeb-Karlsson, S., Ford, L. B., Belesova, K., Bowen, K., Cai, W., Callaghan, M., Campbell-Lendrum, D., Chambers, J., van Daalen, K. R., Dalin, C., Dasandi, N., Dasgupta, S., Davies, M., ... & Costello, A. (2022). The 2022 report of the *Lancet* Countdown on health and climate change: Health at the mercy of fossil fuels. *Lancet, 400*(10363), 1619–1654. https://doi.org/10.1016/S0140-6736(22)01540-9

Rural Health Information Hub. (2024). *Policy, systems, and environment.* https://www.ruralhealthinfo.org/toolkits/health-promotion/2/strategies/policy-systems-environmental

Skin Cancer Foundation. (2022). *UV radiation.* https://www.skincancer.org/risk-factors/uv-radiation/

Scott, S. (2022). *Public health and overpopulation.* https://hir.harvard.edu/public-health-and-overpopulation/

Svarstad, H., Jornet, A., Peters, G., Griffiths, T., & Benjaminsen, T. (2023). Critical climate education is crucial for fast and just transformations. *Nature Climate Change, 13,* 1274–1275. https://doi.org/10.1038/s41558-023-01875-2

Tobin, M., Hajna, S., Orychock, K., Ross, N., DeVries, M., Villeneuve, P. J., Frank, L. D., McCormack, G. R., Wasfi, R., & Steinmetz-Wood, M. (2022). Rethinking walkability and developing a conceptual definition of active living environments to guide research and practice. *BMC Public Health, 22,* 450. https://doi.org/10.1186/s12889-022-12747-3

Today Show. (2021). *Microplastics.* https://x.com/todayshow/status/1385923933388648452?s=12

United Nations. (n.d.a.). *Background—Desertification and its effects.* https://www.un.org/en/observances/desertification-day/background

United Nations. (n.d.b.). *Climate action: Fast Facts.* https://www.un.org/sites/un2.un.org/files/2021/08/fastfacts-health.pdf

United Nations. (n.d.c.). *Causes and effects of climate change.* https://www.un.org/en/climatechange/science/causes-effects-climate-change

United Nations. (n.d.d.). *Forests, desertification and biodiversity: Goal 15.* https://www.un.org/sustainabledevelopment/biodiversity/

United Nations. (n.d.e.). *What is climate change?* https://www.un.org/en/climatechange/what-is-climate-change

United Nations. (2024). *Goal 15: Life on land.* https://www.unep.org/explore-topics/sustainable-development-goals/why-do-sustainable-development-goals-matter/goal-15

U.S. Department of Agriculture. (n.d.a.). *Food and nutrition.* https://www.usda.gov/topics/food-and-nutrition

U.S. Department of Agriculture. (n.d.b.). *Food safety is everyone's business.* https://www.usda.gov/media/blog/2023/06/07/food-safety-everyones-business

U.S. Department of Agriculture. (n.d.c.). *Food security.* https://www.usda.gov/topics/food-and-nutrition/food-security#

U.S. Department of Agriculture. (n.d.d.). *Research and science.* https://www.usda.gov/topics/research-and-science

U.S. Department of Labor. (n.d.). *DOL workplace violence program.* https://www.dol.gov/agencies/oasam/centers-offices/human-resources-center/policies/workplace-violence-program

U.S. News and World Report. (2024). *10 tips for home safety in 2024.* https://www.usnews.com/360-reviews/services/home-security/tips-for-home-safety

USAFacts.org. (2024). *What environmental challenges and opportunities does the U.S. face?* https://usafacts.org/state-of-the-union/environment/

Waterall, J., Rhodes, D., & Exley, K. (2021). Why air pollution is an important issue for all nurses. *British Journal of Nursing, 30*(16). https://doi.org/10.12968/bjon.2021.30.16.982

World Health Organization. (2020). *Climate change: Land degradation and desertification.* https://www.who.int/news-room/questions-and-answers/item/climate-change-land-degradation-and-desertification

World Health Organization. (2024a). *Air pollution.* https://www.who.int/health-topics/air-pollution#tab=tab_1

World Health Organization. (2024b). *Environmental health.* https://www.who.int/health-topics/environmental-health#tab=tab_1

World Health Organization. (2024c). *Environmental health inequalities.* https://www.who.int/europe/news-room/fact-sheets/item/environmental-health-inequalities

World Health Organization. (2024d). *Food safety.* https://www.who.int/news-room/fact-sheets/detail/food-safety

World Health Organization. (2024e). *Health and the environment.* https://www.who.int/westernpacific/about/how-we-work/programmes/health-and-the-environment

World Health Organization. (2024f). *One Health.* https://www.who.int/health-topics/one-health#tab=tab_1

Xu, Y., & Zhao, F. (2023). Impact of energy depletion, human development, and income distribution on natural resource sustainability. *Resource Policy, 83*, 103531. https://doi.org/10.1016/j.resourpol.2023.103531

Yang, M., Chen, L., Wang, J., Msigwa, G., Osman, A., Fawzy, S., Rooney, D., & Yap, P. (2023). Circular economy strategies for combating climate change and other environmental issues. *Environment Chemistry Letters, 21*, 55–80. https://doi.org/10.1007/s10311-022-01499-6

Credits

Fig. 9.1: Adapted from Pacific Public Health Foundation, https://pacificpublichealth.ca/resources/upstream-101-decoding-public-health/. Copyright © 2020 by Pacific Public Health Foundation.

Fig. 9.1a: Copyright © 2021 Depositphotos/A-Y-N.

Fig. 9.2: Jamie Waterall, David Rhodes and Karen Exley, "Air Pollution Affects Across the Lifespan," *British Journal of Nursing*, vol. 30, no. 16. Copyright © 2021 by MA Healthcare, Ltd.

Fig. 9.3: Copyright © 2023 by Mingyu Yang et al. (CC BY 4.0) at https://link.springer.com/article/10.1007/s10311-022-01499-6.

CHAPTER 10

Global Health

"There is no one size that fits all. We must work country by country, region by region, community by community, to ensure the diversity of needs are addressed to support each reality."

—Amina J. Mohammed, deputy secretary-general, United Nations

Learning Outcomes

After reading this chapter, students should be able to:

1. Compare and contrast various global health agencies
2. Describe the components of the 17 Sustainable Development Goals (SDGs)
3. Understand current global healthcare trends and issues
4. Discuss a global health framework
5. Understand how to manage global diseases
6. Understand health policy, advocacy, and global health

Keywords and Concepts

Advocacy; health policy; International Council of Nurses (ICN); Pan American Health Organization (PAHO); Sustainable Development Goals (SDGs); United Nations Children Fund (UNICEF); World Bank; World Health Organization (WHO)

Definitions of the Keywords

Advocacy: Act or process of supporting a cause or proposal (Merriam-Webster, 2024)

Health policy: Keeping people safe and healthy through laws and policies at the local, state, territorial, and federal levels (Office of Disease Prevention and Health Promotion [ODPHP], n.d.c.)

ICN: Federation of more than 130 national nurses associations, representing the more than 28 million nurses worldwide (ICN, n.d.c.)

PAHO: Specialized international health agency for the Americas working to improve people's health (PAHO, n.d.)

SDGs: Adopted by the United Nations (UN) in 2015 to provide a shared global blueprint for everyone (UN, n.d.b.)

UNICEF: An organization that focuses on the most disadvantaged children to improve their well-being and survival (UNICEF, n.d.a.)

World Bank: Global partnership working for sustainable solutions that reduce poverty and prosperity in developing countries (World Bank, 2024)

WHO: An organization with professional individuals worldwide who are experts in public health knowledge (WHO, 2024b)

Introduction

Understanding what is happening around the world is critical for all nurses. The ability to travel quickly to other countries makes it extremely easy for infectious diseases to spread. This was apparent in how quickly COVID-19 became a pandemic.

The U.S. Census Bureau's world population clock estimated that the global population as of September 2022 was 7,922,312,800. This total far exceeds the 2015 world population of 7.2 billion. The world's population continues to increase by roughly 140 people per minute, with births outweighing deaths in most countries (World Population Review, 2024).

Global health is a worldwide approach to improving health care by preventing, detecting, and responding to public health concerns and events (ODPHP, n.d.b.). The need to continue to advocate current conditions while preparing for upcoming situations is vital for the well-being of all individuals in all countries. Those countries that do not have the resources necessary to respond to public health issues must have assistance from others. To do so, training others to help in times of need while focusing on decreasing adverse health outcomes is a significant component of understanding how global health affects everyone. Global health can facilitate methods to provide surveillance and uses of diagnostic testing, keep current with effective communication to allow awareness, and, overall, provide detection and prevention of health-related illnesses and improve health (ODPHP, n.d.b.). This chapter will discuss global trends and issues, investigate pertinent global organizations, and apply global health policy and advocacy.

Background of the Concepts

Monitoring global health issues is crucial for everyone. Areas include life expectancy and mortality, women's and children's health, communicable diseases, and noncommunicable diseases (NCDs). As several national and international countries cannot effectively participate in disease outbreaks or other situations such as disasters, globalization is vital to allow the sharing of knowledge and resources to assist those individuals. With the wide variety of global and international healthcare organizations, incorporating the 17 SDGs shows a commitment to achieving significant health-related gains (WHO, 2018).

The WHO stresses the need for healthcare professionals, especially nurses, to be involved in local, national, and international efforts to meet significant workforce demands. This must include being well-educated and willing to assist with striving to meet the SDGs. The recent pandemic has damaged the professional interests in nursing recruitment in several countries. This has led to the need to encourage nurses to make career choices to help the world not only work on diversity but will be able to incorporate such areas as race and religion into sharing all aspects of inclusivity toward the goals of all peoples (Adhikari & Smith, 2023).

Siegal (2024) identifies specific issues needed to help global healthcare. Included are the aspects of transforming healthcare with artificial intelligence (AI), addressing cost and affordability, responding to the looming global shortfall in healthcare workers, the role of social care, and a sustainable future. Health inequities contribute to the globalization challenges, especially the post-COVID-19 pandemic. AI and advanced technologies must be incorporated to assist with administrative concerns, diagnosis, treatment, and overall client care. Using electronic health records will effectively enhance the entire delivery of healthcare, allowing for incorporation into worldwide means to assist many resources for positive patient outcomes (Siegal, 2023).

Global health encompasses many issues and concerns for people worldwide. Health equity, environmental, social, and governance strategies leading to resilience; improvements to mental health and well-being; the use of virtual technology to meet healthcare needs; the research of improvements and new medical resources; and the development of future guidelines, policies, and procedures to meet the needs of global communities better are all important (World Economic Forum, 2022).

Without the inclusion of the levels of prevention, diseases will continue to proliferate, and morbidity and mortality will increase. Despite persisting health inequities, healthcare needs must be restored and available to everyone (Abdul-Raheem, 2023). Healthcare professionals use evidence-based resources (EBRs) for global health, looking at specific scientifically proven methods as resources to process effective health methods, prevent diseases, and decrease health disparities. In doing so, there is the ability to provide more inclusivity and social engagement, allowing for a more excellent and diverse picture of the studied issues (Hayman et al., 2023). From there, EBRs are used to plan specific programs and policies, assisting with the knowledge to include interventions for positive healthcare methods (ODPHP, n.d.a.).

Voss and Yasobant (2024) describe globalization as impactful for healthcare and whether the outcomes are positive or negative. Positive effects allow for the minimization of the gaps related to inequalities with wealth in various areas of the world. Adverse effects can focus on infectious diseases and their spread caused by individuals' mobility. To positively affect global healthcare, changes need to be made with all organizations and expert individuals involved. Using research methods to provide vulnerable nations with resources, including technology, is vital.

Population health nurses are encouraged to become involved in global issues. This can be accomplished by participating in the guidance of other healthcare professionals and governmental agencies. Organizations such as Sigma Theta Tau International (STTI) and the ICN are two examples. These organizations are influential by representing nursing worldwide to accelerate involvement through direct service, leadership, education, mentorship, and advocacy (STTI, 2024; ICN, n.d.a.).

Global Organizations

The United States has a specific global health policy that includes many different aspects. The policy aims to improve people's health in low- and middle-income countries while contributing to broader U.S. global development goals, foreign policy priorities, and national security concerns (KFF, 2022). Many other international and national organizations work with the United States to meet this policy (Figure 10.1).

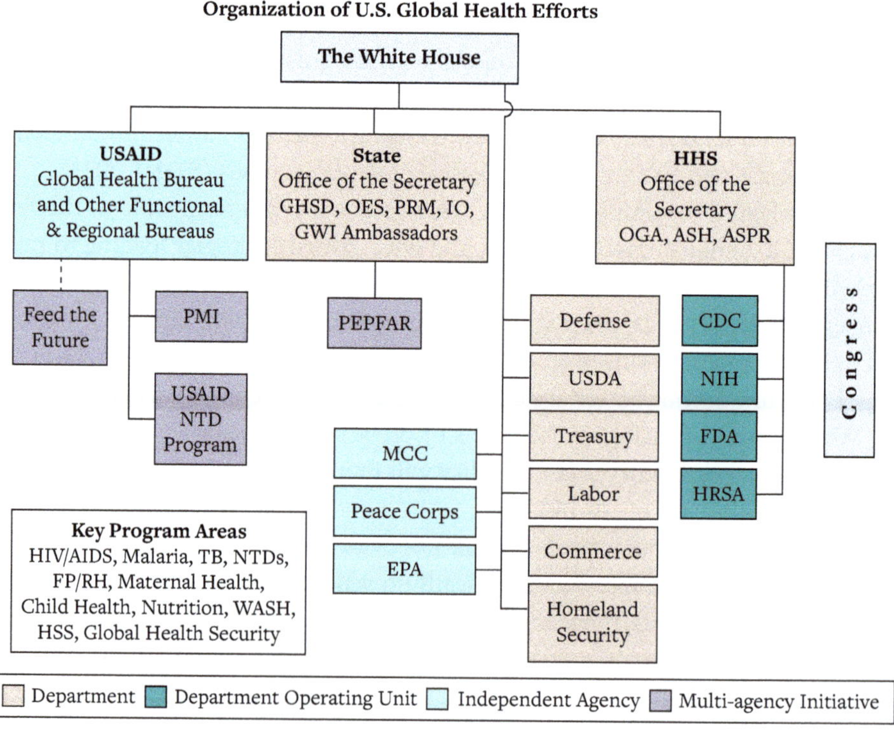

FIGURE 10.1 The U.S. Global Health Policy Efforts

United Nations and Sustainable Development Goals

The UN has an overall responsibility for global health. The UN is an international organization founded in 1945 and comprises 193 member states. Eight Millennium Development Goals were established as foundational goals until 2016. Now, 17 goals are the premise for the overall agenda for 2030 (UN, n.d.a.; UN, n.d.b.).

SDGs are goals developed to assist in ending health inequality and helping meet individuals' needs. In addition, these goals enhance resources for health and education while considering the needs of climate change and care of the oceans and forests (UN, n.d.b.). The 17 goals provide developed and developing countries the opportunity to interact globally. They include decreasing poverty, enhancing health and education, providing equality, and increasing economic growth. Other areas to include are reducing the effects of climate change; protecting the environment (e.g., water, oceans, and forests); focusing on sustainable energy; and using technology (UN, n.d.c.; Figure 10.2).

Studying economic, social, and environmental factors is significant in identifying sustainable development when considering the SDGs. Bali Swain and Yang-Wallentin (2020) concluded that developing countries would be best helped by examining their limitations in resources, policies, economic status, and social factors, while the conclusions for developed countries identified the benefits of social and environmental factors. It is vital to promptly act in these identified areas to address the need for socio-economic development.

Even now, the work completed has yet to be significantly met due to global crises, including COVID-19, security issues, governance concerns with coordination throughout the nations, climate changes, and financial problems that have

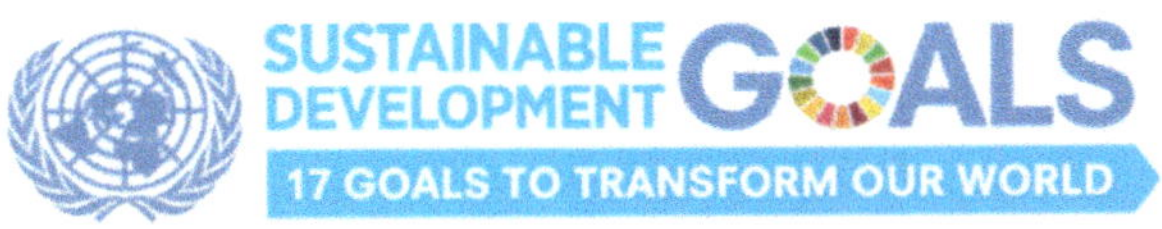

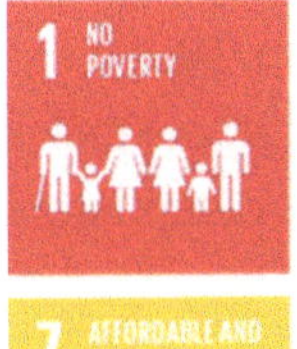

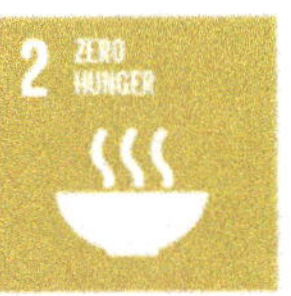

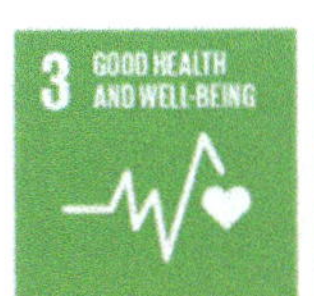

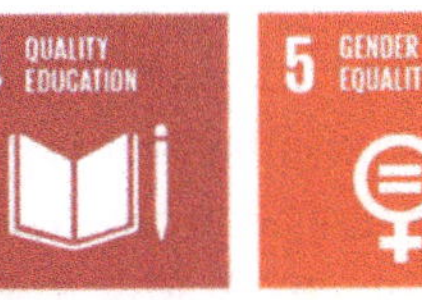

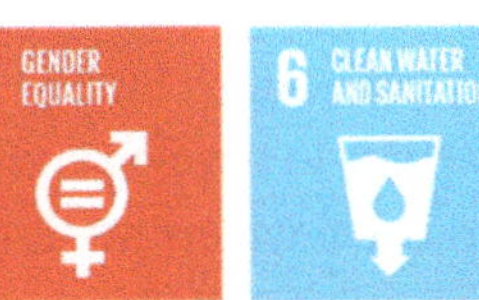

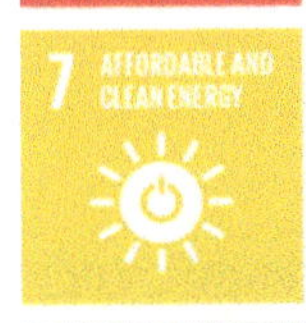

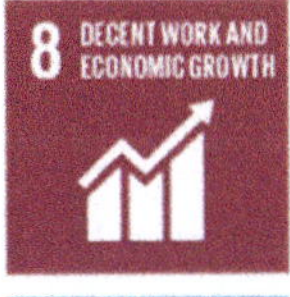

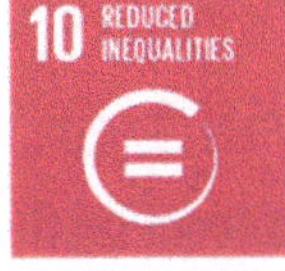

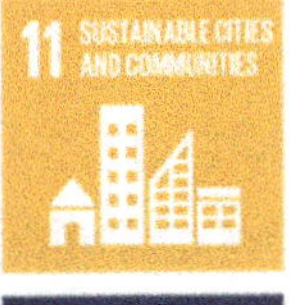

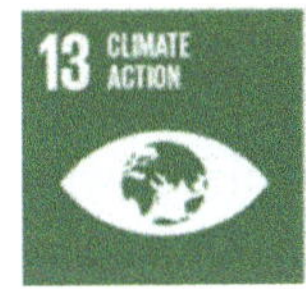

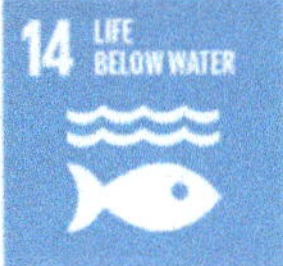

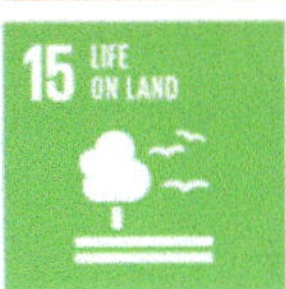

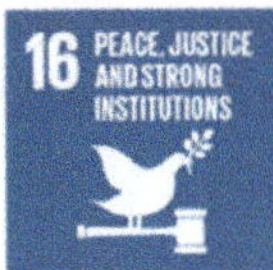

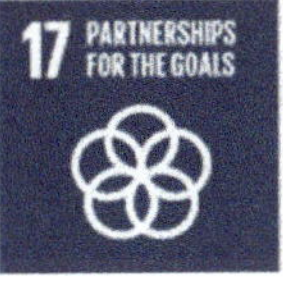

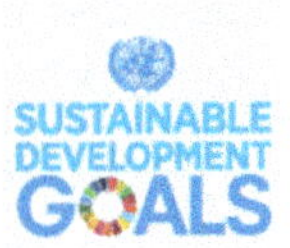

FIGURE 10.2 SDGs

BOX 10.1 ACTIVE LEARNING REFLECTION ACTIVITY

The SDGs and Data Analysis

Monitoring health statistics is critical to noting progress for the SDGs. Use the following link and note the latest report on world health statistics related to the SDGs: https://www.who.int/data/gho/publications/world-health-statistics. Specifically, note the life expectancy discussion post–COVID–19. Answer the reflection questions and do the follow-up assignment.

1. What are three critical impacts from COVID-19 and life expectancy?
2. Note one of the tables and discuss two things you noted with its analysis.
3. Give some examples of specific data you noted from the current report.
4. Discuss two ways this could affect the SDGs.

Your clinical instructor requests a one-page response that reflects and summarizes what you learned by doing this assignment. Include at least five key elements that could be applied to your future nursing practice.

Essentials: Domains: #1; #3; #4; #6; #8; #9

- Competencies: 1.1; 1.2; 1.3; 3.1; 3.6; 4.2; 6.3; 6.4; 8.3; 9.4
- Subcompetencies: 1.1b; 1.2a; 1.2c; 1.3a; 3.1b; 3.1c; 3.1d; 3.1e; 3.6a; 4.2c; 6.3a; 6.4d; 8.3a; 9.4b

Spheres of Care: Chronic disease management

Concepts: Evidence-based practice; Social determinants of health (SDOH); Clinical judgment; Communication

Source: WHO, 2024k.

had deleterious effects on individuals. Due to these concerns, the availability to continue to develop and enhance the goals effectively has been affected by obstacles and has been stunted. The problem lies in how these goals can be accomplished promptly (Filho et al., 2023; Box 10.1).

United Nations Children's Fund

UNICEF focuses on children from birth to adolescence to save lives, protect their rights, and assist with fulfilling their ability to meet their full potential (UNICEF, n.d.b.). The importance of protecting children and enhancing their early development is crucial. The need for developing countries to meet the essentials for children who are disadvantaged through disasters, poverty, violence, exploitation, and affected by wars and disabilities is essential. UNICEF states in its mission the need to have equal rights for women and girls and to provide peace (Ahun et al., 2023; UNICEF, n.d.b.).

UNICEF and the WHO have combined efforts to provide innovative activities for children to enhance childhood development, which is called the *Care for Child Development* (CCD) *package*. In this program, age-specific programs for children ages 0 to 5 years were assembled using evidence-based information and focused on play and communication while interacting with the children and their caregivers. Caregivers were supported with practical caregiving skills along with activities in early learning. Globally, CCD was offered primarily in low- and middle-income countries and territories (Ahun et al., 2023).

Ahun et al. (2023) research findings addressed the opposing concerns of many individuals and environmental settings using CCD. Difficulties were found with specific training techniques, support from the various governments, and the actual benefits obtained from the children and families. Positive effects were supported for those younger than age 3 years and the mothers of targeted disadvantaged families living in rural areas. Specific recommendations going forward included the inclusion of premature births and caregivers; those born with visual, physical, or cognitive forms of disabilities; nutritional deficiencies; and mothers' potential to develop depression. The complete CCD program can continue to evolve through review after the evaluation of each session. Working through the challenges, although frustrating, may result in involving more individuals and policymakers with futuristic ideas to participate while continuing to facilitate effective results.

World Health Organization

The WHO is a vital organization that works to provide universal health services to offset worldwide situations. The primary focus is to work on world health needs, providing safety and ensuring the highest level of care to all individuals, especially the most vulnerable and low-income countries (WHO, 2024b). As the efforts are enormous, the WHO continues to work on several challenges to meet its goals. Three significant areas fall into this: mandate and scope; structure, governance, and money; and tensions between domestic and international measures. In the area of mandate and scope, the WHO must review its strengths and weaknesses while developing the means to reform what changes need to be implemented. As the WHO is a leading international health organization, other global entities must use their influence to continue to support the work of the WHO while following the guidelines put into place (Wenham & Davies, 2023).

As for the issues related to structure, governance, and money, the WHO has many aspects to incorporate into the actual functioning of the organization. Many different concerns need to be considered, including many countries, rules, policies, procedures, and laws. With this in mind, accepting a final decision or plan can be confusing, resulting in negativism, unacceptable interactions with others, financial concerns, and effective methods of analyzing and completing projects (Wenham & Davies, 2023).

BOX 10.2 ACTIVE LEARNING REFLECTION ACTIVITY

Application to the WHO

At the following websites, there are three foundational essential newborn care courses that could be used at a global level:

- https://www.who.int/tools/essential-newborn-care-course
- https://globalhealthmedia.org/videos/

Reflect on the following questions:

1. Is there an availability to get these materials in another language?
2. Name three situations in which you could use this course's information.

Essentials: Domains: #1; #2; #3; #4; #6; #9

- Competencies: 1.1; 1.2; 1.3; 2.2; 3.1; 3.2; 3.3; 3.4; 4.2; 6.1; 9.2; 9.4
- Subcompetencies: 1.1b; 1.2a; 1.3a; 1.3b; 2.2b; 2.2c; 3.1a; 3.1b; 3.1c; 3.1h; 3.2a; 3.3b; 3.4e; 4.2c; 6.1c; 9.2d; 9.4a

Spheres of Care: Wellness/Disease prevention

Concepts: Clinical judgment; Evidence-based practice; SDOH; Communication; Diversity, equity, and inclusion (DEI); Health policy

Sources: Global Health Media, n.d.; WHO, 2024e.

Rapid recognition must be encouraged, limiting the lag of notification length for any form of reporting, including disasters, fires, and weather-related situations. The degree of governmental power and financial stability present can affect the overall global health activities of the WHO. The achievement of having states supportive of what needs to be practiced for good global health is the overall goal for success (Wenham & Davies, 2023; Box 10.2).

World Bank

The World Bank is focused on having a poverty-free place to live globally. There is a need for all individuals to have financial stability in the world to provide every person with effective means to deal with crises, disasters, negative situations, and pandemics. Doing so can maintain appropriate lives through financial means, employment, food security, and environmentally safe settings. The relationships with various governments and the private sector allow it to provide strength for many (World Bank, 2024).

The World Bank provides various financial products and technical assistance to help countries share and apply innovative knowledge and solutions to their challenges. The three priorities that guide its work to promote prosperity for the poorest people are helping create sustainable economic growth, investing in people, and building resilience to shocks and threats that could impede previous progress (World Bank, 2024).

Pan American Health Organization

The PAHO functions as an international healthcare group, improving and protecting health needs, especially those of communicable and noncommunicable causes, and responding to emergencies and disasters (PAHO, n.d.). Used during emergencies such as a disaster, the PAHO offers quality healthcare to all people as needed. Wherever the need, the PAHO shares technological measures with countries, governmental agencies, community groups, and public health organizations to facilitate health needs without discrimination. The actions related to the mobility of resources are enhanced using evidence-based information to make effective decisions and promote positive health outcomes (PAHO, n.d.).

Monteiro et al. (2023) tackled the effects of alcohol consumption that soared during the COVID-19 pandemic. With the WHO sharing specific information through various types of social media, the PAHO additionally took on the topic while providing an interaction using digital conversations to educate the participants. The objectives were to decrease drinking and its complications using evidence-based information in three languages. A conversational agent named *Pahola* was used to distribute the information, reaching more than 1.6 million people (Monteiro et al., 2023).

International Council of Nursing

The ICN is the global voice for nursing. Their mission is to influence and inform the implementation of health, social, educational, and economic policies at global and regional levels to promote health for all. The ICN focuses on several projects that amplify the voices of nurses around the globe by providing high-level global health policies (ICN, n.d.b.).

The ICN provides evidence-based education and training through funds from the WHO. Its goal is to provide up-to-date and relevant knowledge and skills to nurses around the globe. The ICN provides these opportunities to nurses to transform healthcare and health systems and improve patient outcomes (ICN, n.d.c.).

Global Health Framework for Nursing Education

Professional nurses are educated in providing positive healthcare outcomes. Global inclusion, including high levels of care and standards, is stressed within nursing curricula. The *State of the World's Nursing 2020* report provides the latest and current evidence-based information for global workers in nursing with a focus on leadership, employment, and educational needs. Members of the National Health Workforce Account state that the upcoming projected number of nurses by 2030 needs to incorporate how the SDGs will affect how health can be improved and made more robust to be able to provide universal health coverage with progression in the areas of education, gender, workplaces and employees, and overall economic growth (WHO, 2020).

Because the quality of nursing education is a critical determinant of the quality of nursing practice, the guidelines for nursing education in the Global Pillars Framework (GPF) have the potential to execute the call to action to enhance nursing education, nursing care, and nursing services, as illustrated in the *State of the World's Nursing 2020* report (WHO, 2020).

The GPF consists of three pillars and includes the assumptions underpinning the global pillars for nursing education, principles guiding their development, and three pillars specifying expectations for graduates, the education program, and the institution. Pillar I consists of learning outcomes using knowledge, attitudes, skills, collaboration, clinical judgment, professionalism, and leadership, much like the American Association of Colleges of Nursing (AACN) essentials. Pillar II addresses nursing education program standards, curriculum, admission criteria, and learning experiences. Pillar III notes educational institution standards concerning faculty/preceptors, resources, leadership/administration, and program outcomes (Baker et al., 2021; Global Alliance for Leadership in Nursing Education and Science, 2019).

Baker et al. (2021) developed professional nursing education, including policy requirements. With nursing mandating that all nurses have their education earned at least at the baccalaureate level, global concerns can more effectively be met. With global diseases, both communicable and noncommunicative; crises; and pandemics are imminent, healthcare burdens have been identified. The critical areas nurses will successfully include in providing care are in the GPF, which reflects international best practices. Using the GPF will strengthen nursing education, nursing care, and nursing services (WHO, 2020).

Nurses' education must include many topics to understand and practice global nursing needs. Some of the various patterns of international issues that can be provided are types of demographics and transitioning of individuals; epidemiological transitions; development of infectious diseases such as the plague and tuberculosis along with death rates; records of death and birth rates and life expectancies, increased with chronic, long-term health conditions; the advent of antibiotics and alterations with increased life expectancy; presentation of social health conditions; neighborhoods, wealth/poverty, housing, crimes, and drugs. The most significant action that can help nursing education internationally is following the *State of the World's Nursing 2020* report to establish methods to promote effective nursing outcomes globally and the promotion of primary care worldwide (WHO, 2020; 2023; Box 10.3).

BOX 10.3 ACTIVE LEARNING REFLECTION ACTIVITY

Global Primary Care

Primary care is an issue around the globe. The WHO has identified three strategic areas of work to strengthen public healthcare worldwide. Using one of the strategic areas, discuss five specific interventions for a community to develop a plan to assist with the issue. Develop a one-page fact sheet to submit. Visit the following website: https://www.who.int/news-room/fact-sheets/detail/primary-health-care. Reflect on the following points:

1. Briefly discuss some of the critical facts that could hinder these strategies.
2. Why is having primary care services so important?
3. What three strategies could be implemented in a developing country to assist with increasing primary care?
4. What two aspects from this assignment will you use in future nursing practice?

AACN *Essentials* (2021): Domains: #1; #3; #5; #6; #9

- Competencies: 1.1; 1.2; 1.3; 3.1; 3.4; 3.5; 5.1; 6.3; 9.2; 9.3
- Subcompetencies: 1.1a; 1.2a; 1.3a; 3.1a; 3.1b; 3.1c; 3.4b; 3.5a; 3.5c; 3.5d; 5.1a; 5.1f; 6.3a; 9.2b; 9.2d; 9.3a

Spheres of Care: Wellness/Disease prevention; Chronic disease management

Concepts: Clinical judgment; Communication; Compassionate care; DEI; Health policy; SDOH

Source: WHO, 2023a.

Global Health Trends and Concepts

The trends and concepts identified in global health include the gambit of health issues, initiatives to be incorporated, and advancements in the scientific field. Sparta Health approaches health concerns such as conditions of heart disease, strokes, cancer, and diabetes as being placed as the current leading causes of death worldwide. In a review of the risk factors associated with these health concerns, the areas of unhealthy and poor eating, physical inactivity, tobacco and alcohol use, and obesity significantly contribute to these developments. There is a significant concern about the following, especially in low- and middle-income countries. Other global health developments may occur from air pollution, tuberculosis, malaria, and antimicrobial resistance due to antibiotics' decreased effectiveness in treating bacteria and/or viruses. Advancements in technology, especially in healthcare, focus on gene immunotherapy, new mRNA vaccines, and studies using biomarkers and liquid biopsies to assist with cancer detection. Other areas being researched are climate change, vaccine/access, health equity, aging, plant-based diets, wearable technology, and mental health awareness. From continued presentations of infectious diseases to new developing conditions, global health is still dynamic and constantly evolving worldwide (Sparta Health, n.d.).

Many perceptions of implementing global health trends are available through various national and international organizations worldwide. The WHO has listed many healthcare topics containing valuable information to provide education and guidance. In the form of toolboxes, there are notable activities for individuals of all ages and backgrounds to participate in. Some examples include the refugee and migrant health toolkit, air quality standards, essential newborn care training courses, occupational hazards in the health sector, and routine health information systems-rehabilitative toolkit (WHO, 2024e; 2024i; 2024j).

Chen et al. (2020) note that improving individual health globally could be enhanced by combining research education, developing policies and laws, and enhancing current and future practices. Looking into these areas will help account for the need to continue learning about future health problems and the necessary interventions to implement. Chen et al. (2020) suggest that social media successfully communicates information to various individuals.

Managing Global Diseases/Global Surveillance

The WHO aims to prevent and control the increased threat of reemerging and new infections. Strategies have focused on yellow fever, cholera, and influenza. The WHO can intervene by providing stockpiled supplies to countries with epidemics or significant outbreaks of infectious diseases (WHO, 2024h).

Global Outbreak Alert and Response Network

The Global Outbreak Alert and Response Network (GOARN) has been vital in assisting during epidemics and pandemics. This group uses technological resources to rapidly recognize, alert others, and verify and respond to emergencies. By processing the situations, the WHO enables the GOARN to take the information and, through international multidisciplinary working efforts, provide adequate support, training, and response to all governmental agencies (GOARN, 2023).

International Health Regulations

The International Health Regulations (IHR) is responsible for legal issues associated with acute public health emergencies. This organization focuses on countries' legal rights and obligations in conducting business when public health emergencies cross countries' borders. An essential role of the IHR is to report any public health events related to more than 196 countries and 194 WHO member states (WHO, 2024g).

Global Health Security Agenda

The Global Health Security Agenda assists with the vision that the world will become safe and free of global health threats and diseases. This group includes several countries, international organizations, nongovernmental stakeholders, and those from the private sector. Working with the IHR, the concerns are to prevent, detect, and respond to any infectious diseases through its guidelines (Department of Health and Human Services, 2023).

Global Influenza Surveillance and Response System

An additional activity of the WHO is that of the Global Influenza Surveillance and Response System (GISRS). This group focuses on global public health concerns specifically related to the possibility of influenza. By doing so, its activities function to work on surveillance, planning, and preparedness in addition to effective responses to any seasonal, pandemic, and zoonotic influenza events; details the specific influenza epidemiology and disease; and is vigilant to the presentation of influenza, including other respiratory pathogens (WHO, 2024f).

Centers for Disease Control and Prevention/ One Health

The Centers for Disease Control and Prevention's (CDC) One Health acknowledges that animals and the environment are connected to people globally. To follow the One Health objectives, a multidisciplinary group of professionals such as physicians, veterinarians, laboratory technicians, and microbiologists play a significant role in examining the health of not just people but also animals, pets, livestock, and various forms of wildlife. Some disease examples include malaria, rabies, Salmonella infection, West Nile virus, anthrax, and Lyme disease (CDC, 2024b).

The CDC assists with foreign and domestic needs to provide healthcare for individuals, from diseases to safety. The agency has many roles, including identifying and working with current and potential health threats, decreasing deaths and disabilities from diseases, using technology for research and interventions, promoting health, and educating and training leaders and professionals to assist with disease knowledge. The importance of protecting the global environment from health threats that can affect humans is the primary mission of the CDC, and it is provided in its functioning response when these arise (CDC, 2024a).

Rahman et al. (2020) discuss zoonotic diseases representing serious public health condition concerns. These conditions result from animals in contact with humans passing bacteria, viruses, fungi, and other pathogens because of climate change, travel, and people's global movement. Cattle, sheep, goats, dogs, cats, horses, pigs, birds, fish, domestic animals, insects, foodborne pathogens, aquatic environments, and companion animals are included with zoonotic diseases.

This connection involves not only the health of individuals but also the health of animals in our environment. People, animals, plants, and the environment interact in many ways. Populations are continuing to grow and relocate. They also interact with animals and pets, which have become part of their nutritional needs and livelihoods. The possibilities of disease transmission have occurred with close contact with animals and their environments. Other aspects of change in the climate and events with the land have caused new issues relating to food production. Changes include climate control, forest clearing, and various farming practices. Most significant is how people, animals, and products travel to other global, international, and national borders (Rahman et al., 2020).

Other Issues Related to Global Health

Evidence-based health policies are made to prevent disease and provide good health outcomes. Informing others about health policies promotes overall effective health practices. Healthy People 2030 aims to disseminate effective health policies to improve health for all (ODPHP, n.d.c.).

Global health advocacy is needed to influence global health practices to address new or diverse health challenges. More considerable systemic changes are required, involving many variables to improve health outcomes. A broader agenda for multiple issues will meet the needs of all diverse and vulnerable populations (Bertram & Pai, 2023).

Health Policy and Advocacy

Advocating for global health is an innate part of being a future nurse. What happens worldwide could affect all individuals, families, communities, and populations. Can there be a conversation about global health without considering health policy?

The new AACN essentials (2021) embed the professional concept of health policy. Nurses should advocate for adequate health policy at all levels, including globally. This also includes the need for nurses to be actively involved in health policy assessment, decisions, and evaluation.

Domain #3 of the AACN essentials (2021) is Competency 3.4, Advance equitable population health policy. Subcompetencies note the importance of future nurses' understanding and involvement in establishing social justice and health equity. Further Competency 3.5, Demonstrate advocacy strategies, notes the importance of knowing stakeholders and the intent of the advocacy need. Both of these competencies are crucial for future nurses to be involved with, including at the global level (Table 10.1; Box 10.4).

TABLE 10.1 AACN Essentials Domain #3, Competencies 3.4, 3.5

3.4 Advance equitable population health policy.

- 3.4a Describe policy development processes.
- 3.4b Describe the impact of policies on population outcomes, including social justice and health equity.
- 3.4c Identify best evidence to support policy development.
- 3.4d Propose modifications to or development of policy based on population findings.
- 3.4e Develop an awareness of the interconnectedness of population health across borders.

3.5 Demonstrate advocacy strategies.

- 3.5a Articulate a need for change.
- 3.5b Describe the intent of the proposed change.
- 3.5c Define stakeholders, including members of the community and/or clinical populations, and their level of influence.
- 3.5d Implement messaging strategies appropriate to audience and stakeholders.
- 3.5e Evaluate the effectiveness of advocacy actions.

Source: AACN, 2021.

BOX 10.4 ACTIVE LEARNING REFLECTION ACTIVITY

Application of the AACN Essentials Domain #3, Competencies 3.4 and 3.5

Watch the following video about health in all policies: https://www.youtube.com/watch?v=LBcK-_mpYkM. After viewing the video, reflect on how you could be involved in global health policy advocacy. Answer the following reflection questions:

1. Address how you could advocate for changes in health policy for one of the following global health topics:
   a. Clean/adequate water
   b. Climate change
   c. Air pollution
   d. Tuberculosis
2. Prepare a proposal with a short background of the issue (provide statistics), where you would like to initiate this proposal (do not pick the United States), five distinct interventions (provide goals and a time frame), and how you will evaluate it as a positive or negative outcome. Ensure that you provide other stakeholders/community participation as part of your proposal and how you will disseminate it.

AACN *Essentials* (2021): Domains: #1; #2; #3; #5; #6; #7; #8; #9

- Competencies: 1.3; 2.4; 2.7; 3.1; 3.3; 3.4; 3.5; 5.1; 6.1; 7.2; 8.1; 8.3; 9.4
- Subcompetencies: 1.3a; 1.3c; 2.4b; 2.7a; 2.7c; 3.1a; 3.1b; 3.1c; 3.3b; 3.4b; 3.4c; 3.5c; 5.1a; 5.1b; 5.1f; 6.1a; 7.2b; 8.1a; 8.3a; 9.4a

Spheres of Care: Wellness/Disease prevention; Chronic disease management

Concepts: Clinical judgment; Communication; Health policy; SDOH

Source: American Public Health Association, 2022.

Urban and Rural Populations and Global Health

Advocating and providing effective global health policies is critical for developing countries. Unfortunately, a global rural research agenda is lacking. People living in rural areas generally experience more adverse health outcomes than their urban counterparts (Bain & Adeagbo, 2022).

Rural communities experience a more significant burden of NCDs, including diabetes, hypertension, and strokes, and have more limited access to healthcare. Specialized healthcare services also need to be improved in rural areas. With more than 90% of the world's rural population living in Africa and Asia, a lack of a global rural health research agenda contributes to increasing health inequalities, given that many receive inadequate care (Bain & Adeagbo, 2022).

Martino et al. (2023) studied the need to assess and identify equitability in how patient care is delivered in rural and urban environments with attention to race and ethnicity. As rural health conditions overpower urban conditions, the addition of ethnic and racial disparities exacerbates social conditions, contributing to adverse health concerns.

As these issues continue to be investigated, telemedicine has been able to help address many of the rural clients' needs in some areas of the globe. With telemedicine, clients can contact healthcare professionals in rural and urban areas through electronic communication and technology and receive healthcare visits and specialty consultations. Providers can reciprocate by communicating with peers and gaining expert knowledge and education needs (Kim & Zuckerman, 2019).

Unfortunately, in many parts of the globe, telemedicine is lacking. The comparison of agents to urban clients shows that rural telemedicine visits are used more frequently than urban visits. Additionally, urban clients use telemedicine differently, especially when accessing various specialties. For both groups, some specialties, such as dermatologists and adolescent psychiatry, are in demand due to a worldwide shortage and can be more effectively used with telemedicine technology. Telemedicine has been and will be significantly implemented to assist with the early diagnosis, implementation, and evaluation of healthcare needs to help all individuals regardless of where they live (Sheets et al., 2020; Box 10.5).

BOX 10.5 ACTIVE LEARNING REFLECTION ACTIVITY

Global Rural Health Issues and the Use of Telemedicine

In global rural areas, poverty and health inequality are huge. Investigate the following website and answer the follow-up questions: https://www.who.int/activities/addressing-health-inequities-among-people-living-in-rural-and-remote-areas.

1. How could investing in telemedicine help a global community?
2. Name three interventions that could be implemented to assist with the use of telemedicine.

Watch the following TEDx Talk and reflect by answering the follow-up questions: https://www.youtube.com/watch?v=bAqhvi8r4Ao.

1. What are your feelings about rural health practitioners?
2. What are three takeaways noted by the video?
3. How could the idea of telemedicine be used in other global rural areas?

Write a two-page reflection on three aspects of global rural healthcare that surprised you and three aspects that concerned you. Include three elements of this video that you will use in your future nursing practice.

AACN *Essentials* (2021): Domains: #1; #3; #5; #7; #8; #9

- Competencies: 1.2; 1.3; 3.1; 3.3; 5.1; 7.2; 8.1; 8.3; 9.2
- Subcompetencies: 1.2a; 1.3a; 3.1a; 3.1b; 3.1c; 3.1e; 3.3b; 5.1f; 7.2b; 8.1b; 8.3c; 8.3d; 8.3e; 9.2d

Spheres of Care: Wellness/Disease prevention; Chronic disease management

Concepts: Clinical judgment; SDOH; DEI

Sources: TEDx Talks, 2018; WHO, 2024c.

Global Health Essentials of Care

The American Public Health Services is helpful to global health endeavors. This organization assists with guiding public health needs. The development of 10 essentials identifies actions to meet the goals effectively. The areas that are stressed are related to health inequity due to poverty, racism, and gender discrimination. It is vital to be fair and equitable in providing health and well-being opportunities to all people (Public Health Accreditation Board, n.d.).

Other global health concerns include armed conflicts, uprisings, wars, infectious diseases, and humanitarian emergencies. These all negatively affect healthcare as the services become disorganized with a shortage of providers, and the performance of care delivered is chaotic. Issues of healthcare inequity and access to treatments occur despite the use of telemedicine. Resources decrease due to supply chains becoming disrupted. Epidemics develop, and care for combatants is prioritized over that of civilians. Climate changes are occurring, and infrastructures fail, families relocate, and children are injured or orphaned and at risk for diseases. Food cultivation, harvest, and distribution are disrupted, causing nutritional concerns and malnutrition (Advisory Board, 2023).

SDOH and Global Health

The SDOH remains a high priority globally. Health is greatly influenced by social and economic factors beyond any country's healthcare system. Some countries, such as the United States and the United Kingdom, have begun to address the issue. Many developing countries are attempting to determine what factors (such as politics, genetics, or education) are some of the driving forces that need to be addressed through healthcare policy (Abdalla et al., 2022).

Most global countries consider healthcare to be what matters most to health. Improving the health of populations requires enacting policies and programs that address the SDOH, which mandates the need for broad public support. Further improved health policies, advocacy needs, and communication to and with the global public are needed for more investment and application of SDOH (Abdalla et al., 2022).

The PAHO notes the overwhelming influence of SDOH factors, including health inequity, on global health. Without addressing all aspects of the cause, health inequalities will persist. Thus, an SDOH conceptual framework was developed that demonstrates the complexity of the issue (PAHO, n.d.; Figure 10.3).

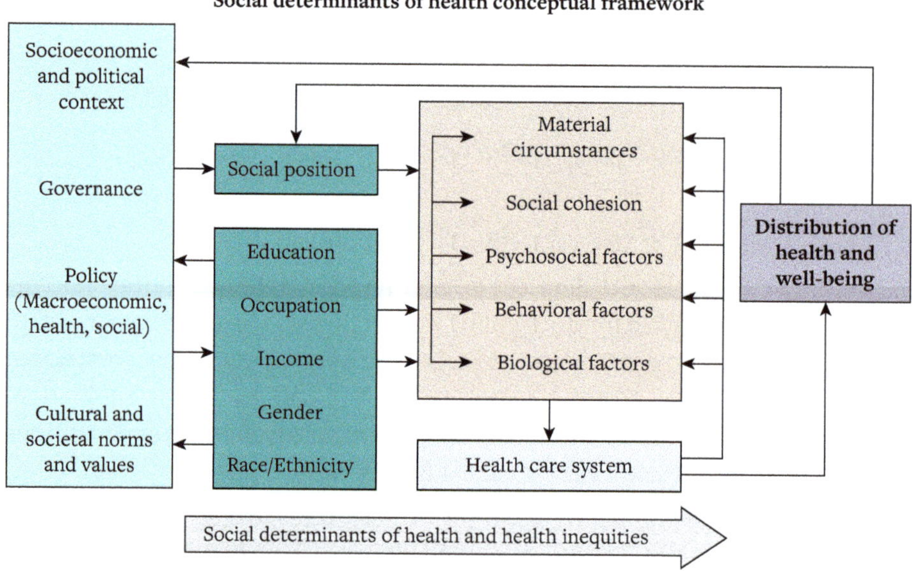

FIGURE 10.3 SDOH Conceptual Framework

Levels of Prevention and Global Health

By globally practicing levels of prevention, healthcare can help make advancements in the following areas: Educate people on how to maintain and promote their health, reduce possible disease risk factors, and promote early identification, prevention, and diagnosis of diseases and complications that may develop. Implementing quaternary prevention, which focuses on limiting medical procedures and interventions that are excessive or unnecessary, is an essential factor. Through the use of preventative measures and the implementation of the various resources available, healthcare professionals can be most effective in assisting in disease prevention and contributing to the health of individuals, families, communities, and countries worldwide (AbdulRaheem, 2023).

Chapter Highlights

- Identification and discussion of global health agencies and their role in global healthcare
- Application of active learning reflection activity on the SDGs
- Application of active learning reflection activity on application to the WHO
- Application of active learning reflection activity on global primary care
- Application of active learning reflection activity on application of AACN Essentials Domain #3, Competencies 3.4 and 3.5
- Application of active learning reflection activity on global rural health issues/ use of telemedicine
- Case study with application of the Minnesota Department of Health intervention wheel
- Case studies related to global surveillance, healthcare advocacy, and the WHO toolkit

Active Learning Exercises

Application to Intervention Wheel

Surveillance is a critical element of public health, especially in global health. Please use the following link (red wedge section/Surveillance) to address the following problem: https://www.health.state.mn.us/communities/practice/research/phncouncil/docs/PHInterventions.pdf.

In Chapter 8, influenza was addressed in the Application to Intervention Wheel activity. One example of a global issue was addressing a pandemic influenza issue.

A great example of the importance of interventions related to surveillance was noted in the Intervention Wheel from Canada.

Nurses in Ontario, Canada, staffed a telephone health helpline to recruit and monitor participants with influenza-like symptoms.

The WHO's site on disease surveillance should help explain the importance of monitoring global disease outbreaks closely: https://www.who.int/westernpacific/emergencies/surveillance.

Using the above information, develop a two-page plan with interventions on using surveillance in a global country of your choice (not Canada or the United States), answering the following questions:

1. How would you find appropriate data on influenza rates?
2. How would you continue surveillance of the issue?
3. How would you disseminate the data to healthcare providers and the general public? Be specific in your interventions.

AACN *Essentials* (2021): Domain: #1; #2; #3; #4; #6; #7; #8

- Competencies: 1.1; 1.2; 1.3; 2,2; 2.5; 2.9; 3.1; 4.2; 6.3; 6.4; 7.3; 8.2; 8.3; 8.5
- Subcompetencies: 1.1b; 1.2a; 1.3a; 2.2b; 2.2e; 2.5a; 2.9a; 3.1a; 3.1c; 3.1d; 3.1e; 3.1h; 4.2c; 6.3a; 6.4d; 7.3b; 8.2b; 8.3a; 8.3d; 8.5f

Spheres of Care: Wellness/Disease prevention; Chronic disease management

Concepts: Communication; DEI; Health policy, SDOH; Evidence-based practice; Clinical judgment

Sources: Minnesota Department of Health, 2019; WHO, 2024d.

Case Studies

Case Study #1

Watch the following videos regarding the 75 years for which public health has cared for the global population. After watching this, think about the next 25 years and produce at least five specific topics that would be beneficial that the global entities could help solve. Under each topic, document four detailed interventions that could be implemented.

- https://www.who.int/campaigns/75-years-of-improving-public-health
- https://www.youtube.com/watch?v=37NMD3u_H8c

AACN *Essentials* (2021): Domains: #1; #3; #4; #6; #7; #8

- Competencies: 1.2; 3.1; 3,2; 3.3; 3.4; 4.2; 6.1; 6.1; 6.2; 6.3; 6.4; 7.2; 7.3, 8.1; 8,2; 8.3
- Subcompetencies: 1.2a; 1.2c; 1.2e; 3.1b; 3.1d; 3.1f; 3.2a; 3.2b; 3.2c; 3.3a; 3.3b; 3.4e; 4.2c; 6.1a; 6.1d; 6.1f; 6.2a; 6.3c; 6.4b; 6.4d; 7.2b; 7.3d; 8.1a; 8.2d; 8.3a

Spheres of Care: Wellness/Disease prevention; Chronic disease management

Concepts: DEI; Communication; Evidence-based practice; SDOH

Sources: WHO, 2023b; 2024a.

Case Study #2

As a student nurse, you should be familiar with how you can participate as a healthcare advocate. One way is to contact governmental representatives (i.e., senators) and encourage them to support a specific global area. Find a representative from your state of residence and write a professional letter asking for their support by presenting the topic and citing the reasons you are asking for support.

AACN *Essentials* (2021): Domains: #1; #3; #6; #7; #9

- Competencies: 1.2; 1.3; 3.1; 3.2; 3.3; 3.4; 3.5; 6.1; 7.2; 9.1; 9.2; 9.3
- Subcompetencies: 1.2a; 1.2c; 1.3a; 3.1c; 3.1e; 3.2a; 3.3a; 3.4d; 3.5a; 6.1a; 6.1d; 6.1f; 7.2b; 7.2d; 9.1g; 9.2d; 9.3a

Spheres of Care: Wellness/Disease prevention; Chronic care management

Concepts: Health policy; SDOH; Clinical judgment; DEI

Case Study #3

Visit https://www.who.int/tools. Choose one toolkit of interest to you and investigate the topics and information presented. Write a blog on your findings based on the chosen topic for the class. Include what is contained in the toolbox, how a nurse could educate individuals about the topic, and the importance of the topic to healthcare needs. Cite sources utilized with proper techniques. Be creative and address additional information about these areas: ages of the participants, sex, educational level, active learning exercises used and developed, and presentation techniques.

AACN *Essentials* (2021): Domains: #1; #2; #3; #4; #8; #9

- Competencies: 1.2; 2.2; 3.1: 3.3; 3.4; 4.2; 8.1; 9.2
- Subcompetencies: 1.2a; 2.2b; 2.2c; 2.2e; 3.1a; 3.1c; 3.3b; 3.4e; 4.2c, 8.1a; 8.3c; 9.2b; 9.2d

Spheres of Care: Wellness/Disease prevention; Chronic disease management

Concepts: Communication; Compassionate care; Evidence-based practice; DEI; SDOH

Source: WHO, 2024j.

NCLEX Questions

1. Which activity would reflect a community health nurse working at the primary prevention level?
    A. Teaching safe sex practices to teenagers
    B. Performing adult hypertension screening
    C. Encouraging women to perform breast self-examination
    D. Helping with a postmastectomy exercise program
2. A family health nurse in the United States is concerned about a recent influenza outbreak in France. What would be the reason for this interest?
    A. Highly infectious diseases can travel quickly due to worldwide traveling.
    B. The United States is relied upon for guidance to address global health issues.
    C. Nurses must follow WHO guidelines when controlling diseases.
    D. A moral obligation of a nurse is to provide safety to clients.

References

Abdalla, S. M., Hernandez, M., Koya, S. F., Rosenberg, S. B., Robbins, G., Magana, L., Nsoesie, E. O., Sabin, L., & Galea, S. (2022). What matters for health? Public views from eight countries. *BMJ Global Health, 7*(6), e008858. https://gh.bmj.com/content/7/6/e008858

AbdulRaheem, Y. (2023). Unveiling the significance and challenges of integrating prevention levels in healthcare practice. *Journal of Primary Care & Community Health, 14*, 21501319231186500. https://doi.org/10.1177/21501319231186500

Adhikari, R., & Smith, P. (2023). Global nursing workforce challenges: Time for a paradigm shift. *Nurse Education in Practice, 69*, 103627. https://doi.org/10.1016/j.nepr.2023.103627

Advisory Board. (2023). *The 13 biggest threats to global health, according to the WHO*. https://www.advisory.com/daily-briefing/2020/01/15/who-health-challenges

Ahun, M., Aboud, F., Wamboldt, C., & Yousafzai, A. K. (2023). Implementation of UNICEF and WHO's care for child development package: Lessons from a global review and key informant interviews. *Frontiers in Public Health, 16*(11), 1140843. https://doi.org/10.3389/fpubh.2023.1140843

American Association of Colleges of Nursing. (2021). *The essentials: Core competencies for professional nursing education*. https://www.aacnnursing.org/Essentials

American Public Health Association. (2022). *What does "health in all policies" mean? Episode 9 of "That's Public Health."* YouTube. https://www.youtube.com/watch?v=LBcK-_mpYkM

Bain, L. E., & Adeagbo, O. A. (2022). There is an urgent need for a global rural health research agenda. *The Pan African Medical Journal, 43*,147. https://doi.org/10.11604/pamj.2022.43.147.38189

Baker, C., Cary, A. H., & da Conceicao Bentoc, M. (2021). Global standards for professional nursing education: The time is now. *Journal of Professional Nursing, 37*(1), 86–92. https://doi.org/10.1016/j.profnurs.2020.10.001

Bali Swain, R., & Yang-Wallentin, F. (2020). Achieving Sustainable Development Goals: Predicaments and strategies. *International Journal of Sustainable Development & World Ecology, 27*(2), 96–106. https://doi.org/10.1080/13504509.2019.1692316

Bertram, K., & Pai, M. (2023). Single-issue advocacy in global health: Possibilities and perils. *PLOS Global Public Health, 3*(9), e0002368. https://doi.org/10.1371/journal.pgph.0002368

Centers for Disease Control and Prevention. (2024a). *About CDC*. https://www.cdc.gov/about/cdc/index.html

Centers for Disease Control and Prevention. (2024b). *About One Health*. https://www.cdc.gov/one-health/about/index.html

Chen, X., Li, H., Lucero-Prisno, III, D. E., Abdullah, A. S., Huang, J., Laurence, C., Liang, X., Ma, Z., Mao, Z., Ren, R., Wu, S., Wang, N., Wang, P., Wang, T., Yan, H., & Zou, Y. (2020). What is global health? Key concepts and clarification of misperceptions. *Global Health Research and Policy, 5*(14). https://ghrp.biomedcentral.com/articles/10.1186/s41256-020-00142-7

Department of Health and Human Services. (2023). *Global health security agenda*. https://www.hhs.gov/about/agencies/oga/global-health-security/agenda/index.html

Filho, W. L., Trevisan, L. V., Rampasso, L. S., Anholon, R., Pimenta Dinis, M. A., Brandli, L.L., Sierra, J., Salvia, A. L., Pretorius, R., Nicolau, M., Eustachio, J. H. P. P., & Mazutti, J. (2023). When the alarm bells ring: Why the UN sustainable development goals may not be achieved by 203o. *Journal of Cleaner Production*, 137108. https://doi.org/10.1016/j.jclepro.2023.137108

Global Alliance for Leadership in Nursing Education and Science. (2019). *Global pillars for nursing education*. https://img1.wsimg.com/blobby/go/97747c23-1877-4faf-a117-708964245689/downloads/Global%20Pillars%20for%20Nursing%20Education.pdf?ver=1668093374817

Global Health Media. (n.d.). *Our videos*. https://globalhealthmedia.org/videos/

Global Outbreak Alert and Response Network. (2023). *About us*. https://goarn.who.int/about

Hayman, D. T. S., Barraclough, R. K., Muglia, L. J., McGovern, V., Afolabi, M. O., N'Jai, A. U., Ambe, J. R., Atim, C., McClelland, A., Paterson, B., Ijaz, K., Lasley, J., Ahsan, Q., Garfield, R., Chittenden, K., Phelan, A. K., & Rivera, A. L. (2023). Addressing the challenges of implementing evidence-based prioritization in global health. *BMJ Global Health, 8*(6), e012450. https://gh.bmj.com/content/8/6/e012450

International Council of Nursing. (n.d.a.). *Education and training*. https://www.icn.ch/how-we-do-it/education-and-training

International Council of Nursing. (n.d.b.). *Mission, vision, constitution and strategic plan*. https://www.icn.ch/who-we-are/mission-vision-constitution-and-strategic-plan

International Council of Nursing. (n.d.c.). *Who we are*. https://www.icn.ch/who-we-are

KFF. (2022). *The U.S. government and global health*. https://www.kff.org/global-health-policy/fact-sheet/the-u-s-government-and-global-health/

Kim, T., & Zuckerman, J. E. (2019). Realizing the potential of telemedicine in global health. *Journal of Global Health, 9*(2), 020307. https://doi.org/10.7189/jogh.09.020307

Martino, S., Elliott, M., Dembosky, J., Haas, A., Klein, D., Gildner, J., & Haviland, A. (2023). *Rural-urban disparities in health care in Medicare*. https://www.cms.gov/files/document/rural-urban-disparities-health-care-medicare.pdf

Merriam-Webster. (2024). *Advocacy*. https://www.merriam-webster.com/dictionary/advocacy

Minnesota Department of Health. (2019). *Public health interventions: Applications for public health nursing practice* (2nd ed.). https://www.health.state.mn.us/communities/practice/research/phncouncil/docs/PHInterventions.pdf

Monteiro, M. G., Pantani, D., Pinsky, I., & Hernandes Rocha, T. A. (2023). Using the Pan American Health Organization digital conversational agent to educate the public on alcohol use and health: Preliminary analysis. *Journal of Medical Internet Research, 7*, e43165. https://doi.org/10.2196/43165

Office of Disease Prevention and Health Promotion. (n.d.a.). *Evidence-based resources*. Healthy People 2030. https://health.gov/healthypeople/objectives-and-data/browse-objectives/global-health/evidence-based-resources

Office of Disease Prevention and Health Promotion. (n.d.b.). *Global health*. Healthy People 2030. https://health.gov/healthypeople/objectives-and-data/browse-objectives/global-health

Office of Disease Prevention and Health Promotion. (n.d.c.). *Health policy*. Healthy People 2030. https://health.gov/healthypeople/objectives-and-data/browse-objectives/health-policy

Pan American Health Organization. (n.d.). *Who are we?* https://www.paho.org/en/who-we-are

Public Health Accreditation Board. (n.d.). *The 10 essential public health services*. https://phaboard.org/center-for-innovation/public-health-frameworks/the-10-essential-public-health-services/

Rahman, T., Sobur, A., Islam, M., Ievy, S., Hossain, J., El Zowalaty, M. E., Rahman, T., & Ashour, H. M. (2020). Zoonotic diseases: Etiology, impact, and control. *Microorganisms*, *8*(9), 1405. https://www.mdpi.com/2076-2607/8/9/1405

Sheets, L. R., Wallach, E., Khairat, S., Mutrux, R., Edison, K., & Becevic, M. (2020). Similarities and differences between rural and urban telemedicine utilization. *Perspectives in Health Information Management*, *7*(18), 1e. https://www.ncbi.nlm.nih.gov/pmc/articles/PMC7883358/

Sigma Theta Tau International. (2024). *About Sigma*. https://www.sigmanursing.org/why-sigma/about-sigma

Siegel, S. (2023). *2024 global health care sector outlook: Navigating transformation*. https://www2.deloitte.com/content/dam/Deloitte/it/Documents/life-sciences-health-care/global-health-care-sector-outlook-2024.pdf

Sparta Health. (n.d.). *Global health challenges in 2024*. https://www.sparta-health.co.uk/global-health-challenges-in-2024

TEDx Talks. (2018). *Bridging the rural healthcare gap | Rubayat Khan | TEDxDhaka*. YouTube, January 18, 2018. https://www.youtube.com/watch?v=bAqhvi8r4Ao

United Nations. (n.d.a.). *About us*. https://www.un.org/en/about-us

United Nations. (n.d.b.). *The 17 Sustainable Development Goals*. https://sdgs.un.org/goals

United Nations. (n.d.c.). *Transforming our world: The 2030 agenda for sustainable development*. https://sdgs.un.org/2030agenda

United Nations Children Fund. (n.d.a.). *About UNICEF*. https://www.unicef.org/about-unicef

United Nations Children Fund. (n.d.b.). *UNICEF mission statement*. https://www.unicef.org/about-us/mission-statement

Voss, J., & Yasobant, S. (2024). *Impact of globalization on healthcare*. MDPI. doi.org/10.3390/books978-3-0365-9507-8

Wenham, C., & Davies, S. (2023). What's the ideal World Health Organization (WHO)? *Health Economics, Policy and Law*, *18*(3), 329–340. doi:10.1017/S174413312300004X

World Bank. (2024). *Who we are*. https://www.worldbank.org/en/who-we-are

World Economic Forum. (2022). *6 issues shaping the future of global health in 2022*. https://www.weforum.org/agenda/2022/02/global-healthcare-2022-mental-health/

World Health Organization. (2018). *Millennium development goals*. https://www.who.int/news-room/fact-sheets/detail/millennium-development-goals-(mdgs)

World Health Organization. (2020). *State of the world's nursing 2020: Investing in education, jobs and leadership*. https://www.who.int/publications/i/item/9789240003279

World Health Organization. (2023a). *Primary health care*. https://www.who.int/news-room/fact-sheets/detail/primary-health-care

World Health Organization. (2023b). *75 years of improving public health*. YouTube, January 13, 2023. https://www.youtube.com/watch?v=37NMD3u_H8c

World Health Organization. (2024a). *75 years of improving public health*. https://www.who.int/campaigns/75-years-of-improving-public-health
World Health Organization. (2024b). *About WHO*. https://www.who.int/about
World Health Organization. (2024c). *Addressing health inequities among people living in rural and remote areas*. https://www.who.int/activities/addressing-health-inequities-among-people-living-in-rural-and-remote-areas
World Health Organization. (2024d). *Disease surveillance*. https://www.who.int/westernpacific/emergencies/surveillance
World Health Organization. (2024e). *Essential newborn care course: 2nd edition*. https://www.who.int/tools/essential-newborn-care-course
World Health Organization. (2024f). *Global Influenza Surveillance and Response System (GISRS)*. https://www.who.int/initiatives/global-influenza-surveillance-and-response-system
World Health Organization. (2024g). *International Health Regulations*. https://www.who.int/health-topics/international-health-regulations#tab=tab_1
World Health Organization. (2024h). *Preparing and preventing epidemics and pandemics*. https://www.who.int/activities/preparing-and-preventing-epidemics-and-pandemics
World Health Organization. (2024i). *Refugee and migrant health toolkit*. https://www.who.int/tools/refugee-and-migrant-health-toolkit
World Health Organization. (2024j). *Tools and toolkits*. https://www.who.int/tools
World Health Organization. (2024k). *World health statistics*. https://www.who.int/data/gho/publications/world-health-statistics
World Population Review. (2024). *World population 2024*. https://worldpopulationreview.com/continents/world-population

Credits

Fig. 10.1: Kaiser Family Foundation (KFF), https://www.kff.org/global-health-policy/fact-sheet/the-u-s-government-and-global-health/. Copyright © 2022 by Kaiser Family Foundation.
Fig. 10.2: Copyright © 2018 by United Nations. Reprinted with permission.
Fig. 10.3: Pan American Health Organization (PAHO), https://www.paho.org/en/topics/social-determinants-health. Copyright © by World Health Organization (WHO).

CHAPTER 11

Community Nursing Roles

"When you are a nurse, you know that every day you will touch a life or a life will touch yours."

—unknown

Learning Outcomes

After reading this chapter, students should be able to:

1. Apply the following community nursing roles: home health, hospice, palliative care, school nurse, faith-based/parish nurse, occupational/employee, correctional/prison, family health, mental health, disability/rehabilitative nursing, forensic nursing/sexual assault nurse examiners (SANEs)
2. Advocate for individuals, families, and community needs through various community health nursing roles
3. Identify how community health nursing roles can assist with providing education and training for any situation, including disasters; providing health preventive and disease promotion; offering social support, counseling, treatment adherence screenings, and direct services, including ethical and cultural assistance; and monitoring and reporting diseases

Keywords and Concepts

Correctional/prison; disability/rehabilitation; faith-based/parish; family; forensic; home health; hospice; mental health; palliative care; occupational; school nursing; sexual assault nurse examiners (SANEs)

Definitions of the Keywords

Correctional/prison nursing: Encompasses all aspects of health and well-being for adults and juveniles who are in the justice system (International Association of Forensic Nursing [IAFN], 2024a)

Disability/rehabilitative nursing: Works with clients of all ages and their families or caregivers soon after the onset of a disabling injury or chronic illness (Association of Rehabilitation Nurses [ARN], n.d.b.)

Faith-based/parish nursing: Focuses on the intentional care of the spirit and the promotion of whole-person health and the prevention or minimization of illness within the context of a faith community (American Nursing Association [ANA], 2017).

Family health nursing: Provides primary healthcare to individuals and families from across the lifespan while using primary, secondary, and tertiary prevention interventions (Nursing-Theory.org, 2023)

Forensic nursing: Provides specialized care for clients who are experiencing acute and long-term health consequences associated with victimization or violence, and provide consultation and testimony in criminal health procedures (IAFN, 2024b)

Home health nursing: Various types of healthcare services that are provided in a home-based setting (Medicare.gov, n.d.)

Hospice nursing: Family-centered services at the end of life for individuals with a decrease in quality of life to enhance treatment and manage disease symptoms (American Cancer Society [ACS], 2023)

Mental health/psychiatric nursing: Provides holistic care to individuals with mental disorders or behavioral problems (American Psychological Association, 2024)

Occupational/employee health nursing: Provides for and delivers health and safety programs and services to workers, worker populations, and community groups (American Association of Occupational Health Nurses [AAOHN], n.d.)

Palliative care: Includes support, symptom management, and comfort to allow a positive and enjoyable end-of-life experience (ACS, 2023)

School nurse: Protects and promotes student health, facilitate optimal development, and advance academic success (National Association of School Nurses [NASN], n.d.)

SANEs: Undergoes specialized education and training to provide holistic care to sexually assaulted individuals (Office of Justice Programs [OJP], n.d.b.)

Introduction

Most nurses choose roles in acute care, prominently in the hospital setting. However, nurses must still provide community and population-based care. Compassionate and skilled nurses are greatly needed to serve people in the community setting (Minority Nurse, 2021).

The COVID-19 pandemic has reset the table for conversations about the concept of public health and the future of nursing. Unfortunately, community-based and public health nurses (PHNs) must actively address the social determinants of health (SDOH) and health disparities/health equality (Pittman & Park, 2021).

The focus of the community/PHN role entails social justice concepts of advocacy, policy development, planning, and allowance for health equity. The scope and standards of practice described by the ANA Public Health Nursing Organization benefit public health by providing for the needs and demands of the public (ANA, n.d.). This chapter focuses on the different specialized community health nursing roles, including home health and home-based care, hospice and palliative care, school, faith-based and parish, occupational/employee health, correctional/prison, forensic, sexual assault nurse examiner, legal nurse consultant, family health, mental health/psychiatric and disability/rehabilitative nursing.

Background of the Concepts

The community/public health nursing role involves several specialties. These include environmental health, data review, evaluation of the need for changes, questions about current practices, active community involvement with processes, organization of specialized groups, and development of interdisciplinary teams to provide methods and training that can be safely implemented. Areas specifically approached include providing immunizations, preventing infections, assessing environmental health needs, and fighting the opioid crisis. Additional roles of the community nurse are disease prevention and promoting health and safety in the community setting. There is a need to visit trending health situations, identify risk factors, and provide healthcare services for all in the community. Most importantly, this nursing specialty helps develop and implement healthcare education for health promotion and disease prevention (ANA, n.d.; Centers for Disease Control and Prevention [CDC] Foundation, n.d.).

To practice in the community/public health nursing role, nurses should have knowledge leading to other clinical, leadership, or research roles. Due to the expanded role in the clinical, leadership, and research positions, excellent communication, interpersonal, analytical, and clinical skills are warranted. The ability to interact with many professionals in other specialties is vital to assimilating effective team relationships, allowing for cooperation and support in the functioning of the needs of the groups (CDC Foundation, n.d.).

Nursing schools must continue to provide a curriculum for students who understand community/public and population-based care. Focusing on acute care and treatments will not produce nursing students who acknowledge the need for specialized community nursing roles (Jones et al., 2022).

Specialized Community Nursing Roles

Nurses frequently specialize within the profession. They move into specific roles and gain additional education to be well-seated in their chosen field of practice. Nursing programs should incorporate specialized community nursing roles so that students understand the importance of community, public health, population-based care, and social factors that can affect health outcomes (Zeydani et al., 2021).

Community-based nursing exists worldwide but is associated with the needs and concerns of the environment in which it exists. Zeydani et al. (2023) supported the focus of the community-based nurse must include individuals and families of all ages working with diseases affecting health, communities, social groups, stakeholders, and social justice; interacting with multidisciplinary professionals; and incorporating cultural diversity (Zeydani et al., 2023). Community-based nurses' interactions are essential with the leaders for the environment's infrastructure and structures, how the community facilitates care with the local schools and universities, healthcare settings, and hospitals. They are professionals educated to be able to participate in educational sessions and assess the needs of the community as well as means of financial support. Community-based nurses must look at the community as a whole, including individuals and families, to increase the degree of healthcare services for all (Zeydani et al., 2023).

Home Health/Home-Based Care

Home health nursing is one of the community-based nursing specializations that are frequently used in healthcare. Care in the home encompasses treating, assisting, and providing services to clients in the home setting, wherever the home may be. Usually, these individuals are older than age 65 and require skilled nursing (U.S. Bureau of Labor Statistics, 2024).

Home health's primary focus is to optimize the quality of life for those experiencing life-limiting, progressive diseases and assist the client and family in remaining in their setting. Home healthcare is usually less expensive, more convenient, and as therapeutic as care provided in a hospital or skilled nursing facility (Medicare.gov, n.d.).

The Homecare Association of America (HCA) reports that between 2020 and 2030, the number of U.S. citizens age 85 or older will double from the current

2.4 million and extend the growth spurt of the shortage of caregivers to more than 12 million. It is reported that more than 25% of potential home care clients are turned away due to staffing issues (HCA, 2023).

The 2022 U.S. National Nursing Workforce Survey indicated that 57% of registered nurses chose employment in the hospital setting; ambulatory care was next with 10.4%, nursing homes at 3.9%, and home healthcare at 3.4% (Smiley et al., 2023). As this indicates growth in the home care field, the continued need for more nurses and workers is necessary, and it has reached crisis levels and continues to grow (HCA, 2023).

Anthony (2024) addresses the need for additional home care nurses due to society's aging, citing the comforts of clients' own homes, prepared foods, familiarity with the setting and individuals around them, and the calming environment. One suggestion to enhance the workforce is to include nursing programs that provide that experience while training.

Home-based care began in the early 19th century, when impoverished individuals lacked access to healthcare and were assisted by religious orders or wealthy women. These women came into the homes and practiced care and comfort measures but were confronted with issues related to care practices. These concerns include determining who needs access to care, how long the care should be provided, who should provide the care, whether the care is for acutely or chronically ill individuals, and the role of the family members (Faster Capital, 2024).

Florence Nightingale and Lillian Wald emerged as leaders for home-based care. They both noted the importance of visiting nursing, using the district nursing approach. Care focused on public health nursing, including social and economic considerations for those needing care (HemoCue, 2021).

As home healthcare has progressed, several changes have facilitated care offered in the home. Modernization of technology and ways to implement special care needs have been incorporated into the provisions for many conditions. Telehealth has been acknowledged as a successful means of communication and compliance techniques with older adults, especially those in rural areas that lack transportation (Eckstadt, 2024; Kowalski & Gifford, 2024; Logan & Zipp, 2024).

Interdisciplinary roles in home health are provided for those with needs identified during the initial assessments and any subsequent changes in condition. Home-based care requires a collaborative approach. The client may require physical therapy, occupational therapy, home health aides, and social workers. Prompt communication and ongoing case conferences will ensure that the client and family meet their health outcomes (Health at Home, 2023; Home Centered Care Institute, 2022).

It is essential to understand that home care includes all three levels of prevention to assist individuals with interventions for recovery, performing self-care and independence, preventing decline, allowing for self-sufficiency, and maintaining the current condition or degree of functioning. Skilled home healthcare interventions may include wound care, education for clients and caregivers, intravenous and/ or other forms of nutritional needs, and assessments and continuous monitoring for declining and unstable health conditions (Medicare.gov, n.d.). Overall, home healthcare's most crucial focus is empowering clients and caregivers to aim for the highest levels of functioning and health.

The Outcome and Assessment Information Set (OASIS) is required if Medicare and/or Medicaid funds are obtained. Currently, OASIS-E is being used as it has been revised to include providing standardization across postacute care conditions, gathering information on the SDOH, and reviewing quality measures to assist in the Improving Medicare Post-Acute Care Transformation Act (Centers for Medicare & Medicaid Services [CMS], 2024).

Outcome measures assess the quality of the care performed on the client. This is determined by how effectively the OASIS data are obtained. For the OASIS tool, the home care agency will initially assess when care is started and then continue at 60-day follow-up and discharge. Any additional assessment activities may need to be included to complete a full review of the client and total health care needs. Criteria specifics are noted in Figure 11.1 (Campbell County Health, 2022; CMS, 2024; National Association for Home Care & Hospice [NAHC], 2024; Box 11.1).

Home Health Care	
Primary Goals:	Recovery from an illness, surgery or injury, or managing a chronic medical condition
Who Is Eligible:	Patients who are homebound, certified by a doctor as being in need of intermittent, skilled care, and under a doctor's plan of care
Care Provided By:	Nurses, physical therapists, speech therapists, occupational therapists, home health aides and medical social workers
Care Provided To:	Patients, with education for caregivers
Who Pays:	Medicare, Medicaid and many private insurance plans
What's Covered:	Nursing care, physical therapy, speech therapy, occupational therapy, medical social worker services, help with bathing, dressing and other daily tasks from a home health aide
When:	Regular visits from the home health team, with 24/7 on-call availability
Where:	Wherever the patient calls home, including a private residence or a facility such as assisted living or senior living
How Long:	As long as a doctor certifies the patient is eligible for home health
Services for Caregivers:	Education and referrals to community resources

FIGURE 11.1 Home Care at a Glance

BOX 11.1 ACTIVE LEARNING REFLECTION ACTIVITY

Application of Home Health/Home-Based Care

A nursing curriculum contains limited exposure to the role and responsibilities of the home healthcare nurse. Home-based nursing is critical to understanding the importance of the continuum of care.

Visit the following links:

- https://www.youtube.com/watch?v=HvAa45mCHGQ
- https://www.youtube.com/watch?v=f7qf7QeUsdM

Then reflect on the following questions:

1. Why is a continuum of care so important for clients and the population? Provide an evidence-based rationale.
2. How should home-based care be implemented in nursing curriculums in the future? Provide an evidence-based rationale.
3. Name three ways to implement home health/home-based principles in your future nursing practice.

Create a one-page handout for future nursing students regarding the roles and responsibilities of home health/home-based nursing.

American Association of Colleges of Nursing (AACN) *Essentials* (2021):
Domains: #1; #3; #4; #6; #7

- Competencies: 1.2; 1.3; 3.1; 3.2; 3.3; 4.2; 6.1; 6.3; 7.1; 7.3
- Subcompetencies: 1.2a; 1.3a; 3.1a; 3.1c; 3.1e; 3.1h; 3.1i; 3.2a; 3.3b; 4.2c; 6.1a; 6.3c; 7.1a; 7.3d

Spheres of Care: Chronic disease management; Regenerative/restorative care

Concepts: Compassionate care; Clinical judgment; Communication; Evidence-based practice

Sources: BAYADA Home Health Care, 2018; VNS Health, 2022.

Hospice

Hospice is Latin and means *guest* and *host* (Hospices of Holland, 2023). Hospices focus on unique settings in the home or specific facilities caring for the terminally ill. London's Dame Cicely Saunders was associated with initiating end-of-life care. By 1963, she emphasized the special needs that occur during the dying process but used the techniques of palliative care to cure conditions, especially cancer. By 1969, Elisabeth Kubler-Ross introduced her research, presenting information from clients experiencing death and dying. Dr. Kubler-Ross found that clients in the home were much more comfortable than in a hospital or nursing home healthcare facility while dying with dignity and being able to make their decisions and wishes known and followed (Hospices of Holland, 2023; National Hospice and Palliative Care Organization [NHPCO], 2024). The United States began funding hospice programs through Medicare in 1982, with the Medicare Hospice Benefit in place by 1986 (Hospices of Holland, 2023; NHPCO, 2024).

Hospice focuses on caring, not curing. Most hospice clients receive care in private homes but can be provided in freestanding hospice facilities, hospitals, nursing homes, assisted living facilities, or other long-term care facilities. Hospice services are available to clients with any terminal illness who has a prognosis of only six months to live. Most people think that cancer is the only diagnosis seen in hospice care, but other terminal issues such as end-stage heart failure, chronic obstructive pulmonary disease, and kidney disease are also represented in hospice care (NHPCO, 2023).

Hospices promote inclusiveness in the community by ensuring equality for all people's access to services. The CDC (2023) noted that in 2020, there were 1.5 million U.S. hospice clients. Unfortunately, one issue is the need for prompt referral for hospice services. NHPCO (2023) reported that in 2020, the length of care was 10% of clients enrolled in hospice for two days or fewer, and 25% enrolled in hospice for five days or fewer.

Hospice is a family-centered service that is specifically focused on allowing families to stay together during the end of life. As the client is close to death, they experience a decrease in their quality of life. There is a specific need to enhance treatment and manage the disease symptoms. Hospice begins as the client's disease process is unable to be controlled by the respective treatment, and through hospice, it is then focused on the ability to manage the symptoms of the disease (ACS, 2023).

In hospice, an interdisciplinary team of various professionals is used to meet the individual needs of the client, family, and caregivers. As the primary focus is on managing the symptoms, other essential aspects include meeting spiritual needs and mental health concerns, supporting client wishes, planning future care, and assisting with critical decision-making for end-of-life activities. The goal is to implement methods to keep the client comfortable and pain-free. The ACS and NAHC help facilitate many of these issues (ACS, 2023).

Initiation of the hospice process may be as difficult as it is challenging for those involved to want to stop care and treatments, abandoning the provision of care and comfort interventions. Cross et al. (2022) researched the timing of the beginning of the admission to hospice. Initially, identifying a terminal diagnosis may not be the best time; however, allowing for the client, family, and caregiver to be able to understand further what is occurring while being supported by healthcare workers through education and emotional support may be optimal.

Assisting with enhancing a client's quality of life is essential for the client, family, and caregivers. Cross et al. (2022) have identified that clients and healthcare professionals need help understanding hospice services and when the best time is for transition to these services to occur. The process is sometimes uncomfortable, and adequate explanations of what hospice can do to assist those involved must be

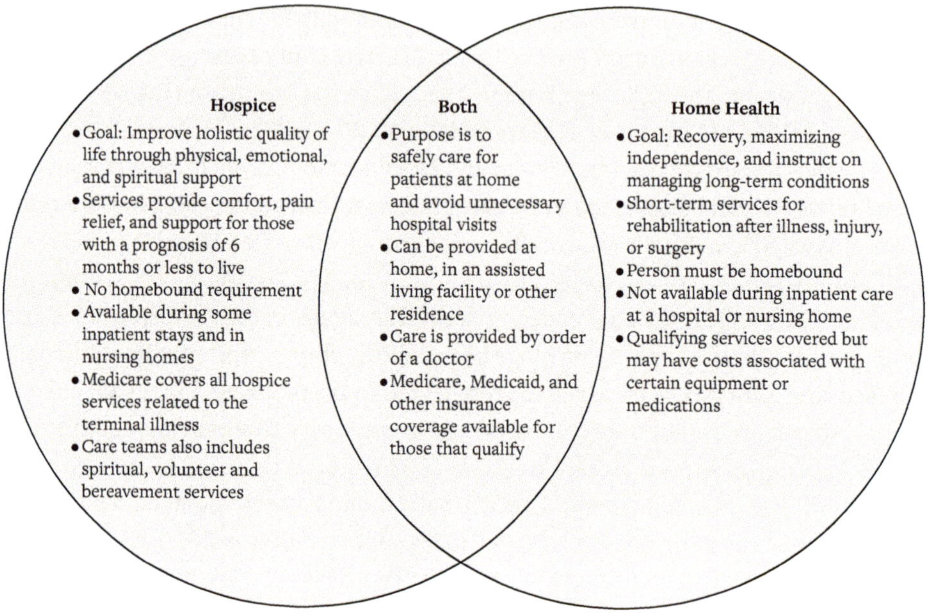

Hospice

- Goal: Improve holistic quality of life through physical, emotional, and spiritual support
- Services provide comfort, pain relief, and support for those with a prognosis of 6 months or less to live
- No homebound requirement
- Available during some inpatient stays and in nursing homes
- Medicare covers all hospice services related to the terminal illness
- Care teams also includes spiritual, volunteer and bereavement services

Both

- Purpose is to safely care for patients at home and avoid unnecessary hospital visits
- Can be provided at home, in an assisted living facility or other residence
- Care is provided by order of a doctor
- Medicare, Medicaid, and other insurance coverage available for those that qualify

Home Health

- Goal: Recovery, maximizing independence, and instruct on managing long-term conditions
- Short-term services for rehabilitation after illness, injury, or surgery
- Person must be homebound
- Not available during inpatient care at a hospital or nursing home
- Qualifying services covered but may have costs associated with certain equipment or medications

FIGURE 11.2 Differences and Similarities Between Home Health and Hospice

shared and placed in a positive context. These misconceptions also relate to those who are employed in the healthcare field, as death is not a topic that many want to broach. The presence of hospice stigma, misconceptions, referral process, and insufficient communication among healthcare workers may lead to difficulties and negative connotations to a well-thought-out form of end-of-life care (Figure 11.2).

Palliative Care

Palliative care is connected with hospice care and begins with variations in client needs. Cicely Saunders observed dying clients and researched using an interdisciplinary group of professionals to relieve pain and provide care and comfort. In 1974, Balfour Mount, a surgical oncologist, coined the term *palliative care* to distinguish it from hospice care. While hospice falls under the umbrella of palliative care, palliative care can be provided from the time of diagnosis of a severe illness and run concurrently with curative or life-prolonging treatment. A later study noted that those clients with lung cancer who received early palliative care and standard oncologic care experienced less depression and increased quality of life and survived for 2.7 months longer than those receiving standard oncologic care (NEJM Resident 360, 2020).

Clients in palliative care may receive medical care for their symptoms and treatment to cure their serious illnesses. Palliative care enhances a person's current care by focusing on their quality of life and their family. Understanding the positive or negative outcomes is freely discussed, and alterations in the care plan can be adjusted or abandoned at times of failure (National Institute on Aging, 2021).

The WHO estimates that globally, 14% of clients needing support for palliative care receive it despite the WHO encouraging universal healthcare following palliative care formatting (WHO, 2024a). Palliative care can be incorporated into a client's comprehensive care during severe illness. This provides full benefits to those needing the interventions and can include various cancer treatments rendered for palliative care or control of symptoms that lead to positive client outcomes. Some examples are chemotherapy, radiation therapy, immunology therapy, and other treatments supporting the intended conditions (ACS, 2023; Hui et al., 2022). The continued usage of various means to assist with support includes mental, physical, emotional, social, and spiritual concerns for all involved. The palliative care team must ensure that all client and family needs are addressed and conducted (ACS, 2023).

Hui et al. (2022) studied the period and identification of those needing this form of care when using standardized referral criteria to assess clients to enter palliative care, which was perceived as beneficial. Using the referral criteria, clients are seen as needing this form of specialized and supportive care where specialists caring for these types of clients can be best used.

Durojaiye et al. (2023) reported that this knowledge should begin during undergraduate nursing education as the graduates must be prepared to deliver this form of care. The research alluded that this education is prominent in high-income countries but limited in low- and middle-income ones. Several barriers were identified, but overall, there needs to be education and involvement with palliative care; there must be education, a positive attitude, self-confidence, and adequate preparation for those caring for those needing this form of care, whether they are still in the educational setting or currently practicing (Figure 11.3; Box 11.2).

Hospice vs. Palliative Care
What Are The Differences?

	Hospice	Palliative
Diagnosis	Terminal	Serious, but not necessarily terminal
Timeframe	Final 6 months of life	Anytime
Treatment	Pain management (no curative treatment)	Pain management + curative treatment
Where	Anywhere you call home	Anywhere you call home
Team	Doctors, nurses, social workers, chaplains, dietitians	Doctors, nurses, social workers, chaplains, dietitians

FIGURE 11.3 Hospice Versus Palliative Care

BOX 11.2 ACTIVE LEARNING REFLECTION ACTIVITY

Application of Hospice/Palliative Care

Watch the following video on palliative care from the WHO and how to assess the appropriateness of this type of care: https://www.who.int/multi-media/details/what-is-palliative-care-and-how-can-it-be-assessed#.

The video explains that palliative care is like "building a house." Take the house plan presented at the end of the session and "build a house" for a client with end-stage lung cancer who is admitted into palliative care. For each building process step, list four ways the nurse can help the client, family, and caregivers. Use your local/state area as a guideline.

Steps to build a house:

1. Provide palliative care.
2. Use essential medications.
3. Provide education and training.
4. Research.
5. Empower people and communities.
6. Promote health policies.

Reflect on two ways to use this learning in your future nursing practice.

AACN *Essentials* (2021): Domains: #1; #2; #4; #6; #7; #8; #9

- Competencies: 1.1; 1.2; 1.3; 2.1; 2.2; 2.3; 2.4; 2.5; 2.8; 2.9; 4.2; 6.1; 7.1; 8.1; 8.2; 9.2; 9.4
- Subcompetencies: 1.1b; 1.2a; 1.3a; 2.1a; 2.1b; 2.1c; 2.2a; 2.2b; 2.2c; 2.2d; 2.2e; 2.3f; 2.4a; 2.4c; 2.5a; 2.5b; 2.5c; 2.5e; 2.5g; 2.8a; 2.8b; 2.8c; 2.8d; 2.8e; 2.9c; 4.2c; 6.1a; 7.1a; 7.1c; 8.1a;8.2c; 9.2c; 9.2f; 9.4b

Spheres of Care: Chronic disease management; Hospice/palliative/supportive care

Concepts: Communication; Compassionate care; Evidence-based practice; Health policy; Clinical judgment

Source: WHO, 2024c.

School Nurse

School nursing came to fruition in the United States sometime in the early 1800s due to population growth. This role began in maternal care due to its relationship to providing compassion and care for newborns, children, and young adults. In 1847, Martha Ballard cared for children in the home, while in 1877, Mary MacKillop established Charity Hospital for Children in Chicago to assist with medical and nursing care to children. As the early 1900s emerged, school nurses became significant members of the healthcare system in schools. While the majority of nurses worked in hospitals, hospital workers were plentiful and began to seek employment in schools. The school nurses assisted students who could not attend school because of an illness or injury and supported and assisted them and their families. In the 1930s and 1940s, the Great Depression and World War II shifted the importance of children and their quality of life. By 1932, school nursing had become a specialized focus, and the National League of Nursing had developed the initial certification examination (EduReaders, 2022).

The popularity of being a school nurse has emerged following specialized education for this outreach of the nursing profession. Currently, school nurse demographics have estimated that more than 25,705 school nurses are employed in the United States (Zippia, 2024d). The majority are women, 93.7%, and 6.3% are men. School nurses are vital to children's health and wellness and assist with their development and academic success (EduReaders, 2022).

The NASN promotes the role of the school nurse. School nurses, grounded in ethical and evidence-based practice, are the leaders who bridge healthcare and education, provide care coordination, advocate for quality student-centered care, and collaborate to design systems that allow individuals and communities to develop their full potential. NASN's mission is to optimize student health and learning by advancing school nursing practice and with core values of working with students and using diversity, equity, and inclusion (DEI; NASN, 2023).

One crucial role found for school nurses is that of health disparities. De Buhr et al. (2020) studied school nurses in Germany and discovered that they positively affected literacy in the school setting in addition to interactions with teachers and parents. Additional help that school nurses provide includes health education, surveillance, and clinical services for public health and health promotion programs involved with all levels of prevention.

The NSAN (2023) noted the disparities in public school nurses between urban and rural areas in the United States. In urban areas, full-time school nurses are employed in 70.3% of schools, whereas rural schools employ full-time nurses in 56.2%. Only 65.7% of all schools have a full-time school nurse, whereas 6.3% still need access to a school nurse.

Implementing and applying the levels of prevention is critical for school nurses to do. Primary prevention consists of teaching healthy lifestyles, promoting healthy activities, and immunizing children for school entry. Secondary prevention is screening for health problems for hearing and vision. States often mandate these screenings for specific grades. Early intervention for ill or injured children and school staff is another prominent function. With the increase in the number of chronic illnesses in children, such as asthma or diabetes, tertiary prevention has become an essential function of school nurses. Providing continuity of care is critical for students to continue school academic needs as school nurses have many roles to facilitate daily (NASN, 2024; Figure 11.4).

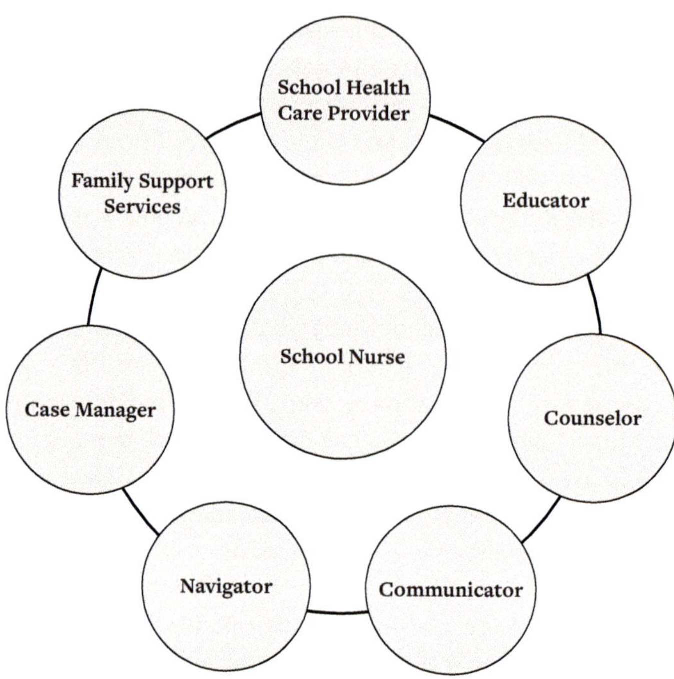

FIGURE 11.4 Many Roles of a School Nurse

Depending on their location, school nurses may need to care for acute or chronic health conditions, mental health concerns, environmental issues, and wellness challenges. In other places, school nurses assist with children's asthma and diabetes. Obesity, mental health, and problems with those living in low socioeconomic backgrounds are not sufficiently researched for adequate analysis, as Pawils et al. (2023) suggest that inadequate research methodologies and standards are being used. The NASN developed a guiding practice framework to support students at school and in the community (NASN, 2024; Figure 11.5; Box 11.3).

Faith-Based/Parish Nursing

Faith-based nursing, previously called *parish nursing*, began in 1973, promoting comprehensive health and wellness in faith-related settings (ANA, 2017). By including clients and their families, the combination of religion and religious beliefs incorporates areas of healthy interventions and plans for compelling care needs.

The work of Nightingale and Wald is grounded in the foundation of faith-based nursing. This type of nursing believes care is based on the body, mind, spirit, or whole person. Faith-based nursing should include prevention, health promotion, maintenance, and acute and chronic conditions (Sessanna et al., 2021).

Faith-based nurses work and interact with clients and their families in homes, religious settings, and nonhospital environments. Their work consists of interacting with individuals holistically through the use of the body, mind, and spirit to assist

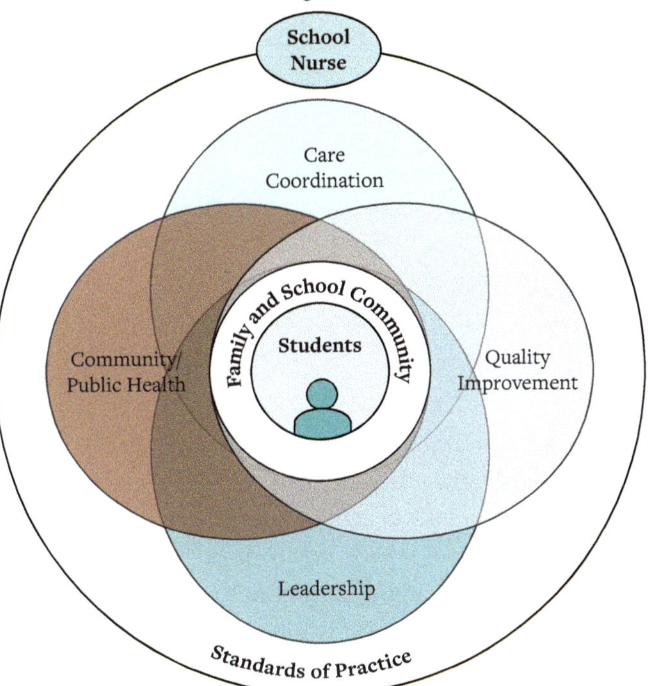

FIGURE 11.5 School Nursing Practice Framework

BOX 11.3 APPLICATION OF SCHOOL-BASED NURSING

Watch the following video about school nurses: https://www.youtube.com/watch?v=ZOC2vGfGHJc. Then watch the following video on the School Nursing Practice Framework: https://www.nasn.org/nasn-resources/framework.

Your community health instructor has made an assignment requiring you to view the previous websites. As a nursing student, prepare a 10-slide PowerPoint presentation (including title and reference slides) describing the roles of a school nurse. The presentation must answer the following proposed questions:

1. What are the five principles mentioned in the school framework video? Briefly describe them.
2. Using the first video on what school nurses do and describe four roles noted in the video that surprised you.
3. In what two ways do you feel that school nursing will evolve in the next 10 years?
4. How will school nurses adapt to the increase in pediatric chronic diseases?
5. Name three ways a school nurse can advocate for children.

AACN *Essentials* (2021): Domains: #1; #3; #4; #6; #8

- Competencies: 1.2; 1.3; 3.1; 3.2; 3.3; 3.4; 4.2; 6.1; 8.1; 8.3
- Subcompetencies: 1.2a; 1.3a; 3.1a; 3.1c; 3.1h; 3.2a; 3.2c; 3.3a; 3.4c; 4.2c; 6.1c; 8.1c; 8.1e; 8.3d

Spheres of Care: Wellness/Disease prevention; Chronic disease management

Concepts: Clinical judgment; Communication; SDOH; Health policy

Sources: NASN, 2024; Spokane Public Schools, 2018.

in positive perceptions of wellness. By collaborating with the client, family, healthcare team, and community, the nurse can have an all-inclusive group with whom to work. They offer support and advocacy for all individuals' religious, cultural, and ethical needs for valuable resources and mentoring others to perform and take over various roles to continue programs for communities (ANA, 2017; Sessanna, 2021).

Schroepfer (2016) reported that faith-based nurses have been identified as significantly helpful in communicating health promotion and disease prevention information in their congregations. This has allowed for not only the educational portion but also consideration of the prevention of hospital readmissions.

Balint and George (2015) significantly discussed the role of the faith-based nurse in helping the uninsured, impoverished, and unhoused. By being available to these groups, a significant ability to work in prevention, health maintenance, and managing chronic disease can be approached. It may be beneficial to coordinate the role of the hospital nurse with the faith-based nurse before hospital discharge. In doing so, nursing plans can be developed for the transitional period. Other interventions for care can include spiritual and mental health needs. They work with not just the provincial topics but also those with chronic health conditions or those who may develop other health deficits that are worsened by the lack of primary care accessibility.

Faith-based nursing has extended to many community settings with increasing healthcare costs and a focus on access and prevention. Ziebarth (2014) noted an updated faith-based community framework that demonstrates holistic care's interconnectedness and global focus. A comparison of parish versus faith-based nursing is displayed in Table 11.1.

Occupational/Employee Health

The Industrial Revolution brought attention to the fact that workers' living environments were poor, families became mobile, finding employment, dirty working conditions, exposure to toxic substances, unsafe settings, use of children workers, contaminated water, and poor access to healthcare needs. Late in the 19th century, the United States and Europe became alerted that illness could be

TABLE 11.1 Parish Nurse Versus Faith-Based

Framework	Parish nurse	Faith-based
Origin	Mid-1980s in Chicago	Reincarnation of faith community nursing outreach done by religious orders in the 1800s
Name	The ANA recognized the name as a specialty in 1997	The ANA changed the name from *parish* to *faith-based* in 2005
Overall concept	Separation of nurse-client relationship from the setting	More holistic in nature, with nurse-client embedded in the role focus
Focus	Caring for members and neighbors in a faith-based setting	Promoting whole-person health and spiritual care in a faith-based community
Interventions	Education, counseling, prayer, presence, active listening, advocacy, referral, and resources	Spiritual care as part of health promotion and education; using evidence-based approach to provide holistic care

Source: ANA, 2017; Ziebarth, 2014.

decreased with proper healthcare practices. Betty Moulder was reported as the first industrial nurse hired, especially to collaborate with the miners and their families regarding their individual health needs. As time passed, the growth of the occupational nurse grew along with their roles and responsibilities. They applied the need to teach safety skills to prevent accidents while keeping workers on the job (AAOHN, n.d.).

Zippia (2024c) states that more than 12,342 occupational health nurses are currently employed in the United States, with 89.0% of all occupational health nurses being women, while 11.0% are men. More than half of the work is for private companies, primarily in healthcare occupational health facilities. The AAOHN is the guiding organization that assists occupational health nurses (Gaines, 2023).

Occupational nurses deliver health and safety programs and services to workers, worker populations, and community groups. The practice focuses on promoting and restoring health, instituting all levels of prevention related to illness and injury, and protecting from work-related and environmental hazards. Education on safety practices is also incorporated into the functions of this nursing role (AAOHN, n.d.). By doing so, organizations and occupational health nurses can offer health services to employees and keep them healthy, decreasing the medical costs an employer spends for their employees and even the number of lost wages due to illness or injury (Gaines, 2023).

Correctional/Prison Nursing

In 1976, the U.S. Supreme Court allowed healthcare to be a constitutional right for U.S. prisoners. Specifically, the areas focused on were the right to access care, the right to care that is ordered, and the right to a professional medical judgment. Thus began the realm and specialty of correctional/prison nursing (Roscoe, 2022).

Correctional health includes the health of families and communities of justice system–involved people and the administrators and staff who work in facilities (CDC, 2024b). These nurses are found in jails, detention centers, prisons, correctional centers, youth custody facilities, and halfway houses (IAFN, 2024a).

Correctional/prison nurses see individuals for their healthcare needs. Beginning with a thorough assessment, the nurse will be able to develop a plan of care that is needed and communicate with a healthcare provider to assess additional care needs. Although the environment is challenging, ensuring safety and security for the staff and inmates comes first (IAFN, 2024a). Everyday situations may relate to the withdrawal of drugs and alcohol, communicable diseases such as sexually transmitted conditions and tuberculosis (TB), and pregnancy of the female population, and mental health conditions, which may have contributed to a legal event, are also commonly present in admission to correctional facilities (CDC, 2024b). Overall, chronic disease conditions, which may have been preexisting for several years, comprise the primary care provided (Lehrer, 2021).

The role of correctional nursing is limited in the nursing curriculum as specific training is needed to deal with nursing care and legal and ethical issues that may be present for this unique client population. Nursing education should cover coping with particular situations when working in this environment. Nurses must be able to assist the inmates with compassionate care and be impartial while working efficiently with prison staff and meeting their unique needs. The potential for ethical conflicts and any prejudice may alter the appropriate level of care by the nurse. Proper education about corrections nursing with specialized training has the potential to have positive care outcomes and portray job satisfaction for the nurses. An important aspect is to have the support of the corrections management to offer adequate care while securing a safe environment (Caro, 2021; IAFN, 2024a).

Health promotion and disease maintenance are critical for corrections nurses. Effective client/inmate education is vital as many have chronic diseases such as heart, diabetes, and liver disease. Providing comprehensive care is imperative for inmates to receive proper and efficient care (IAFN, 2024a; National Commission on Correctional Healthcare [NCCHC], n.d.; Box 11.4).

BOX 11.4 APPLICATION OF CORRECTIONS NURSING

Nursing students need to have more exposure to correctional/prison nursing. Watch the following video: https://www.youtube.com/watch?v=xufwbLTm_fw.

After watching this video, reflect on your feelings about working in this community nursing role by documenting a two-page, double-spaced paper discussing how to prepare for employment in a juvenile detention center.

1. What additional education and training would you request to be offered during the orientation period?
2. Specifically, focus on the following areas and give at least two examples and interventions that you may experience/intervene within this role: potential violent events; confidentiality; refusal of care, including medication administration; abuse of/by juveniles by staff members; resident advocacy; stressful situations involving nurses; and inappropriate behavior.
3. How would you manage the care of a pregnant teen inmate?

AACN *Essentials* (2021): Domains: #1; #2; #3; #4; #5; #6; #7; #8; #9

- Competencies: 1.1; 1.2; 1.3; 2.1; 2.1b; 2.1; 2.8; 2.9; 3.1; 3.3; 4.2; 5.2; 6.1; 6.3. 6.4; 7.1; 7.2; 8.5; 9.2
- Subcompetencies: 1.1b; 1.2a; 1.2e; 1.3a; 1.3c; 2.1a; 2.1c; 2.8a; 2.9a; 2.9d; 3.1a; 3.1c; 3.1e; 3.1h; 3.3b; 4.2c; 5.2a; 5.2c; 6.1d; 6.1f; 6.3a; 6.4d; 7.1c; 7.2b; 8.5a; 9.2c; 9.2d

Spheres of Care: Wellness/Disease prevention; Chronic disease management

Concepts: Communication; Compassionate care; Ethics; DEI; SDOH; Clinical judgment

Source: NCCHC, 2024.

Forensic Nursing

In 1991, Virginia Lynch acknowledged the concept of forensic nursing. As this field was not yet considered a discipline or even a specialty, Lynch noted the issues with individuals who globally experienced forms of violence, death, legal concerns, collection of criminal evidence, and evaluation of the meaning of the evidence. Lynch began to relate the incidences of trauma with police and had concerns about the care and, hence, legal outcomes of contributing causes to the actual legal events (Valentine et al., 2020).

In the United States, forensic nurses most frequently work in hospitals, community antiviolence programs, coroner's and medical examiners' offices, corrections institutions, and psychiatric hospitals. Forensic nurses may also be called in regarding mass-casualty events or community crises. They also provide

BOX 11.5 APPLICATION OF FORENSIC NURSING

Watch the following videos:

- https://www.youtube.com/watch?v=ipgfPGPLeSw&t=79s
- https://www.forensicnurses.org/page/WhatisFN/

After watching the videos, respond to the following questions:

1. Choose a state or county and research the presence of forensic nurses.
2. Research a forensic nursing program in the United States. Discuss the program's curriculum.
3. Develop an informational pamphlet on forensic nurses' functions, roles, and responsibilities for high school students in a career course.

AACN *Essentials* (2021): Domains: #1; #3; #4; #5; #8

- Competencies: 1.1; 3.1; 3.2; 3.3; 4.2; 5.2; 8.1; 8.3
- Subcompetencies: 1.1b; 3.1a; 3.1b; 3.1c; 3.1e; 3.2a; 3.3b; 4.2c; 5.2a; 5.2c; 8.1a; 8.1e; 8.3e

Spheres of Care: Wellness/Disease prevention; Regenerative/restorative care

Concepts: Communication; Compassionate care; Evidence-based practice

Source: Island Health, 2021.

consultation and testimony for civil and criminal proceedings relative to nursing practice, care given, and opinions rendered regarding findings, including legal training. Forensic nursing care is not separate from other types of nursing care but integrated into the client's overall care (IAFN, 2024b).

Valentine et al. (2020) developed the Constructed Theory of Forensic Nursing Care Model Framework. By combining such areas of nursing practice, education, and research, nurses could work on increasing knowledge through research and evidence-based practice. Through the theory, nurses can approach means to enhance client outcomes and expand the services that forensic nurses can provide (Valentine et al., 2020; Box 11.5).

Sexual Assault Nurse Examiner Nursing

As nurses cared for victims of all ages related to trauma crimes, the awareness of the need for specialized standard policies and procedures was warranted. The IAFN was formed in 1992, and in 1995, the ANA was instrumental in viewing SANE as a subspecialization in nursing. These nurses required additional education to support their roles and responsibilities and needed support for their findings by working with other healthcare providers, such as legal professionals (IAFN, 2024c).

Specific roles and responsibilities include providing healthcare solutions for those involved in interpersonal violence. Skills include documenting injury, including taking photos, collecting and preserving forensic evidence, testifying about the injury and evidence collected, providing trauma-informed care, and collaborating with community partners. However, SANE training could expand to use unique abilities to evaluate and treat trauma by providing care for other populations and not just sexually specific ones (OJP, n.d.a.).

The IAFN reports that in 2021, it had a global membership in more than 30 countries. In 2024, 2720 SANE nurses were certified, with some certified for adults or pediatrics and some dual-certified (IAFN, 2024d). The scope of practice and legalities for SANE nurses differ in every state (Figure 11.6).

Legal Nurse Consultant

The legal nurse consultant (LNC) became recognized after it was noted that physicians and not nurses were testifying in cases involving the nursing profession. Legal nurse consultancy is the application of additional knowledge acquired through education and experience regarding applicable legal standards and/or strategies to evaluate medical-legal cases or claims. Further education is needed to understand nurses' unique perspectives on a legal matter involving healthcare issues (American Association of Legal Nurse Consultants [AALNC], 2024).

The LNC career path started growing in the 1980s as the demand for nurse experts in legal healthcare grew (Arshad, 2022). In 1989, the AALNC was founded. By the 1990s, the scope and standards of practice statements were developed, and the LNC Certification examination was offered. Legal nurse consultants are in high demand by practicing attorneys. It has been estimated that more than 4,685 LNCs work in the United States, and 89% tend to work in private companies such as attorney's offices, although some do independent consultations (Zippia, 2024a).

LNCs have many tasks and responsibilities, such as examining cases for merit, reviewing medical records, identifying appropriate standards of care, acting as expert witnesses, and assessing the cost of care and damages. LNCs are not attorneys and must remain in their scope of practice as licensed nurses with specialized training in the law (Arshad, 2022).

Who is a SANE?

A Sexual Assault Nurse Examiner (SANE) is a Registered Nurse

Their responsibilities include:

- Regular nursing care
- Medical/forensic evaluation and treatment
- Evidence collection
- Documentation of any injuries
- An analysis of the findings
- The ability to testify to those findings as a fact or expert witness

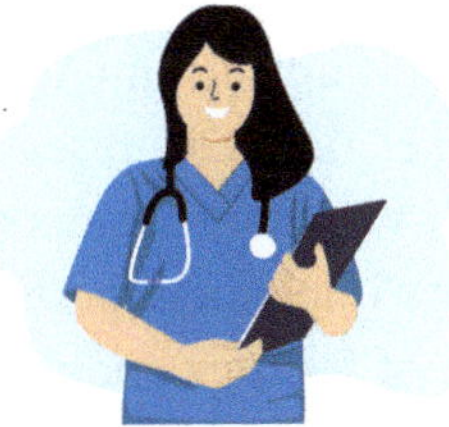

FIGURE 11.6 Who Is a Sexual Assault Nurse Examiner?

Family Health

Family health nursing developed as families were the key stakeholders in caring for ill family members. Specific nurses and methods for initiating and implementing this nursing care must be well documented. As nurses were seen as the caregivers for many, especially family members, the role became entwined with this type of client care delivery. The perception of family health nursing is that it can provide support through communication skills and providing consistent care within the family. This may include their culture, religious orientation, parenting practices, leadership, beliefs, and how these areas function in the family circle through evidence to provide effective healthy practices and outcomes (Thürlimann et al., 2022).

Family health nursing provides primary healthcare to individuals and families from birth to older people while using primary, secondary, and tertiary prevention interventions. By caring for the entire family, nurses can coordinate care and identify any family issues, risk factors, or concerns. Communication within the family circle can allow for robust and positive relationships (Petriprin, 2023).

Dellafiore et al. (2022) identified five areas where the family health nurse shows strength. These include clinical practice, core competencies, outcomes, organizational and educational models, and advanced training programs. Overall, family health nurses contribute to a better understanding of a family's needs as a cohesive group. By incorporating the family into the community, primary services can focus on health promotion and disease prevention.

Broekema et al. (2020) discuss the use of family health nursing while providing home healthcare interventions in the home. Several benefits were identified, especially those in long-term care situations. A chronic illness affects both the client and the family, and working with the family health nurse will make the relationship more impactful.

The Family Health Conversations (FamHC) intervention model may give the family tools that support healthier family functioning. The FamHC model allows nurses to interact with families at various intervals, working to solve problems in routine care. Goals for these interactions include promoting resilience in the family and effective collaboration with all family members and healthcare workers and eliminating any burden on the caregivers. Families need to be flexible and make changes as their needs occur. By supporting themselves, they can be connected in many ways and support each other's needs through appropriate resources and effective communication (Ahlberg et al., 2020).

Ahlberg et al. (2020) researched the use of family health conversations. Nurses in this study were more understanding of the family as a whole, allowing families and nurses to implement better interventions to support all involved. Open communication of feelings and needs was focused on the positive experiences of all the individual family members, assisting in promoting the healthy functioning of the family unit.

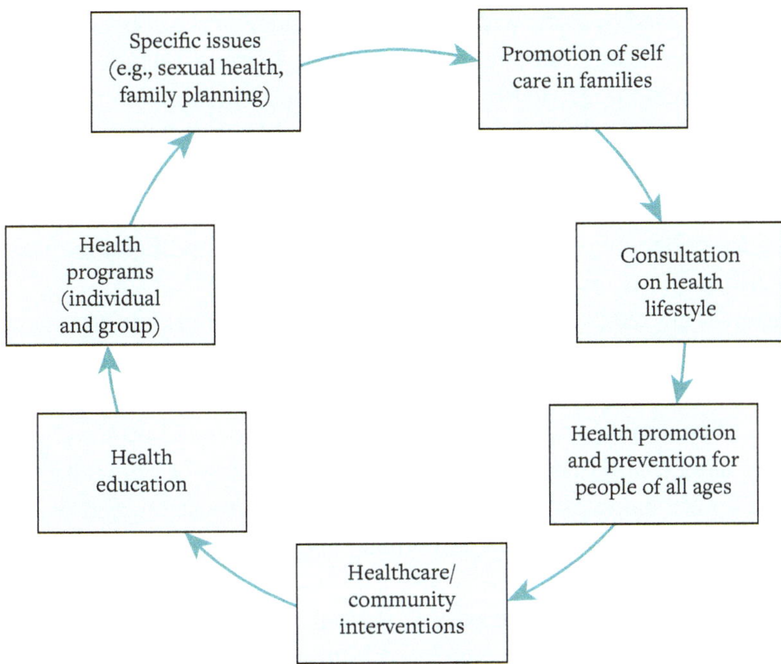

FIGURE 11.7 Roles and Responsibilities of Family Health Nursing

Educational requirements for this role are presented in all nursing curricula for the registered nurse with effective learning strategies related to self-reflection and personal values. Nursing courses incorporate content from birth to death, while the addition of caring, empathy, therapeutic communication, active listening, and compassion is presented in undergraduate studies (Montiel et al., 2020; Figure 11.7).

Mental Health/Psychiatric Nursing

The mental health nursing role began in the late 19th century by William Sweetzer in 1843. J. B. Gray proposed providing mental hygiene in a community-based setting incorporating education, social culture, and religion (Raeburn et al., 2023).

Educational content was added to nursing program curriculums after World War I by the National League for Nursing Education. By 1973, the ANA developed the Nursing Standards of Psychiatric Nursing Practice and Psychiatric-Mental Health Clinical Nurse Specialist Exams (American Psychiatric Nursing Association, 2024). Zippia (2024b) reports that more than 27,693 mental health nurses are employed in the United States. Mental health nurses are 78% more likely to work at private companies than government companies.

Mental health nursing is a specialty group that focuses on providing total care to those with mental disorders or behavioral problems. During the interactions between the client and the mental health nurse, therapeutic communication techniques are used to assist with gaining knowledge of the concerns or stresses with which the individual has been afflicted in their lifetime. Inclusion of the effects of the environmental factors that may contribute to mental health issues along with specific concerns that may stem from an individual's childhood, stresses, and traumas, leading to various mental health situations, are also part of the mental health nurse's concerns. Safety is a significant concern that needs to be addressed, allowing for enhancing a positive and practical understanding of mental health presentations (American Psychological Association [APA], 2024).

Hurley et al. (2022) discussed the demand for mental health nurses, who are frequently underused. This research has identified that the participation of the mental health nurse is not well understood and lacks the intensiveness of activities of the nurse within this specialty. Roles focused on psychotherapy, consumer safety, and diagnosis, and then the inclusion of nontechnical roles, including emotional intelligence, therapeutic communication, and reduction of power differentials or where one individual portrays more authority, knowledge, or agency than another.

Mental health nurses participate in various roles to work on many needs of their clients, including those considered highly technical. The administration and continued follow-up of psychiatric medications and the identification of any potential side effects are critical to educating both clients and families. Other activities include dealing with crisis management situations, including aggression reduction and suicide prevention; providing safety; offering support and direction while dealing with mental health concerns; participating in various forms of therapies; and assisting with learning to live with mental health challenges (APA, 2024; Hurley et al., 2022).

Happell and Gaskin (2022) have identified that nursing students do not view mental health nursing as an area in which to be employed. Whether the positive impression of this practice is not highlighted in nursing programs, the overall negative perceptions in this specialty need to be shifted to a positive outcome.

The activities of mental health nurses include many challenges. Cranage and Foster (2022) present such findings as challenges in the workplace, specifically related to mental health and aggressive behaviors that may occur. Despite the reasons for distress, threats and unwanted behaviors from others are reflected onto the mental health nurse and other staff members in which to provide safety and provide interventions to reduce the stressors that are present. The mental health nurse must be able to provide leadership in many aspects of caring for mental health conditions, including those of the staff involved in assisting the mental health nurse's role.

Registered nurses concentrating on mental health have a primary education in the field. Despite the many practice environments, such as psychiatric hospitals, correctional facilities, and community mental health facilities, mental health nurses will work with multidisciplinary groups of healthcare workers to provide a continuum of care. Focusing on the levels of prevention is also essential for the community mental health nurse to educate on the primary prevention of mental health issues. Early screening with the identification of specific mental health issues is critical in secondary prevention to provide early interventions (APA, 2024; Parkes, 2024; Figure 11.8).

Community Mental Health Nurse (CMHN)

- Community mental health nursing is the application of knowledge of psychiatric nursing in preventing mental illness, promoting & maintaining mental health of the people.
- It includes early diagnosis, appropriate referrals, care & rehabilitation of mentally ill people.

FIGURE 11.8 Roles and Responsibilities of Mental Health Nursing

Disability/Rehabilitative Nursing

In 1974, Susan Novak established the ARN. The ANA established the ARN as a specialty nursing organization two years later. Rehabilitation nursing roots evolved as a subspecialty due to wartime young soldiers, young men who survived injury but faced severe disability. As a result, military hospitals established rehabilitation units that focused extensive efforts on returning these young men to society (ARN, n.d.a.).

Globally, 2.41 billion individuals have benefited from rehabilitative nursing care, especially for those with lower back pain, one of the most prevalent needs (Cieza et al., 2019). Disability/rehabilitation nursing is designed to optimize functioning and reduce disability in individuals with health conditions in interaction with their environment (WHO, 2024b). This individualized nursing specialization focuses on many aspects of clients' needs from birth to the end of life, including participation in health promotion and disease prevention. The client and the family can be assisted in many ways after surgery, a disease process, or an injury, including age-related functioning. By doing so, an individual can be as independent as possible in all aspects of life. Depending on the required needs and resources, the care setting may range from inpatient or outpatient facilities to occupational care centers, an individual's home, the workplace, school, or other community establishments (WHO, 2024b).

Gutenbrunner et al. (2021) and Shirozhan et al. (2022) have supported evidence that the goal for optimum rehabilitative outcomes must include multiprofessionals, especially rehabilitative nurses. As this nursing role has evolved throughout the years, the need for the process is guided by assisting the client in performing self-care independently. In this setting, many other multidisciplinary professionals may be required to deal with disability/rehabilitation needs, such

BOX 11.6 ROLES AND RESPONSIBILITIES OF A REHAB/ DISABILITY NURSE

Read the following RESTART Recovery pages for "Starting Rehabilitation, Participating in Rehabilitation, What's next: Transitions," and financial and legal sections on this website (https://restartrecovery.org/). Additionally, read the information about "Your Advocate" and "The Right Decision."

Develop a 10-slide PowerPoint presentation supported by information from the RESTART Recovery content and the ARN for family caregivers and prospective clients about the topics discussed on the pages. Answer the following questions:

1. What concerns do you think the audience will have after you complete the educational session?
2. How can the nurse better assist the caregivers and client with understanding the rehabilitation process, its application, and interventions?
3. What other healthcare professionals may be needed to assist in rehabilitation and why? Explain their specific roles.
4. What other community organizations may be available for resources and support? What will they be able to contribute?
5. How will you use the learnings from this assignment in your future nursing practice?

AACN *Essentials* (2021): Domains: #1; #2; #4; #5; #6; #7; #8; #9

- Competencies: 1.1; 1.2; 2.1; 2.2; 2.4; 2.8; 4.2; 5.1; 6.3; 7.1; 7.2; 8.3; 8.4; 8.5; 9.3
- Subcompetencies: 1.1b; 1.2a; 1.2b; 1.2c; 2.1a; 2.1b; 2.1c; 2.2a; 2.2b; 2.2c; 2.4b; 2.4c; 2.8c; 2.8d; 4.2c; 5.1c; 6.3a; 7.1c; 7.2a; 7.2b; 7.2d; 7.2e; 8.3a; 8.4b; 8.5c; 9.3a

Spheres of Care: Chronic disease care; Regenerative/restorative care

Concepts: Communication; Compassionate care; Evidence-based practice; SDOH

Source: RESTART, 2024.

as occupational therapists, communication therapists, audiologists, orthotists/prosthetists, clinical psychologists, rehabilitation doctors and nurses, surgeons, and other community health workers (WHO, 2024b).

Shirozhan et al. (2022) additionally researched barriers not only to rehabilitation team members but also to clients, professional caregivers, and family members. These concepts are related to knowledge and skills, mentoring, professional communication, nurses' performance, the nursing workforce, client participation in nursing care, client adaptation, and the efficiency of formal caregivers. The inclusion of these concerns must be rectified to promote positive outcomes and facilitate the professional and comprehensive care needed for those requiring specialized needs (Box 11.6).

Chapter Highlights

- Application of several community nursing roles and responsibilities
- Discussions required for individuals, families, and community needs through various community health nursing roles
- Application of how specialized community health nursing roles can assist with providing education and training for multiple situations
- Application of active learning reflection activity on home-based/home health nurse
- Application of active learning reflection activity on hospice/palliative care nursing
- Application of active learning reflection activity on school-based nursing
- Application of active learning reflection activity on correctional nursing
- Application of active learning reflection activity on rehabilitation/disability nursing
- Case study with application of the Minnesota intervention wheel
- Case studies related to home care violence, comparison of home health agencies, and correctional nursing

Active Learning Exercises

Application to Intervention Wheel

Case management and delegation are critical components of effective home health management. Reference https://www.health.state.mn.us/communities/practice/research/phncouncil/docs/PHInterventions.pdf to assist with the following questions. Pay specific attention to the green wedge and information in "Case Management and Delegation."

As a home health case manager, how would you address the following?

Improved Quality of Life Among Older Adults. A review of nurse-led public health interventions demonstrated that case management, along with other public health nursing interventions, contributed to improved quality of life among older adult populations living in the United States and other countries.

1. Name two goals/objectives to improve the quality of life for the older adult population.
2. For each goal/objective, provide two specific interventions based on evidence-based practice that could be implemented to improve the quality of life for the older adult population.
3. What two specific case management practices would provide an improved quality of life for the older adult population?

Delegation. Delegated functions focus on a single aspect of nursing practice: delegation. The intervention occurs in two ways: with the PHN as the initiator of delegated functions to others (i.e., the delegator) and as the recipient of delegated functions from other health professionals (i.e., the delegatee). PHNs whose assignment involves delivering home health services or other healthcare functions under delegation from a medical provider, the concept of the nurse as the delegatee is undoubtedly very familiar. The role of PHNs as delegators or initiators of delegated functions deserves further examination. Delegation at this level is more at the individual/family level.

You have a new home health client who has been hospitalized for seven days with a hip replacement, uncontrolled diabetes, and severe rheumatoid arthritis and who has a daughter who will stay with the client postdischarge. Using pages 116–125 as guidance, reflect on the following questions:

1. What are the five rights of delegation, and how would you apply them in the scenario? Be specific in terms of other disciplines.
2. What are some of the functions of care that you delegate? To whom would you delegate providing evidence-based support?
3. What are three barriers to delegating to the daughter and why?
4. What are two critical components of adequate and appropriate delegation?

AACN *Essentials* (2021): Domains: #1; #2; #5; #6; #8; #9; #10

- Competencies: 1.1; 1.2; 1.3; 2.1; 2.2; 2.6; 2.9; 5.1; 5.2; 6.2; 8.1; 8.3; 9.2; 10.3
- Subcompetencies:1.1b; 1.2a; 1.3b; 2.1b; 2.1c; 2.2a; 2.2b; 2.2e; 2.6c; 2.6d; 2.9a; 2.9c; 2.9e; 5.1f; 5.2c; 6.2b; 8.1a; 8.3a; 8.3c; 9.2b; 10.3c

Spheres of Care: Chronic disease management; Regenerative/Restorative care

Concepts: Compassionate care; Clinical judgment; Ethics; Communication

Source: Minnesota Department of Health, 2019.

Case Studies

Case Study #1: Home Care Violence

Watch home care threat case study #3 at the following website: https://wwwn.cdc.gov/WPVHC/Nurses/Course/Slide/Unit11_2. This case study concerns a home healthcare nurse familiar with a client who suddenly threatens her. She tells the details of this event to her therapist.

1. Part 1: The story of the client's rage unfolds at 2:02 minutes, and then you must document your responses to the questions. When completed, compare your responses to those provided.
2. Part 2: Exiting the Situation, 2:10 minutes: Document responses to the questions. When completed, compare your responses with those provided.

3. Review the expert analysis. Overall, write a one-page paper comparing your comments with those of the expert by reflecting on three things you learned from completing the case study.

AACN *Essentials* (2021): Domains: #1; #2; #5; #6; #9

- Competencies: 1.2; 2.1; 2.2; 2.3; 2.5; 5.1; 5.2; 5.3; 6.1; 9.2
- Subcompetencies: 1.2a; 2.1a; 2.1b; 2.2d; 2.3a; 2.3c; 2.5c; 5.1a; 5.2a; 5.2c; 5.3a; 5.3b; 6.1a; 9.2b

Spheres of Care: Chronic disease management; Regeneration/restorative care

Concepts: Communication; Clinical judgment; Compassionate care

Source: CDC, 2024a.

Case Study #2: Comparison of Home Health Agencies Using Home Health Compare

A 70-year-old man needs home healthcare services after breaking his ankle. The area has several agencies, but the family is uncertain which agency to choose upon the client's discharge to his daughter's home. The client has Medicare. Please refer to the following website to make an informed decision: https://www.medicare.gov/care-compare/.

The following are instructions on how to educate the client and family on how to navigate the site. You have been asked to assist the client and family with the education. The client lives in Atlanta.

On the home page, you need to review the content under "More Resources," which discusses the areas of this tool, resources and information, and information for health care providers. Under this section is an area titled "Looking to explore and download provider data?" Visit the data catalog at https://data.cms.gov/provider-data/.

Directions:

1. Open the above website and click on "Home Health Services." Look up ZIP code 30327. Leave the optional name of the agency blank.
2. Select "Search." A listing of home health agencies will come up.
3. Select "WellStar Home Health" and two other home health agencies of your choice. You will select the three sites by clicking "Compare" by each agency.
4. Now, choose the white "Compare" button at the top right of the screen, and the screen will open with the comparisons.
5. Compare the following items and analyze who has the best outcomes/results:

    a. Quality ratings
    b. Patient survey ratings
    c. Services offered for each one

d. How often patients got better at walking or moving around
e. How often the home health team began their patients' care in a timely manner
f. How often patients experienced one or more falls with a major injury
g. How often home health patients had to be admitted to the hospital
h. How often patients remained in the community after discharge from home health
i. How often the home health team gave care in a professional way
j. How patients rated the overall care from the home health agency

6. Document for your faculty a short synopsis of each facility, summarize which facility you would choose, and give support for your decision.

AACN *Essentials* (2021): Domains: #1; #2; #5; #6

- Competencies: 1.2; 1.3; 2.1; 2.2; 2.3; 2.5; 5.1; 5.2; 5.3; 6.1
- Subcompetencies: 1.2a; 1.3a; 2.1a; 2.1b; 2.2d; 2.3a; 2.3c; 2.5c; 5.1a; 5.2a; 5.2c; 5.3a; 5.3b; 6.1c

Spheres of Care: Chronic disease management; Regeneration/Restorative care

Concepts: Communication; Clinical judgment; Compassionate care

Sources: CMS, n.d.; Medicare.gov, 2024.

Case Study #3: Correctional Nursing

George is a registered nurse, and John is one of the inmates at the state correctional facility.

John is a long-term offender, serving a lifetime sentence, who entered the facility at age 35 and is now age 61. He is a problematic inmate who is always hostile, bitter, and resentful and harasses the staff constantly.

John has several chronic health conditions, including insulin-dependent diabetes, cirrhosis of the liver, hypertension, a history of TB, and coronary artery disease. His mental health issues include major depressive disorder. He required the use of a wheelchair for mobility and was prescribed several medications for his health conditions.

Answer the following questions:

1. How are the medical and mental conditions of elderly inmates different from or similar to those of the older adult population not incarcerated?
2. Describe three factors that affect healthcare delivery in correctional institutions.
3. What unique challenges would the corrections nurse face in providing John's care?
4. Develop a comprehensive physical, mental, emotional, and spiritual plan of care for John.

AACN *Essentials* (2021): Domains: #1; #2; #3; #4; #5; #6; #7; #8

- Competencies: 1.1; 1.2; 1.3; 2.1; 2.2; 2.2; 2.3; 2.4; 2.5; 2.8; 2.9; 3.1; 3.2; 4.2; 4.3; 5.1; 6.1; 6.3; 6.4; 7.2; 8.3; 8.5
- Subcompetencies: 1.1a; 1.2a; 1.3b; 2.1a; 2.1b; 2.2b; 2.2d; 2.3a; 2.3b; 2.4a; 2.5a; 2.8e; 2.9b; 3.1e; 3.2a; 4.2a; 4.2c; 4.3d; 5.1a; 5.1f; 6.1a; 6.3a; 6.4a; 6.4d; 7.2b; 7.2d; 8.3e; 8.5c; 8.5d

Spheres of Care: Chronic disease management; Regenerative/Restorative care

Concepts: Communication; Compassionate care; DEI; Ethics; Evidence-based practice; Clinical judgment

Source: Developed by authors.

NCLEX Questions

1. In a single day, the school nurse may engage in all three levels of preventive practice. Below is a list of activities she participated in yesterday. Which one represents secondary prevention?
    a. Touched base with a homebound student and her mother about the child's needs
    b. Created and distributed take-home pamphlets about an after-school vaccination program
    c. Helped teach a substance abuse prevention class
    d. Conducted visual screening tests for second graders
2. The client has been recently diagnosed with stage 4 liver cancer with metastasis to the bones. The client asks the nurse what will be included in his plan of care as time passes to help him better manage his condition. Which would be the best response from the nurse?
    a. Hospice care can be used anytime, as it is for anyone with a terminal illness.
    b. When a client develops intensive pain, they will meet the criteria for hospice services.
    c. What the client requests for their advanced directives will determine their chance to be accepted into hospice care.
    d. Hospice care can begin when end of life is determined to be within six months.

References

Abraham, P. (2021). *Unit 1 role of psychiatric nurse*. https://www.slideshare.net/slideshow/unit-1-role-of-psychiatric-nurse/244952904

Agran, P. (n.d.). *School nurses are critical to the safety of our students.*https://irvinecommunitynewsandviews.org/school-nurses-are-critical-to-the-safety-of-our-children/

Ahlberg, M., Hollman, F. G., Berterö, C., & Ågren, S. (2020). Family health conversations create awareness of family functioning. *Nursing in Critical Care, 25*(2), 102–108. https://doi.org/10.1111/nicc.12454

American Association of Colleges of Nursing. (2021). *The essentials: Core competencies for professional nursing education.* https://www.aacnnursing.org/Essentials

American Association of Legal Nurse Consultants. (2024). *About AALNC.* https://www.aalnc.org/About/About-AALNC

American Association of Occupational Health Nurses. (n.d.). *About.* https://www.aaohn.org/About/What-is-Occupational-and-Environmental-Health-Nursing

American Cancer Society. (2023). *What is hospice care?* https://www.cancer.org/cancer/end-of-life-care/hospice-care/what-is-hospice-care.html

American Nursing Association. (n.d.). *Public health nursing.* https://www.nursingworld.org/practice-policy/workforce/public-health-nursing/

American Nursing Association. (2017). *Faith community nursing scopes and standards of practice* (3rd ed.). ANA/Health Ministries Association.

American Psychiatric Nursing Association. (2024). *History of psychiatric-mental health nursing.* https://www.apna.org/history/

American Psychological Association. (2024). *APA definition of psychiatric nursing.* https://dictionary.apa.org/psychiatric-nursing

Anthony, M. (2024). Attracting nurses to home care. *Home Healthcare Now, 42*(2), 71. https://doi.org/10.1097/nhh.0000000000001252

Arshad, S. (2022). *Legal nurse consultant—A flourishing field.* https://nursingcecentral.com/legal-nurse-consultant/

Association of Rehabilitation Nurses. (n.d.a.). *History.* https://rehabnurse.org/about/history

Association of Rehabilitation Nurses. (n.d.b.). *Roles of the rehab nurse.* https://rehabnurse.org/about/roles-of-the-rehab-nurse

Balint, K., & George, N. (2015). Faith community nursing scope of practice: Extending access to healthcare. *Journal of Christian Nursing, 32*(1), 34–40. https://doi.org/10.1097/cnj.0000000000000129

BAYADA Home Health Care. (2018). *What is home care?* YouTube, November 6, 2018. https://www.youtube.com/watch?v=HvAa45mCHGQ

Broekema, S., Paans, W., Roodbol, P. F., & Luttik, M. L. A. (2020). Nurses' application of the components of family nursing conversations in home health care: A qualitative content analysis. *Scandinavian Journal of Caring Sciences, 34*(2), 322–331. https://doi.org/10.1111/scs.12731

Campbell County Health. (2022). *What is home health care?* https://www.cchwyo.org/news/2022/march/what-is-home-health-care-/

Canadian Nursing Association. (2013). *Nurses in occupational and environmental health: Overview of nursing role.* https://nursesinoccupationalhealth.weebly.com/overview-of-nursing-role.html

Caro, A. (2021). The role of prison nursing: An integrative review. *Journal of Spanish Prison Health, 23*(2), 76–85. https://doi.org/10.18176/resp.00034

Centers for Disease Control and Prevention. (2023). *FastStats—Hospice care.* https://www.cdc.gov/nchs/fastats/hospice-care.htm#

Centers for Disease Control and Prevention. (2024a). *Case study 3: Home care threat.* https://wwwn.cdc.gov/WPVHC/Nurses/Course/Slide/Unit11_2

Centers for Disease Control and Prevention. (2024b). *Public health considerations for correctional health*. https://www.cdc.gov/correctionalhealth/about/?CDC_AAref_Val=https://www.cdc.gov/correctionalhealth/default.htm

Centers for Disease Control and Prevention Foundation. (n.d.). *Career spotlight: Public health nurse*. https://www.cdc.gov/scienceambassador/documents/module-7-career-spotlight-infection-public-health-nurse.pdf

Centers for Medicare & Medicaid Services. (n.d.). *Provider data catalog*. https://data.cms.gov/provider-data/

Centers for Medicare & Medicaid Services. (2024). *OASIS-E manual 2024 update*. https://www.cms.gov/files/document/oasis-emanual2024-update.pdf

Cieza, A., Causey, K., Kamenov, K., Hanson, S., Chatterji, S. & Vos, T. (2019). Global Estimates of the need for rehabilitation based on the Global Burden of Disease study 2019: A systematic analysis for the Global Burden of Disease study 2019. *The Lancet*, *396*(10267). https://doi.org/10.1016/S0140-6736(20)32340-0

Constellation. (2022). *What is the difference between home health and hospice?* https://constellationhs.com/articles/what-is-the-difference-between-home-health-and-hospice/

Cranage, K., & Foster, K. (2022). Mental health nurses' experience of challenging workplace situations: A qualitative descriptive study. *International Journal of Mental Health Nursing*, *31*(3), 665–676. https://doi.org/10.1111/inm.12986

Cross, S. H., Ramkalawan, J. R., Ring, J. F., & Boucher, N. A. (2022). "That little bit of time": Transition-to-hospice perspectives from hospice staff and bereaved family. *Innovation in Aging*, *6*(1), igab057. https://doi.org/10.1093/geroni/igab057

de Buhr, E., Ewers, M., & Tannen, A. (2020). Potentials of school nursing for strengthening the health literacy of children, parents and teachers. *International Journal of Environmental Research and Public Health*, *17*(7), 2577. https://doi.org/10.3390/ijerph17072577

Dellafiore, F., Caruso, R., Cossu, M., Russo, M., Baroni, I., Barello, S., Vangone I., Acampora M., Conte, G., Magon, A., Stievano, A., & Arrigoni, C. (2022). The state of the evidence about the family and community nurse: A systematic review. *International Journal of Environmental Research and Public Health*, *19*(7), 4382. https://doi.org/10.3390/ijerph19074382

Durojaiye, A., Ryan, R., & Doody, O. (2023). Student nurse education and preparation for palliative care: A scoping review. *PLoS ONE*, *18*(7), e0286678. https://doi.org/10.1371/journal.pone.0286678

Eckstadt, K. (2024). Structured telephone support for heart failure patients: A literature review. *Home Healthcare Now*, *42*(1), 36–41. https://doi.org/10.1097/nhh.0000000000001221

EduReaders. (2022). *History of school nursing in the United States*. https://edureaders.com/history-of-school-nursing-in-the-united-states/#

Faster Capital. (2024). *Home health care history: The history and evolution of home health care*. https://fastercapital.com/content/Home-Health-Care-History--The-History-and-Evolution-of-Home-Health-Care.html#Origins-of-Home-Health-Care

Gaines, K. (2023). *5 steps to becoming an occupational health nurse*. https://nurse.org/resources/occupational-health-nurse/

Gutenbrunner, C., Stievano, A., Stewart, D., Catton, H., & Nugraha, B. (2021). Role of nursing in rehabilitation. *Journal of Rehabilitation Medicine—Clinical Communications*, *14*(4), 1000061. https://doi.org/10.2340/20030711-1000061

Happell, B., & Gaskin. (2022). The attitudes of undergraduate nursing students towards mental health nursing: A systematic review. *Journal of Clinical Nursing*, *22*(1–2), 148–158. https://doi.org/10.1111/jocn.12022

Health at Home. (2023). *The collaboration and strength of interdisciplinary care in home health*. https://healthathome.care/careers-in-caring/interdisciplinary-care-in-home-health/#

HemoCue. (2021). *National nurses month: Honoring the history of heroes.* https://www.hemocue.us/national-nurses-month/

Home Centered Care Institute. (2022). *The importance of interdisciplinary care for homebound clients.* https://www.hccinstitute.org/the-importance-of-interdisciplinary-care-for-homebound-patients/

Homecare Association of America. (2023). *The home care workforce crisis: An industry report and call to action.* https://www.hcaoa.org/uploads/1/3/3/0/133041104/workforce_report_and_call_to_action_final_03272023.pdf

HospiceWise. (2024). *What's the difference between palliative care and hospice?* https://hospicewise.org/palliative-hospice-differences/

Hospices of Holland. (2023). *A brief history of hospice.* https://understandhospice.org/brief-history-hospice/

Hui, D., Heung, Y., & Bruera, E. (2022). Timely palliative care: Personalizing the process of referral. *Cancers, 14*(4), 1047. https://doi.org/10.3390/cancers14041047

Hurley, J., Lakeman, R., Linsley, P., Ramsay, M., & Mckenna-Lawson, S. (2022). Utilizing the mental health nursing workforce: A scoping review of mental health nursing clinical roles and identities. *International Journal of Mental Health Nursing, 31*(4), 796–822. https://doi.org/10.1111/inm.12983

International Association of Forensic Nurses. (2024a). *Correctional nursing.* https://www.forensicnurses.org/page/CorrectionalNursing/

International Association of Forensic Nurses. (2024b). *Forensic nursing.* https://www.forensicnurses.org/page/WhatisFN/

International Association of Forensic Nurses. (2024c). *SANE certification central.* https://www.forensicnurses.org/page/Certification/

International Association of Forensic Nurses. (2024d). *Sexual assault nurse examiner.* https://www.forensicnurses.org/page/aboutSANE

Island Health. (2021). *Introduction to forensic nursing.* YouTube, September 1, 2021. https://www.youtube.com/watch?v=ipgfPGPLeSw&t=79s

Jones, K., Edwards, L., & Alexander, G. (2022). Shoring up the frontline of prevention: strengthening curricula with community and public health nursing. *American Journal of Public Health,* S237–S240. https://ajph.aphapublications.org/doi/full/10.2105/AJPH.2022.306739

Kowalski, S., & Gifford, S. (2024). In-home management of diabetes and obesity. *Home Healthcare Now 42*(1), 6–12. https://doi.org/10.1097/nhh.0000000000001223

Lehrer, D. (2021). Compassion in corrections: The struggle between security and health care. *Journal of Correctional Health Care, 27*(2), 81–84. https://doi.org/10.1089/jchc.20.07.0061

Logan, D., & Zipp, G. (2024). Home care nurses' knowledge and attitudes regarding telehealth to promote medication compliance among older adults. *Home Healthcare Now, 42*(1), 31–35. https://doi.org/10.1097/nhh.0000000000001230

Martin, P., Duffy, T., Johnston, B., Banks, P., Harkess-Murphy, E., & Martin C. (2013). Family health nursing: A response to the global health challenges. *Journal of Family Nursing, 19*(1), 99–118. https://doi.org/10.1177/1074840712471810

Medicare.gov. (n.d.). *What's home health care?* https://www.medicare.gov/what-medicare-covers/whats-home-health-care

Medicare.gov. (2024). *Find & compare providers near you.* https://www.medicare.gov/care-compare/

Minnesota Department of Health. (2019). *Public health interventions: Applications for public health nursing practice* (2nd ed.). https://www.health.state.mn.us/communities/practice/research/phncouncil/docs/PHInterventions.pdf

Minority Nurse. (2021). *Careers for nurses who like working in the community.* https://minoritynurse.com/careers-for-nurses-who-like-working-in-the-community/

Montiel, T. C., Leal, A. A., & Baltazar, N. (2020). Family-centered practice in nursing education. *Nursing, 50*(7), 61–62. https://journals.lww.com/nursing/citation/2020/07000/family_centered_practice_in_nursing_education.16.aspx

National Association for Home Care & Hospice. (2024). *NAHC resources.* https://nahc.org/nahc-resources/

National Association of School Nurses. (n.d.). *About NASN.* https://www.nasn.org/about-nasn/about

National Association of School Nurses. (2023). *Public school nurses in the U.S.* https://higherlogicdownload.s3.amazonaws.com/NASN/8575d1b7-94ad-45ab-808e-d45019cc5c08/UploadedImages/PDFs/Advocacy/2023-08-03-Public_School_Nurses-Final.pdf

National Association of School Nurses. (2024). School Nursing Practice Framework™. *NASN School Nurse, 0*(0). https://www.nasn.org/nasn-resources/framework

National Commission on Correctional Healthcare. (n.d.). *Health promotion and maintenance.* https://www.ncchc.org/correctional-nursing-practice-what-you-need-to-know/health-promotion-and-maintenance/

National Commission on Correctional Healthcare. (2024). *Discover a career in correctional nursing.* YouTube, February 14, 2024. https://www.youtube.com/watch?v=xufwbLTm_fw

National Hospice and Palliative Care Organization. (2023). *NHPCO facts and figures 2023.* https://www.nhpco.org/wp-content/uploads/NHPCO-Facts-Figures-2023.pdf

National Hospice and Palliative Care Organization. (2024). *History of hospice.* https://www.nhpco.org/hospice-care-overview/history-of-hospice/

National Institute on Aging. (2021). *What are palliative care and hospice care?* https://www.nia.nih.gov/health/hospice-and-palliative-care/what-are-palliative-care-and-hospice-care

NEJM Resident 360. (2020). *Brief history of palliative care.* https://resident360.nejm.org/content-items/history-of-palliative-care

New Hampshire Coalition Against Domestic and Sexual Violence. (n.d.). *Who is a SANE?* https://www.nhcadsv.org/sane.html

Nursing-Theory.org. (2023). *Family nursing.* https://nursing-theory.org/theories-and-models/family-nursing.php

Office of Justice Programs. (n.d.a.). *SANE program development and operational guide: Expanding forensic nursing practice.* https://www.ovcttac.gov/saneguide/expanding-forensic-nursing-practice/

Office of Justice Programs. (n.d.b.). *What is a SANE?* https://www.ovcttac.gov/saneguide/introduction/what-is-a-sane/

Parkes, C. (2024). *Psychiatric mental health, part 12: Primary, secondary, tertiary prevention of mental health disorders.* https://leveluprn.com/blogs/psychiatric-mental-health/principles-12-primary-secondary-tertiary-prevention

Pawils, S., Heumann., S, Schneider, S., Metzner, F., & Mays, D. (2023). The current state of international research on the effectiveness of school nurses in promoting the health of children and adolescents: An overview of reviews. *PLoS ONE, 18*(2), e0275724. https://doi.org/10.1371/journal.pone.0275724

Petriprin, A. (2023). *Family nursing.* https://nursing-theory.org/theories-and-models/family-nursing.php

Pittman, P., & Park, J. (2021). *Rebuilding community-based and public health nursing in the wake of COVID-19.* https://ojin.nursingworld.org/table-of-contents/

volume-26-2021/number-2-may-2021/rebuilding-community-based--public-health-nursing-wake-of-covid-19/

Raeburn, T., Bradshaw, J., & Cleary, M. (2023). Mental health history—It matters. *Issues in Mental Health Nursing, 44*(1), 3–5. https://doi.org/10.1080/01612840.2022.2138437

RESTART. (2024). *RESTART: Key information for your rehab journey.* https://restartrecovery.org/

Roscoe, L. (2022). *Legal history of correctional nursing: Estelle v. Gamble.* https://correctionalnurse.net/history-of-correctional-nursing-part-i/

Schroepfer, E. (2016). Professional issues: Renewed look at faith community nursing. *MEDSURG Nursing, 25*(1), 62–67. https://www.pnmny.org/articles/ARenewedLookatFaithCommunityNursingMSN%20J-F16.pdf

Sessanna, L., Askew, Y. D., & Pomeroy, S. H. (2021). Faith community nursing practice and holistic nursing practice: A comprehensive and inclusive comparison of both specialties. *Journal of Holistic Nursing, 39*(1), 85–102. https://doi.org/10.1177/0898010120928620

Shirozhan, S., Arsalani, N., Maddah, S. S. B., & Mohammadi-Shahboulaghi, F. (2022). Barriers and facilitators of rehabilitation nursing care for patients with disability in the rehabilitation hospital: A qualitative study. *Frontiers in Public Health, 10*, 931287. https://doi.org/10.3389/fpubh.2022.931287

Smiley, R., Allgeyer, R., Shobo, Y., Lyons, K., Letourneau, R., Zhong, E., Kaminski-Ozturk, N., & Alexander, M. (2023). *The 2022 National Nursing Workforce Survey.* https://www.journalofnursingregulation.com/article/S2155-8256(23)00047-9/pdf

Spokane Public Schools. (2018). *What do you do? School nurses.* YouTube, March 21, 2018. https://www.youtube.com/watch?v=ZOC2vGfGHJc

Thürlimann, E., Verweij, L., & Naef, R. (2022). The implementation of evidence-informed family nursing practices: A scoping review of strategies, contextual determinants, and outcomes. *Journal of Family Nursing, 28*(3), 258–276. https://doi.org/10.1177/10748407221099655

U.S. Bureau of Labor Statistics. (2024). *Home health and personal care aides.* https://www.bls.gov/ooh/healthcare/home-health-aides-and-personal-care-aides.htm#tab-1

Valentine, J., Sekula, L. K., & Lynch, V. (2020). Evolution of forensic nursing theory—Introduction of the constructed theory of forensic nursing care: A middle-range theory. *Journal of Forensic Nursing, 16*(4), 188–198. https://doi.org/10.1097/jfn.0000000000000287

VNS Health. (2022). *Why home care nursing is special.* YouTube, September 6, 2022. https://www.youtube.com/watch?v=f7qf7QeUsdM

World Health Organization. (2024a). *Palliative care.* https://www.who.int/news-room/fact-sheets/detail/palliative-care

World Health Organization. (2024b). *Rehabilitation.* https://www.who.int/news-room/fact-sheets/detail/rehabilitation#

World Health Organization. (2024c). *What is palliative care and how can it be assessed?* https://www.who.int/multi-media/details/what-is-palliative-care-and-how-can-it-be-assessed#

Zeydani, A., Atashzadeh-Shoorideh, F., Abdi, F., Meimana, H., Zohari-Anboohi, S., & Skerrett, V. (2021). Effect of community-based education on undergraduate nursing students' skills: A systematic review. *BMC Nursing, 20*, 233. https://bmcnurs.biomedcentral.com/articles/10.1186/s12912-021-00755-4

Zeydani, A., Atashzadeh-Shoorideh, F., Hosseini, M., & Zohari-Anboohi, S. (2023). Community-based nursing: A concept analysis with Walker and Avant's approach. *BMC Medical Education, 23*(1), 762. https://bmcmededuc.biomedcentral.com/articles/10.1186/s12909-023-04749-5

Ziebarth, D. (2014). Evolutionary conceptual analysis: Faith community nursing. *Journal of Religious Health, 53*, 1836–1837. https://link.springer.com/article/10.1007/s10943-014-9936-x

Zippia. (2024a). *Legal nurse consultant nurse demographics and statistics in the U.S.* https://www.zippia.com/legal-nurse-consultant-jobs/demographics/

Zippia. (2024b). *Mental health nurse demographics and statistics in the U.S.* https://www.zippia.com/mental-health-nurse-jobs/demographics/

Zippia. (2024c). *Occupational health nurse demographics and statistics in the U.S.* https://www.zippia.com/occupational-health-nurse-jobs/demographics/

Zippia. (2024d). *School nurse demographics and statistics in the U.S.* https://www.zippia.com/school-nurse-jobs/demographics/

Credits

Fig. 11.1: Adapted from Campbell County Health, https://www.cchwyo.org/news/2022/march/what-is-home-health-care-/. Copyright © 2022 by Campbell County Health.

Fig. 11.2: Adapted from Constellation Health Service, https://constellationhs.com/articles/what-is-the-difference-between-home-health-and-hospice/. Copyright © 2022 by Constellation Health Service.

Fig. 11.3: Hospice Wise, https://hospicewise.org/palliative-hospice-differences/. Copyright © 2024 by Hospice Wise.

Fig. 11.4: Phyllis Agran, https://irvinecommunitynewsandviews.org/school-nurses-are-critical-to-the-safety-of-our-children/. Copyright © by Irvine Community News & Views (ICNV).

Fig. 11.5: National Association of School Nurses (NASN), https://www.nasn.org/nasn-resources/framework. Copyright © 2024 by National Association of School Nurses (NASN).

Fig. 11.6: New Hampshire Coalition Against Domestic and Sexual Violence, https://www.nhcadsv.org/sane.html. Copyright © by New Hampshire Coalition Against Domestic and Sexual Violence.

Fig. 11.6a: Copyright © 2023 Depositphotos/enway_studio.

Fig. 11.7: Paul Martin et al, *Journal of Family Nursing*, vol. 19, no. 1. Copyright © 2013 by SAGE Publications.

Fig. 11.8: Adapted from Princy Abraham, https://www.slideshare.net/slideshow/unit-1-role-of-psychiatric-nurse/244952904. Copyright © 2021 by Princy Abraham.

Index

A

B

C

S

T

U

V

W

Z

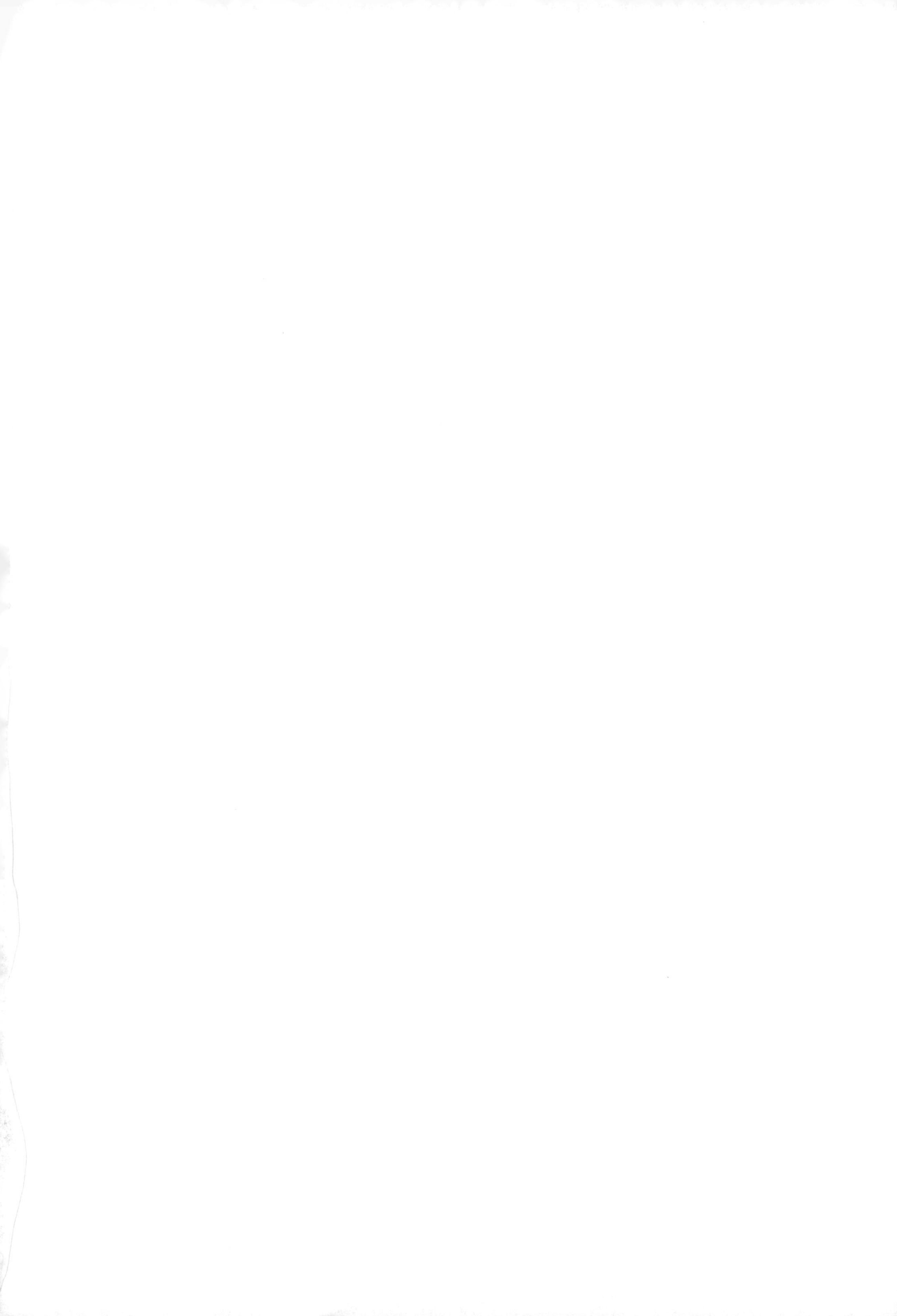

www.ingramcontent.com/pod-product-compliance
Ingram Content Group UK Ltd.
Pitfield, Milton Keynes, MK11 3LW, UK
UKHW050140280726
14058UKWH00006B/742